Preterm Birth

Preterm Birth

Mechanisms, Mediators, Prediction, Prevention and Interventions

Edited by

FELICE PETRAGLIA MD

Obstetrics and Gynecology, Department of Pediatrics, Obstetrics and Reproductive Medicine, University of Siena, Siena, Italy

JEROME F STRAUSS III MD PhD

Virginia Commonwealth University Health System, Richmond, VA, USA

STEVEN G GABBE MD

Department of Obstetrics and Gynecology, Vanderbilt University School of Medicine, Nashville, TN, USA

GERSON WEISS MD

Department of Obstetrics, Gynecology and Women's Health, New Jersey Medical School of UMDNJ, Newark, NJ, USA

Published in association with The Society for Gynecologic Investigation

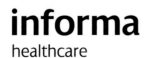

First published in the United Kingdom in 2007 by Informa Healthcare, 4 Park Square, Milton Park, Abingdon, Oxon OX14 4RN. Informa Healthcare is a trading division of Informa UK Ltd. Registered Office: 37/41 Mortimer Street, London W1T 3JH. Registered in England and Wales number 1072954.

Tel: +44 (0)20 7017 6000
Fax: +44 (0)20 7017 6699
Email: info.medicine@tandf.co.uk
Website: www.informahealthcare.com

A CIP record for this book is available from the British Library.

Library of Congress Cataloging-in-Publication Data

Data available on application

ISBN-10: 0 415 39227 6
ISBN-13: 978 0 415 39227 3

Distributed in North and South America by
Taylor and Francis
6000 Broken Sound Parkway, NW, (Suite 300)
Boca Raton, FL 33487, USA

Within Continental USA
Tel: 1 (800) 272 7737; Fax: 1 (800) 374 3401
Outside Continental USA
Tel: (561) 994 0555; Fax: (561) 361 6018
Email: orders@crcpress.com

Distributed in the rest of the world by
Thomson Publishing Services
Cheriton House
North Way
Andover, Hampshire SP10 5BE, UK
Tel: +44 (0)1264 332424
Email: tps.tandfsalesorder@thomson.com

Composition by Exeter Premedia Services Private Ltd, Chennai, India
Printed and bound in India by Replika Press Pvt. Ltd.

Contents

Contributors

A López Bernal MD DPhil
Division of Obstetrics and Gynaecology
University of Bristol and
Department of Clinical Science at South Bristol
St Michael's Hospital
Bristol
UK

Andrew M Blanks PhD
RCUK Fellow in Reproduction
Warwick Medical School
Clinical Sciences Research Institute
University Hospital – Walsgrave Hospital
Coventry
UK

John RG Challis PhD FRCOG FRSC
Vice-President, Research and
    Associate Provost
University of Toronto
Toronto, ON
Canada

Jennifer C Condon PhD
Department of Biochemistry
North Texas March of Dimes Birth Defects Center
University of Texas Southwestern
    Medical Center at Dallas
Dallas, TX
USA

Sharon M Cooley MRCOG MRCPI
Specialist Registrar Obstetrics and Gynaecology
National University of Ireland Galway
University College Hospital
Galway
Ireland

Xuesen Dong PhD
Centre for Women's and Infant's Health
Samuel Lunenfeld Research Institute
    at Mount Sinai Hospital
University of Toronto
Toronto, ON
Canada

Anna Dorogin
Centre for Women's and Infant's Health
Samuel Lunenfeld Research Institute
    at Mount Sinai Hospital
University of Toronto
Toronto, ON
Canada

Pasquale Florio MD PhD
Department of Pediatrics, Obstetric and
    Reproductive Medicine
University of Siena
Siena
Italy

Letizia Galleri PhD
Department of Pediatrics
Obstetrics and Reproductive Medicine
University of Siena
Siena
Italy

Robert E Garfield PhD
Department of Obstetrics,
    Gynecology and Reproductive Sciences
University of Texas Medical Branch
Galveston, TX
USA

Alessia Giovannelli PhD
Department of Pediatrics,
    Obstetrics and Reproductive Medicine
University of Siena
Siena
Italy

Laura T Goldsmith PhD
Department of Obstetrics,
    Gynecology and Women's Health
New Jersey Medical School of UMDNJ
Newark, NJ
USA

Daniel B Hardy PhD
Department of Biochemistry
North Texas March of Dimes Birth Defects Center
University of Texas Southwestern Medical Center
    at Dallas
Dallas, TX
USA

Brian R Heaps MD
Department of Obstetrics,
    Gynecology and Reproductive Sciences
University of Texas – Houston Health Science Center
Houston, TX
USA

Michael House MD
Assistant Professor
Division of Maternal-Fetal Medicine
Department of Obstetrics and Gynecology
Tufts University
Boston, MA
USA

B Lowell Langille PhD
University Health Network
Toronto General Research Institute
Toronto, ON
Canada

Phyllis Leppert MD PhD
Professor and Vice Chair of Research
Department of Obstetrics and Gynecology
Duke University School of Medicine
Durham, NC
USA

Xiang-Hong Li MS
Division of Reproductive Endocrinology
Department of Obstetrics and Gynecology
University of Texas Southwestern Medical Center
Dallas, TX
USA

Charles J Lockwood MD
Anita O'Keefe Young Professor of Women's
    Health and Chair
Department of Obstetrics, Gynecology and
    Reproductive Sciences
Yale University School of Medicine
New Haven, CT
USA

Stephen J Lye PhD
Centre for Women's and Infant's Health
Samuel Lunenfeld Research Institute
    at Mount Sinai Hospital
University of Toronto
Toronto, ON
Canada

Daniel MacPhee PhD
Division of Basic Medical Sciences
Memorial University of Newfoundland
St John's, NF
Canada

William L Maner
Department of Obstetrics, Gynecology and
    Reproductive Sciences
University of Texas Medical Branch
Galveston, TX
USA

Paul J Meis MD
Department of Obstetrics and Gynecology
Wake Forest University
Winston-Salem, NC
USA

Carole R Mendelson PhD
Departments of Biochemistry and
    Obstetrics and Gynecology
North Texas March of Dimes Birth Defects Center
University of Texas Southwestern Medical Center
    at Dallas
Dallas, TX
USA

Jennifer Mitchell
Centre for Women's and Infant's Health
Samuel Lunenfeld Research Institute
    at Mount Sinai Hospital
University of Toronto
Toronto, ON
Canada

John J Morrison MD MRCOG FRCPI BSC DCH
Professor and Head
Department of Obstetrics and Gynaecology
National University of Ireland Galway
University College Hospital
Galway
Ireland

Timothy JM Moss PhD
School of Women's and Infants' Health
University of Western Australia and
Women and Infants Research Foundation
Perth, WA
Australia

John P Newnham MD FRANZCOG
Professor of Obstetrics and Gynecology
    (Maternal Fetal Medicine) and
    Head, School of Women's and Infants' Health
University of Western Australia
King Edward Memorial Hospital
Perth, WA
Australia

Jane E Norman MD FRCOG
Professor (Honorary Consultant) in Obstetrics
    and Gynaecology
University of Glasgow
Glasgow
UK

Alexandra Oldenhoff
Centre for Women's and Infant's Health
Samuel Lunenfeld Research Institute
    at Mount Sinai Hospital
University of Toronto
Toronto, ON
Canada

Inass Osman MB ChB PhD
Specialist Registrar in Obstetrics and Gynaecology
West of Scotland Deanery
Glasgow
UK

Felice Petraglia MD
Obstetrics and Gynecology
Department of Pediatrics, Obstetrics
    and Reproductive Medicine
University of Siena
Siena
Italy

Fernando M Reis MD PhD
Associate Professor
Department of Obstetrics and Gynecology
University of Minas Gerais
Belo Horizonte
Brazil

Filiberto Severi MD
Department of Pediatrics, Obstetrics and
    Reproductive Medicine
University of Siena
Siena
Italy

Oksana Shynlova
Centre for Women's and Infant's Health
Samuel Lunenfeld Research Institute
    at Mount Sinai Hospital
University of Toronto
Toronto, ON
Canada

Roger Smith FRACP PhD
Mothers and Babies Research Centre
University of Newcastle
Callaghan, NSW
Australia

Simona Socrate PhD
d'Arbeloff Assistant Professor of Mechanical
  Engineering
Department of Mechanical Engineering
Massachusetts Institute of Technology
Cambridge, MA
USA

Jerome F Strauss III MD PhD
Executive Vice President for Medical Affairs
VCU Health System and
Dean School of Medicine
Virginia Commonwealth University
Richmond, VA
USA

Steven Thornton DM FRCOG
Professor of Obstetrics and Gynaecology
Warwick Medical School
University of Warwick
Coventry
UK

Paolo Boy Torres MD
Department of Pediatrics, Obstetrics and
  Reproductive Medicine
University of Siena
Siena
Italy

Michela Torricelli MD
Department of Pediatrics, Obstetrics and
  Reproductive Medicine
University of Siena
Siena
Italy

Prudence Tsui
Centre for Women's and Infant's Health
Samuel Lunenfeld Research Institute
  at Mount Sinai Hospital
University of Toronto
Toronto, On
Canada

Gerard HA Visser MD
Department of Obstetrics
University Medical Center
Utrecht
The Netherlands

Kenneth Ward MD
Department of Obstetrics and Gynecology
University of Hawaii
Kapiolani Hospital
Honolulu, HI
USA

Gerson Weiss MD
Professor and Chair
Department of Obstetrics, Gynecology
  and Women's Health
New Jersey Medical School of UMDNJ
Newark, NJ
USA

R Ann Word MD
Professor of Obstetrics and Gynecology
Divisions of Reproductive Endocrinology
  and Urogynecology
University of Texas Southwestern Medical Center
Dallas, TX
USA

Preface

It is with great pleasure that we introduce the first volume of the 'SGI Summit' series. These volumes will each address important topics in the fields of reproductive and women's health in a multidisciplinary fashion, encompassing both basic and clinical science. It represents the Proceedings of the Meeting on Preterm Birth held in Siena on November 10–12, 2005.

Preterm birth was chosen because it is the most critical obstetric syndrome. Given the immense societal impact of prematurity, there is an on-going need to assess the state of current knowledge and the direction of future research. The aim of the present volume is to provide the reader with an understanding of the innovations and complex mechanisms regulating preterm birth and to illustrate the immense progress that has been made. The combination of basic science and clinical implications are the guideline of the book. The present volume includes not only the latest information but is rich in diagrams, figures and references which will also be useful to scientists and physicians.

While the role of the myometrium, cervix, placenta and membranes in initiating labor is clear, the series of events has not yet been established. These opening chapters contain the most up-to-date information on the anatomical and functional aspects of this process.

The new development in the knowledge of the extracellular matrix, hormones, cytokines, prostaglandins and growth factors is the major content of the Section II.

New mediators are often discovered and their role in the pathogenesis of preterm labor is suggested.

Section III on the methods of prediction and prevention is more clinically oriented and refers to the new tools offered to understand the predisposition of pregnant women for preterm birth. The genetic or biochemical studies on populations are innovative.

The treatment of women with preterm labor is the last topic in this volume. Drug development is challenging, not only because it is difficult to combine both efficacy and safety, but because we are still seeking to understand the causes of preterm birth. There are several drugs now under investigation, and the future will undoubtedly bring new therapies.

The SGI will pursue this series and will do the best to remain a great source of new scientific knowledge in obstetrics and gynecology. Meetings and publications will generate an incredible exchange and development of reproductive science in the service of women's health. We hope this monograph will set the standard for those to come.

Felice Petraglia
Jerome F Strauss III
Gerson Weiss
Steven G Gabbe

Acknowledgments

The SGI and the SGI Summit Organizing Committee wishes to gratefully acknowledge Adeza, Ferring, Schering Italia, Organon Italia, and Solvay, for educational grants that helped sponsor the first SGI Summit, and the March of Dimes National Foundation for support. We also thank Ava Tayman, Linda Gildersleeve, Franca Fantacci, Annalisa Simi, Giuliana Pasquini, and Roberta Corsi for their secretarial help.

SECTION I

MECHANISMS

1

Myometrial programming: a new concept underlying the regulation of myometrial function during pregnancy

Stephen J Lye, Prudence Tsui, Xuesen Dong, Jennifer Mitchell, Anna Dorogin, Daniel MacPhee, Alexandra Oldenhoff, B Lowell Langille, John RG Challis, and Oksana Shynlova

INTRODUCTION

In this review a new model to explain the regulation of myometrial function during pregnancy and labor is described (see Figure 1.1). It is proposed that the myometrium undergoes dramatic changes in phenotype from early pregnancy until the onset of labor, characterized by an early proliferative phase, an intermediate phase of cellular hypertrophy and matrix elaboration, a third phase in which the cells assume a contractile phenotype, and a final phase in which cells become highly active and committed to labor. It is further proposed that phenotypic modulation of these uterine myocytes is the result of integration of endocrine signals and mechanical stimulation of the uterus by the growing fetus. Our previous studies have shown that these signals are important in regulating the onset of labor, and we now also have indications that they regulate earlier myometrial smooth muscle differentiation. The high rate of myometrial cell proliferation in early pregnancy recapitulates important aspects of many smooth muscle populations during development. We have drawn upon our understanding of smooth muscle differentiation to suggest that the subsequent phenotypic modulation of uterine smooth muscle cells during pregnancy also revisits developmental changes common to smooth muscle cell populations, until term when a myometrium-specific conversion commits these cells to labor. Our data are obtained mostly from the rat but we believe that they are generally applicable across species.

THE PROBLEM: PRETERM LABOR

Preterm birth is an immense problem; it occurs in 5–10% of all pregnancies, and is associated with 70% of neonatal deaths and up to 75% of neonatal morbidity. Preterm neonates are 40 times more likely to die than are term infants, and are at increased risk of cerebral palsy, blindness, deafness, and respiratory illness. In 2002 over 60% of twins were preterm compared with 10.4% among singletons; this led to 4–11-fold greater mortality and morbidity in twins compared to singletons.[1] The cost of prematurity is estimated at over $13 billion for neonatal care alone in the USA.[1] Furthermore, most children who weigh <800 g at birth and reach the age of 7 years have neurological or developmental measures in the suspect or abnormal range, and require rehabilitation or early intervention services. Unfortunately, decades of research directed to the development of drugs to inhibit myometrial contractile activity have not reduced the incidence of preterm birth.[2] Clearly, new approaches are needed.

STUDIES OF THE INITIATION OF LABOR

It is not surprising that research directed toward preterm delivery has focused on the onset of labor. Indeed, the vast majority of research investigations relating to myometrial function, including our own, have focused on events during the last few hours of pregnancy. Over the past decade our knowledge of the mechanisms leading to the onset of labor has increased dramatically (see ref 3 for detailed review). We have proposed that the fetal genome ultimately regulates the timing of parturition, and that this is accomplished through two separate but integrated pathways; an endocrine cascade comprising the fetal hypothalamic–pituitary–adrenal-placental axis, and a mechanical pathway in which fetal growth imposes tension of the uterine wall inducing biochemical and molecular changes within

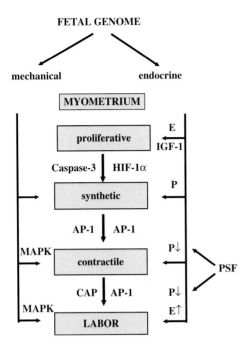

Figure 1.1 A model for the control of myometrial programming during pregnancy. Uterine myocytes exhibit a program of differentiation from proliferative to synthetic and to contractile, and to labor phenotypes. The mechanisms controling these differentiation events involve an integration of mechanical and endocrine signals originating in the fetus. Mechanical forces influence the expression of transcription factors (HIF-1α, AP-1), growth factors, extracellular matrix proteins and contraction-associated protein (CAP) genes, but this is dependent on the endocrine environment (primarily the presence or absence of progesterone (P) or estrogen (E) at specific period of gestation). (See text for detailed explanation.)

the myometrium. Both of these pathways are required in order to increase the expression of a cassette of contraction-associated proteins (CAP; e.g. the gap junction protein Cx43, receptors for agonists such as oxytocin and stimulatory prostaglandins, and Na^+/Ca^+ ion channels that control myometrial excitability) that induce activation of the myometrium. We now believe that these signals modulate the expression of a much wider cadre of genes including extracellular matrix (ECM) proteins, cell-matrix adhesion complexes[5] and contractile proteins,[6] and thus control the contractile phenotype of uterine myocytes at labor. Once activated, the myometrium can optimally respond to the increased production of uterine agonists (e.g. oxytocin, stimulatory prostaglandins), which in turn drive myometrial contractions required for delivery of the fetus.

While there is limited information, the myometrial events associated with term labor are believed to operate during preterm labor, while the underlying causal events may be quite different.[2] However, this knowledge has not been translated into the development of effective tocolytic agents that have positively impacted on the incidence of preterm birth. Indeed, data suggest that rather than decreasing there has been an increase in the incidence of preterm birth (see ref 1 for details). In general, the tocolytic agents – even those that have been developed based on our understanding on myometrial activation such as oxytocin antagonists, ion-channel blockers or prostaglandin synthesis inhibitors – have not been shown to result in effective blockade of preterm delivery. In this review it is suggested that the activation of the myometrium represents a terminal differentiation of uterine myocytes. At this time, stimulatory pathways within the myocytes are upregulated, and pathways that might lead to myometrial inhibition [e.g. cyclic adenosine monophosfate (cAMP) pathway] are downregulated. Consequently, effective tocolysis at this stage is problematic. It is further suggested that during pregnancy the myometrium undergoes a program of differentiation phases or phenotypes, characterized by an early proliferative phase, an intermediate phase of cellular hypertrophy and matrix elaboration, a third phase in which the cells assume a contractile phenotype, and a final phase in which cells become highly active and committed to labor. It is suggested that in order to fully control the contractile function of the myometrium during labor, this myometrial program, and the mechanisms that control it, must be understood.

MYOMETRIAL PROLIFERATIVE PHENOTYPE

During early pregnancy, uterine myocytes proliferate very rapidly – as measured by increased incorporation of BrdU into myocytes and of proliferating cell nuclear antigen (PCNA) expression – predominantly in the longitudinal muscle layer of both gravid and nongravid horns of unilaterally pregnant rats. This suggests that this proliferative phenotype is controlled by endocrine rather than mechanical signals.[7] In addition to proliferation there is increased expression of anti-apoptotic factors such as Bcl-2 (see Figure 1.2), which contributes to the overall increase in cell number. Data from nonpregnant rodents suggest that myometrial proliferation is induced by estrogen-regulated growth factors such as insulin-like growth factor (IGF) 1 and epidermal growth factor (EGF).[8] Our preliminary data indicate dramatic changes in IGF-1 and IGF binding proteins (IGFBP) expression associated with the proliferative phenotype during early pregnancy. In particular, high

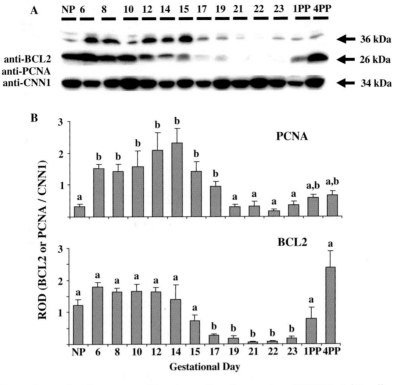

Figure 1.2 The effects of gestational age on proliferating cell nuclear antigen (PCNA) and B-cell lymphoma/leukemia 2 (BCL2) protein expression in the pregnant rat myometrium. Representative Western blots (A) and densitometric analysis (B) of PCNA and BCL2 protein levels throughout normal gestation and post-partum normalized to calponin (CNN1). The bar graphs showing the mean ± SEM ROD (n = 4 at each time point). Data labeled with different letters are significantly different from each other (P < 0.05). (Modified from Shynlora et al.[7])

levels of expression of IGF-1, and IGFBP-1 and IGFBP-3 were observed during days 6–14. Of considerable interest, it was observed that the expression of IGFBP-1, -2, -3, -5 and -6 is remarkably restricted to specific phases of myometrial differentiation, raising the possibility that they might exert IGF-independent actions to control myometrial phenotype.

TRANSITION TO THE SYNTHETIC PHENOTYPE

Around day 14, proliferation ceases and the expression of the anti-apoptosis factor Bcl-2 begins to decline (see Figure 1.2). At this point myocyte growth switches from proliferation to a phase of hypertrophy, termed the synthetic phase due to its association with increased synthesis of matrix and cellular growth. The cause of the switch in phenotype is unknown, but it coincides with dramatic activation of the intrinsic apoptotic

cascade that involves expression of initiator caspase-9 and effector caspase-3, -6 and -7 (see Figure 1.3). An increased cleavage of the caspase substrate poly (ADP-ribose) polymerase-1 (PARP) was detected but, surprisingly, no evidence of wide-scale apoptosis was found (by terminal deoxynucleotidyl transferase-mediated 2-deoxyuridine-S triphosphate nick end labelling (TUNEL) staining or DNA laddering), suggesting that this cascade may act to regulate other processes.

We have been very interested in determining the mechanisms that induce this temporally discrete activation of the caspase cascade in the myometrium. Our attention was thus drawn to the classic treatise on the pregnant uterus by SRM Reynolds in 1949.[9] Reynolds commented upon a process called 'uterine conversion' that occurs around mid-pregnancy. He reported that, "Soon after implantation, the accumulation of fluid in the tiny conceptus forces the uterus to bulge locally in order to accommodate it. The shape of the conceptus is . . . spheroidal. The process continues until, at a specific

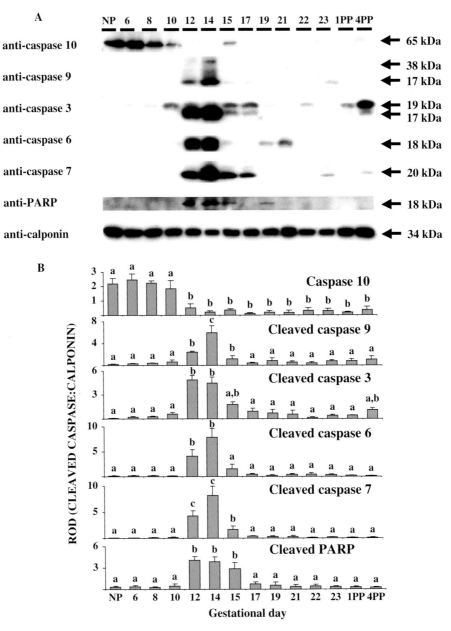

Figure 1.3 Expression of cleaved caspase 3–9, caspase-10 proteins and their poly(ADP-ribose) polymerase 1 (PARP-1) substrate in the pregnant rat myometrium. (A) Representative Western blots show the expression of caspase family proteins (cleaved caspase 3, 6, 7, 9, and caspase 10) and cleaved PARP-1 throughout normal gestation. (B) Densitometric analysis of caspase protein levels (in relative units) were normalized to calponin. The bars represent mean ± SEM ROD (n = 4 at each time point). Data labeled with different letters are significantly different from each other (P < 0.05). (Reproduced with permission from Shynlova et al.[7])

time critical for each species, a maximum radius is attained. Then within a space of time marked in hours the conceptus elongates. Thereafter it grows as a cylinder. This change from one pattern of growth to another has been called *uterine conversion*." We were interested to determine whether this process might be linked to the differentiation of the myometrium from the proliferation to synthetic phase. We assessed embryo

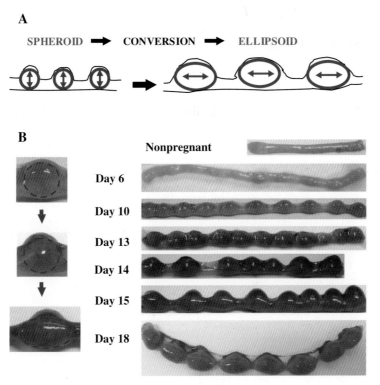

Figure 1.4 A composite figure showing (A) schematic and (B) photographic representation of 'uterine conversion' in rats (the transition in embryo shape from spheroid to ellipsoid that occurs around day 12–14 of rat gestation). (Reproduced with permission from Shynlova et al.[7])

shape between days 6 and 18 of gestation, and noted that there was indeed a switch from spheroidal to elipsoid growth, which in the rat occurred around day 14, coincident with the activation of the caspase cascade within the myometrium (see Figure 1.4). In his report, Reynolds suggested that uterine conversion was induced by an ischemic insult within the myometrium. He stated that, "As the conceptus approaches its maximum spheroidal size ... the uterine tissues begin to be stretched, and tension develops within them. This tension is so great that an ischaemia amounting to almost complete circulatory stasis takes place, except in the neighborhood of the placenta ... Conversion from sphere to cylinder, which requires only a few hours, causes a release of uterine tension and, with this, there is reestablishment of the maternal blood flow throughout the uterus."

Our data indicated that it was the extrinsic (or stress-induced) caspase cascade that was activated in the myometrium on day 14. One of the stressors that can activate this pathway is hypoxia, and so we sought evidence of myometrial hypoxia at this time. Through two different markers – hypoxia-inducible factor-1α (HIF-1α), and the hydroxyprobe pimonidazole hydrochloride – we demonstrated the presence of hypoxia, primarily in the circular layer of the myometrium, on day 14. Importantly, we demonstrated that activation of the caspase cascade on day 14 only occurred in the gravid horn of unilaterally pregnant rats, supporting the suggestion that uterine tension as a result of the growing embryo might be responsible. In preliminary studies we have recently been able to demonstrate that stretch does indeed precipitate activation of the caspase cascade. In these experiments, we implanted small cylinders (0.2 × 3 cm) of expandable material (dehydrated laminaria, used obstetrically to elicit cervical dilatation, or superabsorbent polymer (TAISAP)) into the nongravid horn of unilaterally pregnant rats. We monitored the expression of caspase-3 in the myometrium over the next 24 h. We found a time-dependent increase in caspase in the stretched horn over the 24 h period. Importantly, sham-operated rats displayed no caspase expression in the nongravid horn, nor did rats in which a 0.1 × 3 cm (nonexpandable) polyvinyl tube was inserted as a control for a nonspecific intrauterine device (IUD) effect. Thus, we have documented an association between the differentiation of uterine myocytes from a proliferative to a synthetic phenotype, a transient period of tissue hypoxia, and a stretch-induced activation of the stress-induced caspase apoptotic pathway. Data that are consistent with Reynolds' description of the mechanisms underlying uterine conversion some 50 plus years ago.

Of significance, our preliminary data show late in pregnancy, when we have shown that uterine stretch induces increased expression of contraction-associated protein (CAP) genes (e.g. the oxytocin receptor and Cx43), there is no increase in expression of caspase-3 in the myometrium. Nor were we able to induce expression of caspase-3 in the myometrium by insertion of cylinders made from expandable material laminaria or TAISAP into the nongravid horn at this time. These data suggest that the environment at day 14 is permissive to activation of this pathway, but that this is not the case at other times of pregnancy. The nature of this permissive environment is unknown at this time, though it is notable that at day 14 progesterone levels are high, whereas they fall to relatively low levels around term.

Despite the dramatic activation of the stress-induced apoptotic cascade, we found no evidence of significant myocyte apoptosis around day 14, suggesting that this pathway may modulate other physiologic processes. Caspase-3 has been reported to induce activation of transcription factors that regulate myocyte differentiation, the so-called myocyte regulatory factors (MRF: MyoD and myogenin). Indeed, it has been shown that this pathway is required for skeletal muscle differentiation.[10] Myocyte differentiation and apoptosis share several key features, e.g. disassembly/restructuring of actin filaments, and activation of myosin light chain kinase (MLCK). It is interesting to speculate that caspase activation initiates myometrial differentiation to the synthetic phenotype. Our initial analysis has not revealed any change in myometrial expression of MyoD/myogenin associated with caspase activation, but the are many MRF so it is quite possible that other members of this family of differentiation factors may be involved.

MYOMETRIAL SYNTHETIC PHENOTYPE

The synthetic phase of myometrial differentiation is characterized by growth which is due to an increase in cell size rather than proliferation, and the synthesis and deposition of interstitial matrix that forms the ground substance of the myometrium. During this period from day 15 to around day 21 there is a dramatic increase in the protein:DNA in the pregnant myometrium, indicative of hypertrophy.[7] Importantly, this myocyte hypertrophy requires a degree of tension on the myometrial wall and the presence of progesterone. Thus, hypertrophy only occurs in the gravid and not in nongravid horns of unilaterally pregnant rats, and administration of the progesterone antagonist RU486 on day 17 induces cessation of hypertrophy. In concert with myometrial cell hypertrophy, a marked increase in the expression of genes encoding structural extracellular matrix proteins that form the interstital matrix – notably collagen I, collagen III and elastin – was noted.[4] As with hypertrophy, expression of the fibrillar matrix proteins is restricted to the gravid horn, suggesting a role for mechanical tension (see Figure 1.5). Moreover, progesterone also seems to be required for their synthesis, since their expression decreases with the fall in progesterone at term or with administration of RU486 on day 19; administration of progesterone to prevent the endogenous fall of this hormone blocked the fall in expression of these matrix proteins. These changes in cell growth and matrix deposition are also associated with data indicating remodeling of cell matrix contacts through structures called focal adhesions – clusters of integrin molecules within the cell membrane. The extracellular domains of the integrin molecules interact with the extracellular matrix surrounding the cell, while their cytoplasmic domains interact with complexes of cytoplasmic and cytoskeletal proteins which control a variety of cellular functions, including cytoskeletal reorganization and cell growth. Focal adhesion kinase and its downstream target paxillin are critical components of the focal adhesion signaling network, and elevated activity of this kinase has been associated with turnover and remodeling of focal adhesions. During the synthetic phase of myocyte differentiation, expression of phosphorylated (activated) focal adhesion kinase and paxillin on the gravid myometrium was found. Thus, it is speculated that as the myocytes grow in size, remodeling of the focal adhesions allows the cells to maintain critical cell matrix interactions. In addition to changes in myocyte growth and matrix synthesis, the synthetic phenotype is also associated with the expression of contractile proteins (e.g. γ-smooth muscle actin) and associated proteins (e.g. l-caldesmon), which are characteristic of a relatively undifferentiated contractile state. The synthetic phase is associated with an elevated expression of IGFBP-6 (Lye and Shynlova, unpublished results), though the significance of this remains to be determined.

TRANSITION TO THE CONTRACTILE PHENOTYPE

Around day 21 the myometrium undergoes further differentiation into a contractile phenotype. At this time the rate of cellular hypertrophy appears to stabilize and there are marked changes within the myocyte.

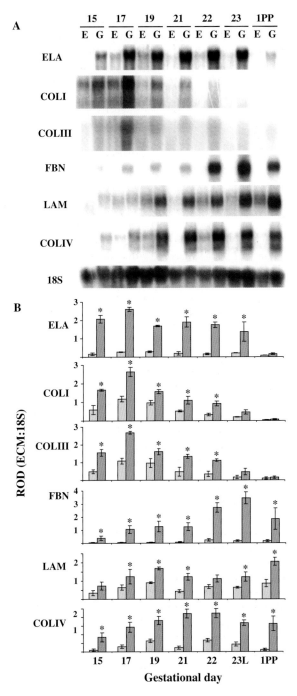

A

| 15 | 17 | 19 | 21 | 22 | 23 | 1PP |

E G E G E G E G E G E G E G

ELA

COLI

COLIII

FBN

LAM

COLIV

18S

B

ROD (ECM:18S)

ELA

COLI

COLIII

FBN

LAM

COLIV

15 17 19 21 22 23L 1PP

Gestational day

There are also changes in the interaction between the myocyte and the underlying matrix as the muscle prepares for the process of labor. The transition to the contractile phenotype is associated with a dramatic change in the synthesis of matrix proteins. The synthesis of interstitial matrix that was characteristic of the synthetic phase gives way to increased expression of matrix proteins that form the basement membrane, the matrix that surrounds the cells, and to which they anchor themselves. Thus, significant upregulation of the expression of fibronectin, laminin β2 and collagen IV, beginning around day 21 and continuing to term, was demonstrated. Again the expression of these genes was restricted to the gravid horn, suggesting (as in the case of the interstitial matrix proteins) that uterine tension may play a role in the regulation of their expression (see Figure 1.5). However, in contrast to the regulation of interstitial matrix gene expression, increased expression of the basement membrane proteins is associated with falling levels of progesterone. Indeed, administration of RU486 on day 19 induced a premature switch in matrix protein synthesis from interstitial to basement membrane subtypes. This suggests that the transition from the synthetic to the contractile phenotype is due to the fall in progesterone levels. This possibility was strengthened by the observation that administration of exogenous progesterone to maintain elevated levels of this steroid blocked the changes in matrix synthesis, and the transition to the contractile phenotype. Furthermore, we have recently obtained preliminary data that cyclic stretch of cultured myocytes reduces the expression of collagen I, increases expression of fibronectin, and causes the cells to assume a mature spindle-shaped morphology. These data provide exciting support for a role for stretch in the switch to the contractile phenotype.

In addition to the switch in extracellular matrix synthesis, there are also marked changes in the contractile protein isoforms within the smooth muscle cells, with increases in the γ-actin isoform more characteristic of a contractile phenotype relative to the α-smooth muscle actin isoform,[6] and smooth muscle-specific forms of tropomyosin and myosin heavy chain relative to the non-contractile isoforms of these proteins. There was

Figure 1.5 Expression of extracellular matrix (ECM) components in the myometrium of unilaterally pregnant rat during gestation. (A) Representative Northern blots show the expression of ECM genes in empty (E) and gravid (G) horns of unilaterally pregnant rats. (B) Densitometric analysis of ECM *(Continued)* mRNA levels in empty (white bars) and gravid (black bars) horns (in relative units) normalized versus 18S mRNA. Values represent mean ± SEM (n = 3 at each time point). A significant difference from the empty horn of the same day is indicated by *(P < 0.05). ELA, elastin; COL, collagen; FBN, fibronectin; LAM, Laminin. (Reproduced with permission from Shynlova et al.[4])

also an increase in h-caldesmon expression, a calcium-binding protein which interacts with the contractile protein machinery within the cell to inhibit uterine contractility at late gestation. As with the other phases of myometrial differentiation, phenotype-specific expression on IGFBF was noted – IGFBP-2 was upregulated over 99-fold during the contractile phase (Lye and Shynlova, unpublished results).

LABOR PHASE

As the influence of progesterone wanes the myometrium undergoes a final switch in phenotype as labor is initiated. We have previously described the series of molecular and biochemical events associated with labor, and the role of endocrine and mechanical signals.[8] At this time the myometrium becomes fully committed to the development of intense coordinated contractions that will bring about the delivery of the fetus(es). This period is associated with a significant increase in myometrial tension as uterine growth ceases but fetal growth continues. This induces the co-incident expression of a cassette of genes – including the sodium channel, oxytocin receptor, prostaglandin F receptor and the gap junction protein (Cx43 – which increase the electrical excitability of myocytes, their responsiveness to uterotonic agonists and their ability to synchronize the contractile waves across the uterine horns. Importantly, the increased expression of these CAP only occurs in the gravid horns of unilaterally pregnant rats. Insertion of a polyvinyl tube into the nongravid horn to induce stretch of that horn is able to induce expression of the CAP genes on the day of labor, providing direct evidence that stretch plays a critical role in the labor-associated expression of these genes. However, while stretch is necessary for CAP gene expression, it is not alone sufficient, since insertion of the tube on day 17 (when progesterone levels are elevated) did not lead to increased CAP gene expression. Moreover, administration of exogenous progesterone beginning on day 20 also blocked the expected expression of CAP genes on day 23 and the initiation of labor. Thus, the terminal differentiation of the myometrium to the labor phenotype requires changes in both endocrine (reduced progesterone) and mechanical (increased stretch) pathways.

In addition to changes in the contractile state of the cell, transition to the labor phenotype is associated with changes in the interaction of the smooth muscle cells and the underlying matrix via the focal adhesions. We observed a dramatic decrease in the level of phosphorylation of focal adhesion kinase and its downstream target paxillin.[5] In other systems, decreased focal adhesion kinase activity is associated with stabilization of focal adhesions and it is speculated that in the laboring myometrium this would enable the myocytes to anchor themselves to the newly synthesized extracellular matrix in basement membrane. This would aid in bringing about a shortening of the uterine horns as the waves of myocyte contraction move across the uterus, thus aiding in delivery of the fetus(es). Again, the critical role of progesterone is apparent in that exogenous administration of progesterone inhibits the decrease in phosphorylated focal adhesion kinase/paxillin and blocks the process of labor.

ROLE OF PROGESTERONE IN THE TRANSITION TO CONTRACTILE AND LABORING PHENOTYPES

Progesterone is required in virtually all species for the establishment and maintenance of pregnancy. Progesterone plays a pleiotropic role during pregnancy, contributing to the preparation of the implantation site, immunologic protection of the fetus, and suppression of uterotonic agonist synthesis to name a few. In addition, progesterone has multiple effects on the myometrium, including support of uterine growth, matrix synthesis and the inhibition of CAP gene expression.[8] As described above, the actions of progesterone suppress the initiation of labor and removal of the source of progesterone during early pregnancy (e.g. by ovariectomy), or administration of a progesterone antagonist (e.g. RU486), causes termination of pregnancy. In virtually all species a fall in tissue/plasma progesterone levels is a critical event prior to the onset of labor. Indeed, administration of exogenous progesterone at term (to prevent the normal withdrawal of this steroid) effectively prevents the initiation of labor. This presents a conundrum in humans since progesterone levels do not fall prior to the initiation of labor in this species. Moreover, even in those species where there is a prepartum fall in progesterone levels (e.g. sheep and rat), the fall is incomplete at the time of labor, and sufficient progesterone is available to saturate the receptor in the absence of a superimposed local withdrawal mechanism. In women where there is no evidence for a prepartum fall in plasma or tissue P4, administration of the progesterone receptor (PR) antagonist RU486 still leads to increased uterine activity, which suggests that progesterone plays a similar role in the human to that in other animals. Conversion of pregnenolone to P4 by placental syncytiotrophoblast, as reflected in levels and expression of 3β-hydroxysteroid dehydrogenase (3βHSD), does not change with labor at term or preterm. It is possible that another P4-like steroid (perhaps a P4 metabolite that interacts with PR) might serve as the active progestagen in human pregnancy, and change prior to labor or displace P4 from its receptor binding. We found that levels of allopregnanolone – the 3α,5α-reduced metabolite of P4 that can bind gamma-amino butyric acid (GABA) A receptors and inhibit smooth muscle – did not decrease at labor.[11] The 5β metabolite blocks oxytocin receptor (OTR) binding and inhibits oxytocin (OT)-induced contractions, but no evidence exists for it changing at term.[12,13] Hardy and Mendelson[14] recently proposed that increased P4 metabolism by upregulation of 20αHSD might induce local P4 withdrawal.

The majority of P4 actions are conferred through a nuclear, ligand-activated transcription factor, the PR. Three isoforms of PR have been described; the full length PR-B, and the truncated isoforms PR-A and PR-C. In mammals, PR-B functions predominantly as an activator of P4-responsive genes. PR-A acts as a modulator or repressor of PR-B function and of other nuclear receptors, including the glucocorticoid receptor (GR), at least in the context of artificial response elements. PR-A lacks one of the three activation function domains (AF3) contained within PR-B and it has been shown that it antagonizes P4 activation of PR-B function in transfected myometrial cells (see Figure 1.6).[15] Thus, antagonism of P4 action may be exerted through changing levels of PR, altered PR-B/PR-A interaction, or changes in levels of co-activator or co-repressor proteins. Controversy exists as to whether an increase in the PR-A:PR-B ratio occurs with human labor. Mesiano demonstrated an increased PR-A:PR-B ratio, inferred from measurements of mRNA levels, possibly mediated by PG.[16]

Recently, Condon et al[17] reported decreased levels of steroid receptor co-activator-1 (SRC-1) and SRC-3 in human fundal myometrium at labor, which may diminish PR function.[17] Our own data suggest that these co-activators are increased in the lower uterine segment (LUS), providing additional evidence for a regionalization of P4 signaling (Dong and Lye, unpublished results). In addition, we recently identified a novel co-repressor of PR that provides an additional mechanism to account for a functional withdrawal of P4.[18] This repressor, polypyrimidine tract-binding protein-associated splicing factor (PSF), blocks PR signaling through two distinct mechanisms. PSF binds to the DNA binding domain (DBD) of PR, inhibiting interaction of the receptor with its response element in target genes (see Figure 1.7). PSF also targets PR for degradation through the proteosomal pathway. Importantly, we have shown that expression of PSF increases in rat myometrium at the onset of labor and in association with a reduction in the level of PR protein (see Figure 1.8). We have preliminary data to show that PSF is expressed in human tissues including myometrium, fetal membranes and placenta; but to date we have no data on changes in expression with the onset of labor. Significantly, the onset of human labor is associated with a reduction in PR binding to progesterone response element (PRE), providing evidence of a functional withdrawal of P4.[19] Since we have demonstrated that PSF binds to the DBD of PR, preventing its interaction with PRE, we propose that PSF might effect this functional withdrawal of P4. Relevant to our investigation of cytokine-induced P4 withdrawal, our preliminary data indicate that tumor necrosis factor (TNF) α can increase PSF expression in mammalian cells; estrogen treatment of MCF7 cells also leads to increased PSF expression. Increased PSF expression at term would likely diminish P4 action in fetal membranes, decidua and myometrium.

Transforming growth factor (TGF) β has also been proposed as an endogenous antagonist of P4 action, as it reduces P4 stimulation of dependent genes.[20] Glucocorticoids may also compete with P4 to regulate expression of genes such as corticotrophin releasing hormone (CRH) and 15-hydroxyprostaglandin dehydrogenase (PGDH). However it is not clear whether these are separate actions through glucocorticoid receptor (GR) and PR, or if there is competition for a similar binding site.[21] Proinflammatory cytokines modulate P4 responsive genes such as PGDH and matrix metalloproteinase (MMP) but the mechanism of this interaction is unknown.

Assuming that a functional withdrawal of progesterone is achieved by one or more of the mechanisms described above, what downstream targets might be impacted in order to induce activation of CAP genes within the myometrium? Our previous data have implicated members of the activator protein-1 (AP-1) family of transcription factors. This family includes members of the Jun subgroup (c-jun, junB and junD), and members of the Fos subgroup (c-fos, Fra-1, Fra-2 and fosB). These transcription factors bind to consensus AP-1 sequences in a large number of target genes, including those important for myometrial function during pregnancy – e.g. CAP genes and genes involved in cell/matrix growth and remodeling. AP-1 family proteins bind AP-1 consensus sequences as dimers; Jun members can bind as homo- or heterodimers, while Fos members must have a Jun partner. In general Jun homodimers are less transcriptionally active than Fos/Jun heterodimers. We have measured the expression of these AP-1 genes in the rat myometrium throughout pregnancy (see Figure 1.9). Expression of Jun members (c-jun, junD) was relatively high (compared to Fos) during the majority of pregnancy, raising the possibility that they might suppress activation of AP-1 responsive genes. However, on the day of labor there was a dramatic increase in the expression of Fos genes (c-fos, fosB, Fra-1 and Fra-2) and of JunB.[22] As was the case for the CAP genes, exogenous administration

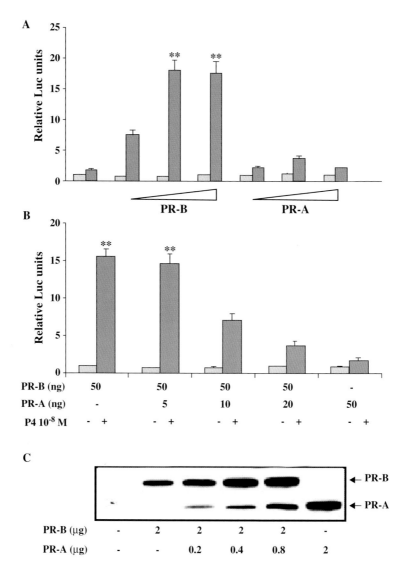

Figure 1.6 Differential transcriptional activities of progesterone recepter (PR) isoforms PR-B and PR-A in myometrial cells. Syrian hamster myometrial (SHM) cells were transfected with increasing amounts of PR-B or PR-A expression vector (10, 20, 50 ng) (A), or with 50 ng expression vector of PR-B with increasing amounts (5, 10, 20 and 50 ng) of PR-A (B). Expression vectors were co-transfected with 300 ng $3\times$ progesterone response element promoter linked to luciferase (PRE-Luc) luciferase report vector and 200 ng cytomegalovirus promoter linked to β-galactosidase (CMV-βGal). Four hours after transfection, the medium was replenished and cells were either untreated (open columns) or treated (filled columns) with 10^{-8} M progesterone (P4) for 30 h. Luciferase activities were normalized to β-galactosidase activities and were plotted as the fold induction over the promoter basal activity in the absence of PR expression vector and P4. Values are shown as means $\pm$SD from three independent experiments. Statistical analysis was performed using two-way ANOVA and a Student–Newman–Keuls test; $**P < 0.001$, n = 3. (C) The expression of PR-A and PR-B derived from expression vectors with indicated amounts of plasmids was tested by transient transfection into SHM cells; the same amount of protein lysates (60 μg) was separated on 8% SDS gel. After transfer, membrane was blotted with anti-PR monoclonal antibody AB-52. (Reproduced with permission from Dong, Challis, Lye, J Mol Endocrinol, 2004; 32(3): 843–57.)

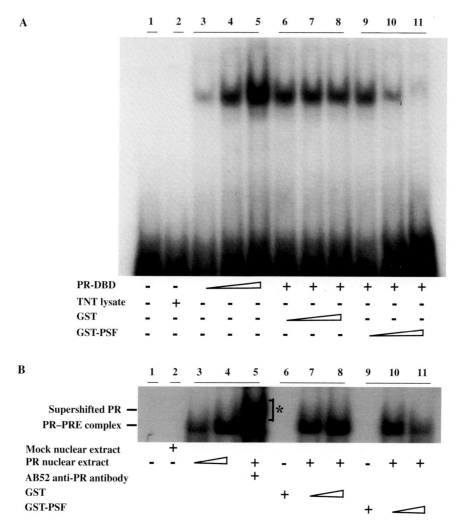

Figure 1.7 Protein-associated splicing factor (PSF) interferes with binding of the progesterone receptor DNA binding domain (DBD) to the progesterone response element (PRE). (A) An electrophoretic mobility shift assay was performed with the ^{32}P-labeled PRE incubated with the in vitro translated PR DBD (1, 2, and 5 μl in, lanes 3–5, respectively, and 2 μl in lanes 6–11), and increasing amounts of bacterially expressed gluthatione-S-transferase (GST) (lanes 6–8) or GST (PSF) (lanes 9–11). The TNT lysate (lane 2) was used as a negative control. (B) The PR nuclear extract (1 and 2 μg) was incubated with the ^{32}P-labeled PRE oligonucleotide in a dose-dependent manner (lanes 3 and 4). 'Mock' indicates the nuclear extract from 293 T cells transfected with the empty mammalian expression vector Sigma (pFLAG-CMV2) vector. Anti-PR antiserum AB-52 (1.5 μg) was added to the incubation mixture (lane 5). The addition of increasing doses of GST or GST-PSF (1 and 2 μl) to the same reaction as lane 4 is shown in lanes 7–8 and lanes 10–11, respectively. In the control experiments (lanes 6 and 9), GST or GST-PSF was incubated with the PRE without adding the PR nuclear extract. All reactions contained 10 nM progesterone. (Reproduced with permission from Dong et al.[18])

of progesterone could suppress the increased expression of these transcription factors on day 23 of pregnancy. Moreover, the increased expression of these genes was restricted to the gravid horn of unilaterally pregnant rats, suggesting a role for mechanical stretch. We have gained

direct evidence for stretch-induced regulation of Fos gene expression through a series of in vitro experiments. Thus, we found that static stretch of primary rat myometrial cells induced a time- and force-dependent increase in c-fos mRNA expression.[23] This stretch-induced increase

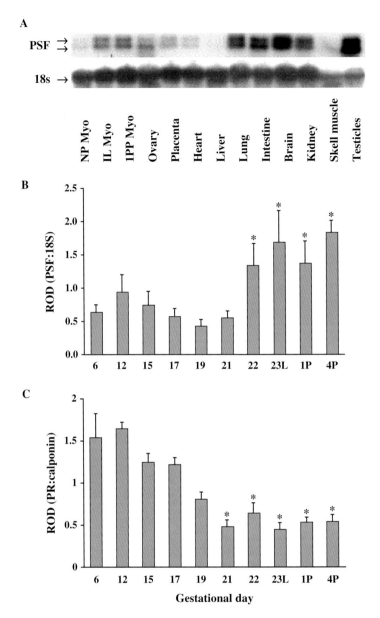

Figure 1.8 Expression profiles of protein-associated splicing factor (PSF) and the progesterone receptor (PR). (A) Tissue distribution of PSF in the rat was analyzed by Northern blotting. Various rat tissues were collected, and total RNA was isolated. PSF transcription was detected by a ^{32}P-labeled PSF probe. NP Myo, non-pregnant myometrium; IL Myo, in labor myometrium; 1PP Myo, day 1 post-partum myometrium; Skel, skeletal. (B) Myometrial tissue was collected during and after pregnancy from rats (n = 5 at each time point). Total RNA was extracted and subjected to Northern blotting to assess PSF expression levels. The intensity of PSF mRNA bands was quantified by densitometry and normalized by 18S mRNA. The bars represent the means ± SEM ROD (n = 5). There was a significant change in PSF expression during gestation (P = 0.03). (C) Myometrial tissue was collected during and after pregnancy from rats (n = 4 at each time point). Total protein was extracted and subjected to Western blotting using anti-PR antibody to assess PR expression levels. Membranes were then stripped and Western blotted with anti-calponin antibody as a loading control. The intensity of PR protein bands was quantified by densitometry and normalized by calponin. The bars represent the means ±SEM ROD. Significant difference is indicated by *. (Reproduced with permission from Dong et al.[18])

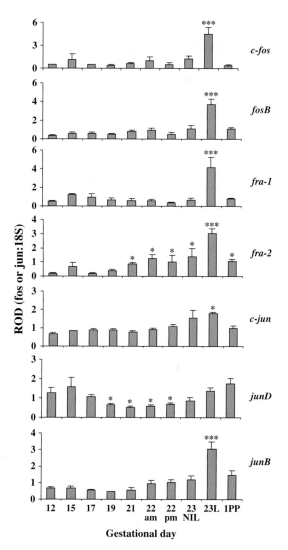

Figure 1.9 Northern blot analysis of the expression of AP-1 family genes in pregnant rat myometrium. Densitometric analysis of fos and jun mRNA levels in rat myometrium during gestation normalized versus 18S mRNA and represented as mean ± SEM ROD, n = 3. A significant difference is indicated by *(P<0.05) or ***(P<0.001). (Reproduced with permission from Mitchell and Lye, Biol Reprod, 2002; 67: 240–6.)

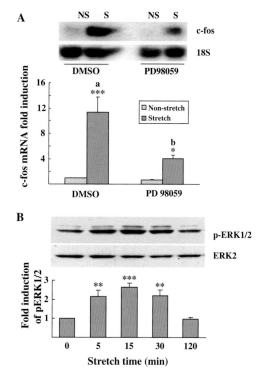

Figure 1.10 Effect of mitogen-activated protein kinase (MAPK) inhibitors on stretch-induced *c-fos* expression. (A) Myometrial smooth muscle cells (SMC) were pre-treated with 25 μM PD98059 for 60 min and subjected to 25% static stretch for 30 min to assess *c-fos* mRNA expression. S, Cells subjected to stretch; NS, non-stretch control cells. Shown are representative Northern blots for *c-fos* (upper panel), and the same membrane stripped and reprobed with 18S (lower panel), and the corresponding bar graph showing the mean ± SE of *c-fos* (relative to 18S), n = 3. (B) Time-course of MAPK phosphorylation by static stretch. Myometrial SMC were subjected to 25% static stretch for the indicated time periods. MAPK phosphorylation was analyzed by Western blot using phospho-specific MAPK antibodies. Shown are representative immunoblots for p-ERK1/2 (upper panels) or a control anti-ERK1/2 antibody (lower panels). The intensity of ERK phosphorylation was quantified by densitometry, normalized to their respective protein levels and represented in the corresponding bar graph as mean ±SEM ROD, n = 4. Data were subjected to two-way (A) or one-way (B) ANOVA followed by all pairwise multiple comparison procedures (Student– Newman–Keuls method). *P < 0.05, **P < 0.01, ***P < 0.001 indicates significant difference from non-stretch controls; 'a' is significantly different from 'b' (P < 0.05). (Modified from Oldenhof et al, Am J Physiol Cell Physiol, 2002; 283: C1530–9.)

could be blocked by prior exposure of the cells to PD98059, an inhibitor of the mitogen-activated protein kinase (MAPK),[24] suggesting a role for this signaling pathway in stretch-induced Fos activation (see Figure 1.10a). This possibility was confirmed when we showed a rapid increase in activated (phosphorylated) extracellular signal-regulated kinase (ERK) following stretch of myometrial cells (see Figure 1.10b). Finally, these in vitro data were confirmed in vivo when we demonstrated an increase in phospho-ERK in the myometrium of gravid (but not empty) horns during labor in the rat (see Figure 1.11). These data suggest that one pathway by which the initiation of labor could be induced would include a functional withdrawal of progesterone, possibly mediated in part by PR co-repressors such as PSF. This in turn would result in stretch-induced activation of ERK signaling, and the increased expression of AP-1 transcription factors which target the expression of genes that contribute to myometrial activation. However, given the complexity of labor it is very likely that multiple pathways exist to regulate this process.

A NEW MODEL FOR THE REGULATION OF MYOMETRIAL FUNCTION DURING PREGNANCY AND LABOR

The data described here have led us to propose that uterine myocytes exhibit a program of differentiation throughout pregnancy, which encompasses at least four distinct cell phenotypes. These include an initial phase of myocyte proliferation, a synthetic phase involving interstitial ECM synthesis, focal adhesion remodeling, myocyte hypertrophy, a contractile phase of upregulation of CAP and downregulation of myometrial inhibitory pathways, and, finally the expression of myometrial labor genes, synthesis of uterotonic agonists and development of the intense, synchronous contractions of labor (see Figure 1. 12). This circle of events is concluded by a phase of postpartum uterine involution characterized by the expression of genes associated with apoptosis, wound repair, and tissue regeneration. We suspect that the final labor stage of differentiation creates a phenotype that may be resistant to tocolytic approaches. It is proposed that efforts should focus on regulators of the myometrial phenotypes. Identification of such regulators will inform studies to generate novel therapeutic agents that can modulate the phenotype functional characteristics of the myocyte, rather than modulating individual biochemical pathways. This may reveal more effective means of preventing preterm birth and prolonging pregnancy.

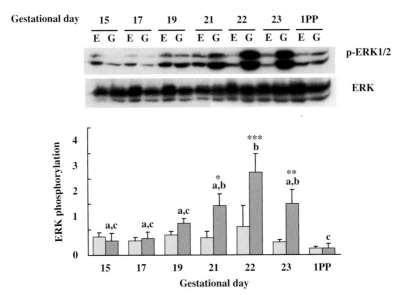

Figure 1.11 MAPK phosphorylation in empty and gravid horns of unilaterally pregnant rats during gestation. Extracellular signal-regulated kinase 1/2 (ERK1/2) phosphorylation was analyzed in gravid (G) and empty (E) horns of unilaterally pregnant rats on the indicated days of gestation by Western blot using phospho-specific p-ERK1/2 antibodies. Shown are immunoblots for phosphorylated ERK1/2 (upper panels) or a control anti-ERK1/2 (lower panels). The intensity of ERK phosphorylation was quantified by densitometry and ERK levels were normalized to their respective protein levels and represented in the corresponding bar graph as mean ± SEM ROD, n = 3. Data were subjected to two-way ANOVA followed by all pairwise multiple comparison procedures (Student–Newman–Keuls method). Data labeled with different letters are significantly different from each other ($P < 0.05$). * $P < 0.05$, **$P < 0.01$, ***$P < 0.001$ indicates significant difference versus empty horn of the same gestational day. (Modified from Oldenhof et al, Am J Physiol Cell Physiol, 2002; 283: C1530–9.)

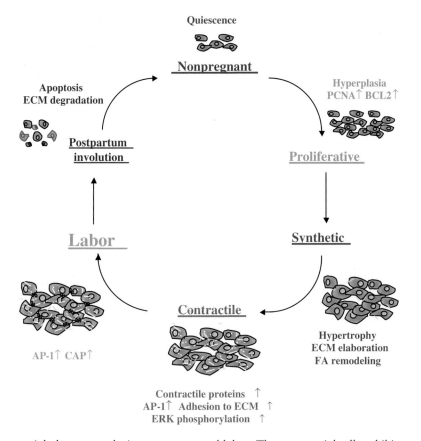

Figure 1.12 Myometrial phenotypes during pregnancy and labor. The myometrial cells exhibit a programmed pattern of distinct phenotypes throughout pregnancy, labor and postpartum. These include: (i) an initial proliferative phenotype in which myocytes undergo hyperplasia; (ii) a synthetic phase involving myocytes hypertrophy and interstitial matrix synthesis; (iii) a contractile phenotype involving upregulation of contractile proteins as well as downregulation of myometrial inhibitory pathways; (iv) a labor phase with expression of myometrial contraction-associated protein (CAP), synthesis of uterotonic agonists, and development of intense, synchronous contractions; and finally (v) a phase of postpartum uterine involution with expression of genes associated with apoptosis, wound repair, and tissue regeneration. This allows the uterus to resume its normal, nonpregnant receptive conditions. The myometrium adapts to pregnancy by changing its molecular biochemistries, functions, and cellular phenotypes across gestation but the mechanisms leading to these changes are largely unknown. AP-1, activator protein 1; BCL2, B-cell lymphoma/leukemia 2; ECM, extracellular matrix; ERK, extracellular signal-regulated kinase; FA, focal adhesion; PCNA, proliferating cell nuclear antigen.

REFERENCES

1. March-of-Dimes, Perinatal Statistics, 2006.
2. Challis JR, Lye SJ, Gibb W et al. Understanding preterm labor. Ann NY Acad Sci 2001; 943: 225–34.
3. Gibb WL, Lye SJ, Challis JRG. Parturition. In: Knobil E and Neill JD, eds. Physiology of Reproduction. New York: Elsevier Inc, 2006: 2925–74.
4. Shynlova O, Mitchell JA, Tsampalieros A et al. Progesterone and gravidity differentially regulate expression of extracellular matrix components in the pregnant rat myometrium. Biol Reprod 2004; 70(4): 986–92.
5. MacPhee DJ, Lye SJ. Focal adhesion signaling in the rat myometrium is abruptly terminated with the onset of labor. Endocrinology 2000; 141(1): 274–83.
6. Shynlova O, Tsui P, Dorogin A et al. Expression and localization of alpha-smooth muscle and gamma-actins in the pregnant rat myometrium. Biol Reprod 2005; 73(4): 773–80.
7. Shynlova O, Oldenhof A, Dorogin A et al. Myometrial apoptosis: activation of the caspase cascade in the pregnant rat myometrium at midgestation. Biol Reprod 2006; 74(5): 839–49.
8. Lye SJ, Mitchell J, Nashman N et al. Role of mechanical signals in the onset of term and preterm labor. Front Horm Res 2001; 27: 165–78.

9. Reynolds SRM. Patterns of uterine growth during pregnancy. In: Hoeber, (ed). Physiology of the Uterus, 2nd edn. New York: Hoeber, 1949: 218–34.

10. Fernando P, Kelly JF, Balazsi K et al. Caspase 3 activity is required for skeletal muscle differentiation. Proc Natl Acad Sci USA 2002; 99(17): 11025–30.

11. Jackson MR, Walsh AJ, Morrow RJ et al. Reduced placental villous tree elaboration in small-for-gestational-age pregnancies: relationship with umbilical artery Doppler waveforms. Am J Obstet Gynecol 1995; 172(2 Pt 1): 518–25.

12. Grazzini E, Guillon G, Mouillac B et al. Inhibition of oxytocin receptor function by direct binding of progesterone. Nature 1998; 392(6675): 509–12.

13. Thornton S, Terzidou V, Clark A et al. Progesterone metabolite and spontaneous myometrial contractions in vitro. Lancet 1999; 353(9161): 1327–9.

14. Hardy DJ, Mendelson CR. Spatial regulation of 20a-hydroxy-steroid dehydrogenase activity and progesterone receptor expression in the myometrium of women in labor. J Soc Gynecol Invest 2004; 11(2 (suppl)): 172A.

15. Dong X, Challis JR, Lye SJ. Intramolecular interactions between the AF3 domain and the C-terminus of the human progesterone receptor are mediated through two LXXLL motifs. J Mol Endocrinol 2004; 32(3): 843–57.

16. Mesiano S. Myometrial progesterone responsiveness and the control of human parturition. J Soc Gynecol Invest 2004; 11(4): 193–202.

17. Condon JC, Jeyasuria P, Faust JM et al. A decline in the levels of progesterone receptor coactivators in the pregnant uterus at term may antagonize progesterone receptor function and contribute to the initiation of parturition. Proc Natl Acad Sci USA 2003; 100(16): 9518–23.

18. Dong X, Shynlova O, Challis JRG et al. Identification and characterization of the protein-associated splicing factor as a negative co-regulator of the progesterone receptor. J Biol Chem 2005; 280(14): 13 329–40.

19. Henderson D, Wilson T. Reduced binding of progesterone receptor to its nuclear response element after human labor onset. Am J Obstet Gynecol 2001; 185(3): 579–85.

20. Casey ML, MacDonald PC. Transforming growth factor-beta inhibits progesterone-induced enkephalinase expression in human endometrial stromal cells. J Clin Endocrinol Metab 1996; 81(11): 4022–7.

21. Karalis K, Goodwin G, Majzoub JA. Cortisol blockade of progesterone: a possible molecular mechanism involved in the initiation of human labor. Nat Med 1996; 2(5): 556–60.

22. Mitchell JA, Lye SJ. Differential expression of activator protein-1 transcription factors in pregnant rat myometrium. Biol Reprod 2002; 67(1): 240–6.

23. Shynlova OP, Oldenhof AD, Liu M et al. Regulation of c-fos expression by static stretch in rat myometrial smooth muscle cells. Am J Obstet Gynecol 2002; 186(6): 1358–65.

24. Oldenhof AD, Shynlova O, Liu M et al. Mitogen-activated protein kinases mediate stretch-induced c-fos mRNA expression in myometrial smooth muscle cells. Am J Physiol Cell Physiol 2002; 283(5): C1530–9.

Cervical function during pregnancy and parturition

R Ann Word and Xiang-Hong Li

CERVICAL FUNCTION DURING PREGNANCY, PARTURITION, AND THE PUERPERIUM

During most of pregnancy, the cervix remains unyielding and reasonably rigid. The function of the cervix is to keep the cervical canal closed so that expansion of the uterine cavity may proceed undisturbed. The cervix and cervical mucus also serve as barriers to invading microorganisms.[1] At the end of pregnancy, however, the cervix must undergo cervical ripening – defined as increased softening, distensibility, effacement, and early dilation of the cervix by digital examination – to allow successful delivery of the fetus through the cervix and vagina. These two functions of the cervix, i.e. maintenance of intrauterine pregnancy and facilitation of delivery, are diametrically opposed, require tight orchestration, and must be coordinated with uterine contractions for successful delivery of a term infant.

Recent studies using serial endovaginal ultrasound measurements of cervical length, dilation, and funneling of the fetal membranes into the cervical canal have contributed significantly to our understanding of cervical function during pregnancy.[2–4] Values for the normal progression of cervical length and dilation during pregnancy have been obtained. However, there is not a clear understanding of the mechanisms by which these changes occur. Furthermore, it is not understood why some women undergo progressive shortening of the cervix during pregnancy without labor while others are at high risk for preterm birth. The precise value of cervical shortening and funneling in the second trimester in terms of predicting preterm labor is controversial. Nevertheless, all studies agree that women with a shortened cervix at 18–22 weeks of gestation are at increased risk for preterm delivery, and that extreme shortening of the cervix, accompanied by funneling of the

membranes at 18–22 weeks is predictive of preterm birth, often prior to 28 weeks of gestation.[5–7] Results from cervical sonography, together with the knowledge that, in term pregnancy, cervical ripening precedes myometrial contractions of labor, suggest that both preterm and term parturition in women is a process of long duration and that uterine contractions of labor are late events in the parturition process. To impact the preterm birth rate, we need to understand the biologic mechanisms that regulate progressive changes in cervical function during pregnancy.

CERVICAL SOFTENING AND MAINTENANCE OF PREGNANCY

Many investigations have yielded important information regarding the cellular, biochemical, and molecular changes during cervical ripening at term in which the soft, but mechanically competent, cervix becomes pliable and distensible at the end of pregnancy. It could be argued, however, that equally dramatic changes in cervical function occur as soon as pregnancy is established. In women, the cervix begins to soften as early as 1 month after conception. These changes result from increased vascularity and edema of the entire cervix, together with hypertrophy and hyperplasia of the cervical glands. The glands of the endocervical canal are not true glands but crypts, i.e. invaginations of the luminal epithelial cells into the cervical stroma. Proliferation of endocervical epithelial cells during pregnancy is remarkable such that, by the end of pregnancy, the endocervical glands occupy approximately 50% of the entire cervical mass. This is in marked contrast to the nonpregnant cervix in which endocervical epithelial cells are relatively scant (Figure 2.1). Endocervical glands are important in providing immunologic protection

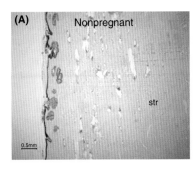 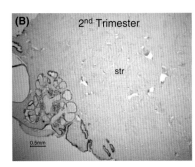 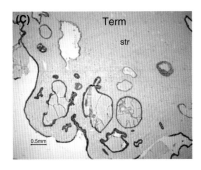

Figure 2.1 Endocervical crypts are increased in the cervix during pregnancy: endocervical epithelial cells were immunostained with an antibody to cyclooxygenase (COX) 2. (A) Endocervical crypts are scant and of superficial depth in nonpregnant women. Hyperplasia and number of crypts are increased in the (B) second and (C) third trimesters. Cervical stroma (str) is counterstained blue.

and secreting copious amounts of thick mucus during pregnancy. Furthermore, these cells may serve other important functions during pregnancy. For example, endocervical epithelial cells are enriched in enzymes involved in prostaglandin biosynthesis,[8] contain high levels of cytokines and chemokines such as interleukin (IL) 8,[9] secrete protease inhibitors,[10-12] and are enriched in enzymes involved in steroid hormone metabolism.[13-14] In a study conducted by Yoshimatsu et al,[15] detection of cervical gland area by cervical sonography correlated with cervical length and cervical rigidity by digital examination. Cervical gland area remained constant until 31 weeks of gestation, but decreased substantially thereafter. In women with threatened preterm labor, the detection rate of cervical gland area was significantly decreased compared with women without threatened preterm labor. Pregnancy outcome was poorer, and preterm birth was increased significantly in the threatened preterm labor group with absence of cervical gland area by sonography.[15] Thus, epithelial endocervical cells appear to play an important role in maintenance of cervical competency. Further studies are indicated to understand the precise regulatory signaling pathways in these cells, and the interactions between the cervical stroma and epithelium.

Under normal resting conditions, the cervix is dynamic, exhibiting occasional opening and closing even in the absence of uterine contractions. From gestational ages of 20–28 weeks, the median normal cervical length is 35 mm, decreasing gradually to 30 mm at term. This modest change in cervical length is associated with increased cervical softening and cervical volume; but, the cervix does not efface before term despite the gravitational forces imposed by the growing fetus, placenta, and increases in amniotic fluid volume. The sonographic terms 'funneling' or 'beaking' occurs in the late third trimester, and indicates that the internal cervical os is visibly separated by the two sidewalls of the upper

end of the cervical canal, thereby producing thinning of the cervix (effacement) by physical examination. The temporal relationship between cervical effacement and onset of labor are in agreement with clinical studies by Bishop,[16] indicating that cervical ripening is first observed near the internal os (effacement), which ultimately progresses to dilation of the internal cervical os as the fetal membranes further distend and protrude into the cervical canal (Figure 2.2).

The lack of compliance of the cervix during most of human pregnancy presents a formidable challenge when pregnancy must be terminated prior to the third trimester of pregnancy. Antiprogestins, together with prostaglandins, are often necessary to bring about sufficient change in cervical compliance for successful termination of a first or second trimester pregnancy. At term, induction of labor prior to cervical ripening is a major risk factor for Cesarean section due to failed induction. Thus, maintenance of cervical rigidity at term is a major obstetrical problem for successful vaginal delivery. On the other hand, preterm cervical insufficiency results in preterm birth even in the absence of uterine contractions.

The maintenance phase of cervical rigidity during pregnancy may be less important in rodents compared with other species. For example, in rats and mice, cervical softening begins early in pregnancy (day 12) and increases progressively throughout gestation.[17-19] An accelerated phase of cervical ripening and rapid increase in cervical distensibility occurs 1–3 h prior to parturition.[20,21] In sheep, the cervix remains long and closed throughout pregnancy until a sharp increase in cervical compliance occurs 12 h prior to uterine contractions of labor.[22] In guinea pigs, progressive softening and dilation of the cervix begins on day 58, with maximum ripening on day 65 of a 68 ± 3 day pregnancy.[23] Thus, it appears that, in some species, the cervix has undergone functional adaptations to preserve

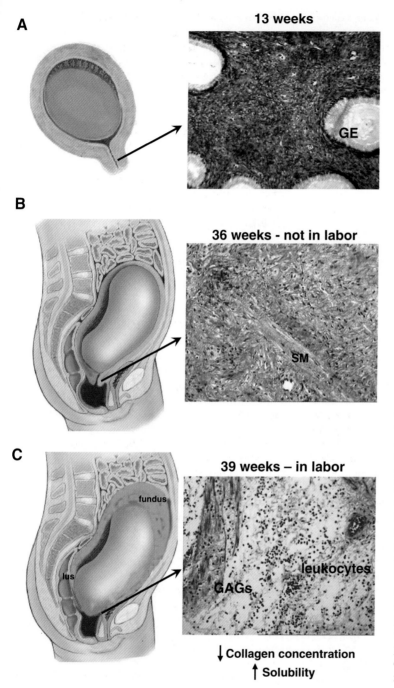

Figure 2.2 Cervical changes during pregnancy and cervical ripening. During early pregnancy (A) and before cervical ripening at term (B), the cervix is characterized by dense, organized, collagen bundles (stained blue), few or rare inflammatory cells, hyperplasia of glandular epithelium (GE), and hypertrophy and hyperplasia of the cervical fibroblasts and smooth muscle (SM). Prior to cervical ripening, there are histologic changes in the stroma, but the cervix is not effaced. (C) During cervical ripening, the cervix undergoes morphologic, anatomic, and structural changes that result in cervical dilation, and incorporation of the cervix into the lower uterine segment (lus) by the contracting fundal myometrium. Cervical collagen bundles are widely dispersed associated with increased amounts of hydrophilic glycosaminoglycans (GAGs) and infiltration of leukocytes. Collagen concentration is decreased and collagen solubility is increased during cervical ripening predominantly due to alterations in GAGs, although leukocyte-derived proteases contribute to collagen degradation during cervical dilation in labor.

cervical rigidity until late pregnancy when cervical ripening begins. Although cervical softening progressively increases from day 12 to the day of parturition in rats and mice, experiments using mouse models of failed cervical ripening indicate that pronounced changes in cervical softening are insufficient to yield to uterine contractions of labor unless the accelerated phase of cervical remodeling (i.e. cervical ripening) occurs.[13,24]

Animals deficient in the matricellular protein thromobospondin-2 (TSP-2) experience preterm cervical softening, although parturition occurs on time in TSP-2 null females.[25] There are several possible explanations for this phenotype. In quadrupeds, lack of uterine contractions, or the short umbilical cords of mice, may allow pregnancy to proceed despite preterm cervical insufficiency. It is also possible that the biomechanical changes of advanced cervical softening are not identical to those of ripening, which occurs in the last few hours of gestation in the mouse. Similar to other studies, Drzewiecki et al[26] found that cervical softening is associated with progressive increases in cervical compliance in the rat cervix throughout gestation. It was suggested that simultaneous changes in cervical volume, hypertrophy, hyperplasia, and geometric change counterbalance the softening effects until term when cervical ripening allows for full cervical dilation in the presence of uterine contractions.

PROCESS OF CERVICAL RIPENING, EFFACEMENT, AND DILATION

Cervical ripening is most obvious during the last few weeks of human pregnancy.[16] The ripe cervix is soft, thin, and easily stretched with examination, which is in marked contrast to the findings in early and mid pregnancy. This change in tissue properties is associated with histologic changes and major alterations in the extracellular matrix and cellular composition of cervical tissue (Figure 2.2). Prior to cervical ripening, cross-linked collagen fibrils are organized in tight bundles which provide tensile strength, rigidity, and stiffness. The predominant extracellular matrix proteins are type I and type III collagen, and total collagen content increases throughout pregnancy in proportion to cervical growth. During cervical ripening at term, the decline in collagen concentration is not due to loss of cervical collagen (per tissue wet weight).[27–29] The rate of collagen synthesis is not decreased, collagen type I and III mRNA levels are not decreased, and the total collagen content is stable.[29] Rather, the decrease in cervical collagen concentration during cervical ripening is primarily due to an increase in cervical tissue hydration which occurs in response to substantial increases in hydrophilic glycosaminoglycans and noncollagenous proteins.[30] Increases in hydrophilic glycosaminoglycans result in dispersal and disorganization of the collagen fibers, increased collagen solubility, and increased susceptibility to endogenous proteases.

The process by which cervical collagen is solubilized and disrupted during cervical ripening is not completely understood. Numerous investigations indicate that changes in glycosaminoglycans are involved. The complex carbohydrate moieties of the proteoglycan or the free carbohydrates in the extracellular matrix exhibit diverse physicochemical properties in the cervical connective tissue.[31,32] The glycoprotein decorin is in great abundance in cervical tissue. Decorin binds and immobilizes collagen fibers. In late gestation, collagen dispersal is promoted by decreases in decorin concentrations and simultaneous increases in hyaluronan (HA).[27] HA is a hydrophilic glycosaminogycan that weakens the interaction of collagen with fibronectin and may thereby contribute to collagen dispersal in late gestation. During cervical ripening, the content of HA is increased, and mRNA for the enzyme HA synthase 2 is upregulated prior to parturition.[31] In mice, the HA content of the cervix is upregulated the day prior to parturition, and progesterone suppresses the temporal increase in cervical HA synthase 2 gene expression.[31] Low molecular weight HA binds to the cell surface receptor CD44, and stimulates macrophages that are recruited to sites of inflammation to produce chemokines that, in turn, maintain the inflammatory response through recruitment of other inflammatory cells.[32,33]

COLLAGEN DEGRADATION DURING CERVICAL RIPENING

Regulation of collagenolytic events during cervical ripening differs from that during cervical dilation. A massive influx of leukocytes occurs during active labor in sheep, women, guinea pigs, pigs, cows, and rats. It is believed that these inflammatory cells are the predominant source of collagenases. It is not clear, however, whether infiltrating leukocytes are necessary for cervical ripening. Studies conducted by Timmons and Mahendroo[34] indicate that neutrophil depletion before term had no effect on timing or success of parturition, suggesting that neutrophils may not play a role in cervical ripening in the mouse. The role of monocytes, eosinophils, or other cell types in the ripening process is not clear, especially in experimentally induced neutrophil depletion. Studies conducted in a mouse model in which a transgene insertion in the mouse genome resulted in impaired cervical remodeling throughout pregnancy, despite an extensive infiltrate of inflammatory cells in the cervix, also supports the idea that factors other than, or in addition to, inflammatory cell recruitment are necessary for cervical ripening. The role of matrix metalloproteases (MMP) and other collagenases in the ripening process are also unclear. Different cell types, and thereby different proteases, may be operative during ripening compared with the dilatation phase of active labor. Remodeling of the collagen bundles caused by HA and hydrophilic proteoglycans may simply increase the susceptibility of solubilized collagen to endogenous proteases, thereby requiring no increase in collagenolytic enzyme expression nor recruitment or activation of inflammatory cells. Increased concentrations of MMP and increased numbers of leukocytes correlate with the extent of cervical dilation after initiation of uterine contractions of labor, but may not be involved in cervical ripening prior to labor.

Much of the difficulty in interpreting studies regarding cervical ripening in women come about due to differences in the sources of clinical material and various sampling techniques. In many studies, tissues from the decidua, fetal membranes, and lower uterine segment are used to investigate the changes in gene expression during the initiation of labor, and results are often extrapolated to the cervix. Investigations using cervical tissues often involve biopsies from nonpregnant women, pregnant women at term prior to labor, and women immediately postpartum. Since cervical ripening occurs during the last weeks of pregnancy in women, it would be expected that most of the biopsies in women at term involve cervical tissue from a ripened cervix. Needle or small punch biopsies may not be of sufficient depth to analyze the stromal collagenous region of the cervix, especially near the cervical os.

Recent studies addressing the roles of IL-8[35] and immune cells[36] in cervical ripening demonstrate that distinct differences exist between cervical ripening prior to labor and cervical dilation during labor. Punch biopsies (6 mm) were obtained from 17 women at term before the onset of labor, 12 before cervical ripening (Bishop score >4) and five with cervical ripening (Bishop score <4). In addition, biopsies were obtained from 11 women after vaginal delivery. Although tissue levels of IL-8 were increased dramatically in the cervix of women after delivery (949 ± 305 pg/mg protein), IL-8 levels were 56.5 ± 13 pg/mg protein in cervical stroma from women with an unripe cervix compared with 71.5 ± 29.1 pg/mg in the ripe cervix. Although the values were not statistically significant in the study by Sakamoto et al,[36] other studies indicate that cervical IL-8 levels are increased in pregnant women at term compared with early pregnant or nonpregnant women,[37] suggesting that progressive increases in cervical IL-8 precede cervical ripening. Using immunohistochemistry, expression of IL-8 receptors is restricted to granulocytes, macrophages, and T-lymphocytes in the cervix of women after vaginal delivery. Expression of IL-8 receptors and neutrophil numbers were increased in cervical tissues after labor, but not before.[35,36] In contrast to the lack of significant infiltration of granulocytes in the ripened cervix before labor, the number of macrophages in the ripened cervix (Bishop score >4) was increased compared with the unripe cervix at term,[36] suggesting that macrophage infiltration or differentiation/ activation in the cervix may play an important role in cervical ripening before labor.

SPATIAL AND TEMPORAL REGULATION OF S100A9 (CALGRANULIN B) IN THE PREGNANT UTERUS

The signals responsible for the initiation of leukocyte recruitment during cervical dilation during parturition are unknown. S100A9 may represent a new chemotactic factor contributing to macrophage and neutrophil migration into myometrium and cervix during the initiation or progression of the parturition process. S100A9 is a myeloid-related protein expressed in activated neutrophils and differentiated macrophages.[38] The two Ca^{2+}-binding proteins S100A8 (calgranulin A, 11 kDa) and S100A9 (calgranulin B, 14 kDa) heterodimerize to form a protein complex that is highly expressed in tissues involved in active inflammatory disease.[38] S100A8 and S100A9 alone are partially antagonistic to function of the Ca^{2+}-dependent heterocomplex. Thus, differing levels of these two gene products gives rise to versatility in regulation of the inflammatory response. S100A8/ S100A9 heterodimers specifically bind fatty acids such as arachidonic acid in a calcium-dependent manner, and the complex also binds to the major fatty acid transporter (CD36) of endothelial cells, and interacts with heparan sulfate proteoglycans via the S100A9 subunit. Thus, secreted S100A8/S100A9 complexes may facilitate arachidonic acid transport and prostaglandin production in certain cell types. S100A9 may be involved in neutrophil migration to the cervix and myometrium because S100A9 enhances monocyte adhesion to endothelial cells through activation of the β2 integrin Mac-1 on neutrophils.[39] S100A8/S100A9 heterodimers also facilitate monocyte migration through the endothelium.[38] Using proteomic analysis, S100A8[40–42] and S100A9[40,42] have been reported to be increased in amniotic fluid and blood[40] in women in labor with intra-amniotic inflammation.

S100A9 mRNA levels are upregulated in the cervix, lower uterine segment, and fundal myometrium of women in labor (Figure 2.3).[43] Utilizing an antibody that recognizes S100A9 alone as well as bound in its heterodimeric complex, the protein is localized to cervical and myometrial neutrophils and, to a lesser extent, tissue macrophages. In cervical tissues from women before labor, S100A9 protein is limited to granulocytes within the vasculature (Figure 2.4B). The number of S100A9-positive cells is increased dramatically in cervical tissues in labor. S100A9 is also expressed in vascular endothelium adjacent to marginating neutrophils and monocytes, suggesting that secretion of the complex onto vessel walls is involved in the migration of leukocytes into the cervical stroma (Figure 2.4D). Intensity of staining and number of positive cells are increased in cervical tissues relative to the lower uterine

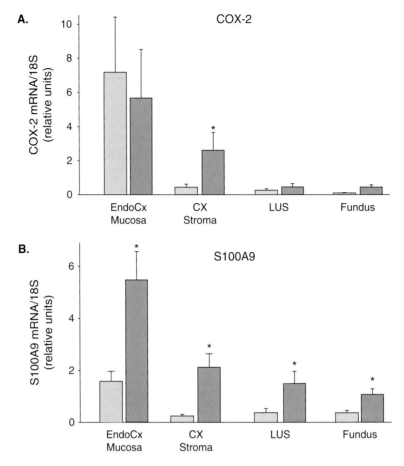

Figure 2.3 Expression of cyclooxygenase (COX) 2 and S100A9 in cervical and myometrial tissues during pregnancy at term. Tissues were obtained from the endocervix (EndoCx Mucosa), cervical stroma (CX Stroma), lower uterine segment (LUS), and uterine fundus (Fundus) in women before (open bar, n = 9–12), or after (solid bar, n = 8–10) the onset of cervical ripening and labor. Expression of (A) COX-2 and (B) S100A9 mRNA was determined by real-time polymerase chain reaction and expressed relative to 18S and an external standard. *P ≤ 0.05 compared with corresponding tissue not in labor (data from Havelock et al.[43])

segment, and myometrial tissues from the same uterine specimens.

EFFECT OF PROSTAGLANDINS ON THE CERVIX

For decades, prostaglandins (or prostaglandin analogs) have been shown to induce ripening of the cervix and initiate labor (depending on the dose, gestational age, and route of administration). The biochemical properties of the extracellular matrix after prostaglandin-stimulated cervical ripening are similar to those of the cervix during physiologic cervical ripening, demonstrating decreased collagen concentrations, increased

collagen solubility, and increased synthesis of hydrophilic glycosaminoglycans.[44–46] Prostaglandin E2 augments the potency of certain chemokines including the major neutrophil chemoattractant IL-8.[47] Whether or not prostaglandins play an obligatory role in spontaneous cervical ripening at term is not clear. For example, exposure of the cervix to high concentrations of prostaglandins in seminal fluid does not induce cervical ripening prior to term.[48] Inhibition of prostaglandin synthesis does not alter antiprogestin-induced cervical ripening, and prostaglandins (PG) E_2 and $PGF_{2\alpha}$ do not increase in cervical mucus during the last third of gestation or during cervical ripening.[49,50] Thus, although there is abundant evidence to support a role for prostaglandins in cervical ripening, additional factors

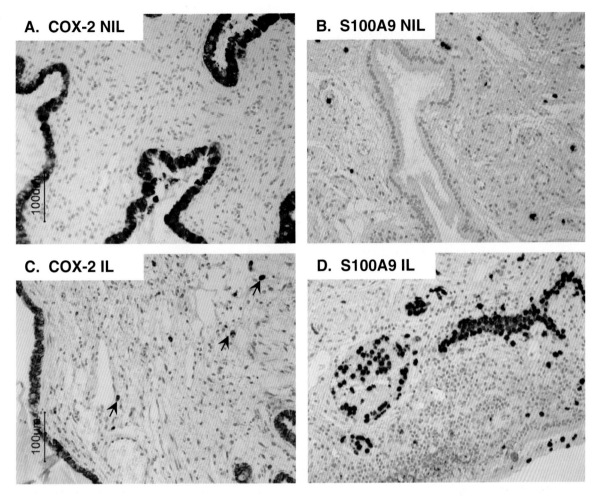

A. COX-2 NIL

B. S100A9 NIL

C. COX-2 IL

D. S100A9 IL

Figure 2.4 Immunolocalization of cyclooxygenase (COX) 2 and S100A9 in human cervical tissues during pregnancy before and after labor. Immunohistochemistry was used to localize expression of COX-2 and S100A9 in tissue sections from women at term before [(A) and (B), respectively] or after the onset [(C) and (D), respectively] of labor. In tissues from women in labor, expression of S100A9 was localized to marginating, rolling, and infiltrating leukocytes, whereas COX-2 was localized to cervical epithelium, stromal cells, and macrophages (arrows).

involving prostaglandin receptors,[51–54] prostaglandin degradative enzymes,[55] chemokines and cytokines,[56–59] estrogen and other steroids,[60,61] and matrix molecules[62] are probably involved in this complex remodeling process during physiologic cervical ripening at term.

PROSTAGLANDIN SYNTHESIS AND CERVICAL RIPENING

Prostaglandins are synthesized from arachidonic acid, and are converted to prostaglandin PGH_2 by prostaglandin endoperoxide H synthase (PGHS) or

cyclooxygenase (COX). Two isoenzymes exist, COX-1, or the constitutive form, and COX-2, the inducible isoenzyme. These enzymes are responsible for the rate-limiting step in prostaglandin biosynthesis. COX-2 is upregulated by various growth factors and cytokines, and has been shown in most studies to be increased in the cervix during parturition.

COX-2 expression is spatially regulated in the human uterus in pregnancy and labor, with increased expression in the cervix and lower levels in the fundus.[43,63] This gradient of expression parallels that of leukocyte migration into the uterus during labor.[23] It has been suggested that this enzyme is also elevated in myometrial tissues from women in labor. We (Havelock et al[43]) and others[63] have shown that COX-2 mRNA is not significantly different in fundal myometrial specimens from laboring and nonlaboring women whether obtained at the time of Cesarean section or Cesarean hysterectomy. COX-2 mRNA levels, however, are increased in the myometrium of women with chorioamnionitis.[43] Studies in a murine model have demonstrated induction of uterine COX-2, but not COX-1, during inflammation-mediated preterm labor caused by lipopolysaccharide (LPS) administration.[32] Furthermore, COX-1-deficient mice, which show delay in the onset of term labor, did not show a delay in onset of preterm labor after administration of LPS. Thus, although induction of COX-2 in the fundal myometrium does not appear to be involved in physiologic labor at term, induction of COX-2 may play a role in parturition complicated by intrauterine infection.

In contrast to the myometrium, COX-2 is increased significantly in the cervical stroma after cervical ripening during labor (Figure 2.3). Increased expression of COX-2 in the cervix is not singularly due to expression of COX-2 in infiltrating immune cells. Enzyme expression is strikingly absent in most infiltrating monocytes and neutrophils.[43,64] Rather, in the laboring cervix, COX-2 is expressed predominantly in cervical epithelial cells, stromal fibroblasts, and activated endothelial cells. The temporal relationship between changes in these cells relative to the onset of cervical ripening is not known, although inhibition of prostaglandin synthesis in the rat results in at least partial inhibition of spontaneous cervical ripening at term.[65]

The spatial pattern of S100A9 gene expression in the pregnant uterus is similar to COX-2, as S100A9 mRNA is increased in endocervical tissues relative to other tissue types in the uterus (Figure 2.3). However, unlike COX-2, S100A9 gene expression is increased significantly in all tissue components of the pregnant uterus from women in labor.

Intense immunostaining of COX-2 in endocervical epithelial cells in pregnant women was studied further using cervical tissues obtained from nonpregnant women and pregnant women earlier in gestation. Interestingly, epithelial cells lining the lumen of the endocervical canal were COX-2-positive in nonpregnant women and pregnant women throughout gestation (Figure 2.1).[10] Intensity of immunostaining in the epithelial cells in the nonpregnant cervix or cervix in early gestation, however, appear to be less than that seen in term pregnancy, suggesting that although COX-2 may be constitutively present in endocervical epithelial cells, the level of expression may be regulated throughout human pregnancy, and that expression of COX-2 in epithelial cells may increase progressively throughout gestation

(prior to induction of COX-2 in the stromal compartment during cervical ripening or labor).

Prior to cervical ripening, epithelial cell-derived prostaglandins may be inactivated by elevated levels of 15-hydroxyprostaglandin dehydrogenase (PGDH) in cervical stromal cells. Significant decreases in PGDH gene expression in the stroma[66] may facilitate prostaglandin action, which leads to induction of IL-8 gene expression and synthesis of IL-8 receptors in the stroma, thereby effecting a feed-forward loop for cervical remodeling by activated fibroblasts and recruited inflammatory cells.

OXYTOCIN RECEPTOR GENE EXPRESSION IN HUMAN CERVIX DURING PREGNANCY

The spatial pattern of oxytocin receptor gene expression in the cervix relative to the lower uterine segment and fundal myometrium has been described.[43,67,68] Enrichment of oxytocin receptor gene expression in the fundus relative to the lower uterine segment and cervix is thought to be one mechanism for the coordinated regulation of contractions that generate the necessary force for cervical dilatation and expulsion of the fetus. Oxytocin signal transduction, however, does not seem to be essential for initiation of labor.[69] In the study by Havelock et al[43] in which tissues were collected at well-defined regions of the uterus rather than surgical incision sites, oxytocin receptor gene expression appeared to be increased in the lower uterine segment and cervix during labor. Although the significance of the labor-associated increase in oxytocin receptor mRNA in the cervix and lower uterine segment is not known, oxytocin stimulates prostaglandin E2 release from cervical tissues and myometrial smooth muscle cells in vitro,[70,71] suggesting that increased oxytocin receptors in the cervix may facilitate cervical ripening through oxytocin-induced increases in prostaglandin biosynthesis. The mechanism of increased oxytocin receptor mRNA in the cervix may occur through stretch and descent of the presenting fetal part. Further, relief of progesterone inhibition in the cervix and lower uterine segment may lead to tissue-specific increases in oxytocin receptors.

ROLE OF PROGESTERONE IN THE MAINTENANCE OF CERVICAL COMPETENCY DURING PREGNANCY

In the majority of mammalian species, the transition from uterine quiescence and cervical competency to increased myometrial excitability and cervical ripening is heralded by a precipitous decline in circulating levels of progesterone. By contrast, in humans, the circulating levels of progesterone during pregnancy are extraordinarily high ($>10^{-7}$ M) and do not decrease prior to parturition. Such levels of progesterone in pregnant women are much greater than those of most other pregnant mammals, and are in huge excess of the K_D for binding to the progesterone receptor ($K_D = 10^{-9}$–10^{-10} M). Thus, even a moderate to pronounced decline in circulating progesterone in pregnant women would have little effect on progesterone-mediated actions. In consideration of the high affinity of progesterone for its receptor, it is questionable whether the marked decline in circulating progesterone that occurs in other mammals is of sufficient magnitude to compromise progesterone receptor function in the cervix.[72–74] In cervical tissues from mice,[13,75] local metabolism of progesterone within the cervix also plays an important role in progesterone withdrawal and the initiation of labor.

Effect of antiprogestins on cervical ripening

In women at term, treatment with the progesterone receptor antagonist mifepristone (RU486) dramatically increases cervical ripening, even though spontaneous labor may not occur for several days or weeks.[76–78] Likewise, in species that do not depend on progesterone withdrawal for initiation of parturition (humans, guinea pigs, old world monkeys, and the tree shrew *Tupaja belangeri*), progesterone receptor antagonists (RU486 and onapristone) are not very effective in inducing parturition when given alone. But they do exhibit conditioning effects on the uterus by increasing sensitivity of the myometrium to oxytocin and prostaglandins, and by induction of cervical ripening.[23] Antiprogestin-induced labor is often complicated by protracted delivery despite full cervical dilation, suggesting that uterine contractions are not fully effective after progesterone receptor antagonism. Contractions in response to antiprogestins (irregular, prolonged contractions of low amplitude) differ from contractions of spontaneous or oxytocin-induced labor (regular, periodic contractions of high amplitude). In contrast to the effects of antiprogestins on myometrium, most human studies conducted to date indicate that progesterone receptor antagonists are effective cervical ripening agents.[23,61,79,80] In preterm pregnant rats (day 14), preterm pregnant guinea pigs (day 49) and preterm pregnant monkeys (day 160), antiprogestins result in dose-dependent increases in cervical distensibility and dilation.[81–83] These effects on the cervix precede the onset of uterine contractions by several hours and do not correlate with

progesterone concentrations in peripheral blood.[23] Interestingly, cervical responsiveness to antiprogestins increases with gestational age, suggesting that progesterone receptor-mediated maintenance of cervical competency progressively declines in advanced pregnancy. The increased sensitivity of the cervix to antiprogestins at term may indicate that progesterone receptor function in the cervix declines progressively during pregnancy. The mechanism for this decline is not clear but increased synthesis of prostaglandins or other bioactive lipid mediators, such as platelet activating factor, in response to stretch or inflammatory stimuli may be involved.

Progesterone receptor isoforms and progesterone metabolism

The mechanism by which antiprogestins induce cervical ripening is also unclear. It has been proposed that prostaglandins mediate the effects of antiprogestins on cervical ripening. However, in guinea pigs, indomethacin fully inhibits LPS-induced cervical ripening,[84] but indomethacin has no effect on antiprogestin-induced cervical ripening in late pregnancy.[83] Likewise, the platelet-activating factor antagonist WEB-2170 inhibits LPS-induced cervical ripening but does not inhibit antiprogestin induction of preterm cervical ripening.[85]

Studies conducted in our laboratory[14,86] and others[87,88] indicate that cervical change during parturition in women is associated with alterations in the expression of progesterone receptor isoforms, and changes in the metabolism of estrogen and progesterone. The relationship between these changes and the onset of cervical ripening or cervical dilation during active labor is not known. Since prostaglandins alter the expression patterns of progesterone receptor isoforms,[89] changes in steroid hormone receptor profiles may occur in response to labor rather than the initial process of cervical ripening. Studies in the mouse cervix indicate that progesterone metabolism by steroid 5α-reductase type I is crucial for cervical ripening (but not cervical softening), and that activation of this enzyme precedes cervical ripening and uterine contractions of labor.[13] In cervical tissues from women, however, progesterone metabolism does not involve steroid 5α reductase type I, but a decline in 17β hydroxysteroid dehydrogenase type II, and increased metabolism of progesterone by 20α-hydroxysteroid dehydrogenase.[14] Whether these changes in steroid hormone metabolizing enzymes are sufficient to induce local progesterone withdrawal in the face of high circulating progesterone concentrations in women has not been proven. Nonetheless, local progesterone metabolism and changes in progesterone receptor isoforms may serve to facilitate cervical ripening or dilation. Further studies in this area are warranted.

Analysis of expression of progesterone receptor-responsive genes in cervical tissues as an index of progesterone receptor functional activity

Oxytocin receptor and COX-2 mRNA transcripts, which are negatively regulated by progesterone, are increased in the cervix in labor,[8] and the most dramatic labor-related changes in expression of these genes occurs in the cervix, not the lower uterine segment or fundal myometrium. Similarly, IL-8 and inducible nitric oxide synthase (iNOS) mRNA transcripts are also downregulated by progesterone, and these genes are also upregulated in the cervix in labor.[90,91] On the other hand, the transcription of PGDH is induced by progesterone.[92] PGDH is highly expressed in cervical stromal cells prior to labor but is downregulated during labor.[55] These results provide support for the idea that progesterone receptor function may be altered in cervical tissues in women in labor with decreased expression of some genes and release of progesterone repression of other genes.

Taken together, results from virtually all mammalian species indicate that progesterone receptors serve an important role in maintaining the structural integrity of the cervix during pregnancy. In mice, rabbits, rats, cows, pigs, and sheep, progesterone receptor function is compromised at term by decreased circulating progesterone and increased progesterone metabolism in progesterone receptor target tissues. In women, however, alterations in progesterone receptor expression, DNA binding properties, and/or transcriptional activity may play an important role in facilitating transition of the cervix from a structurally competent barrier that resists the gravitational forces of the fetus and amniotic sac to an easily stretchable, compromising elastic organ that allows delivery of the fetus.

REGULATION OF PROGESTERONE RECEPTOR FUNCTION: TRANSFORMING GROWTH FACTOR (TGF) β

Several lines of evidence suggest that TGF-β acts as a gene- and tissue-specific antiprogestin, and its biological effects would oppose myometrial relaxation and pregnancy maintenance possibly leading to induction of inflammatory response pathways and activation of nuclear factor κB (NFκB), a transcription factor that further antagonizes progesterone receptor function.[93–95] TGF-β acts in progesterone-responsive cells to inhibit

the actions of progesterone to modify levels of mRNA for connexin43 (Cx43), parathyroid hormone-related protein (PTH-rP), endothelin (ET-1), and enkephalinase.[96–99] In addition, TGF-β acts in several tissues to: (i) decrease the synthesis of a variety of Gαs-linked receptors; (ii) inhibit adenylyl cyclase activity; (iii) inhibit the action of cyclic adenosine monophosfate (cAMP), possibly at the level of protein kinase A; and (iv) decrease the number of natriuretic peptide receptors.[98] The molecular mechanisms for the antiprogestational effects of TGF-β have not been elucidated.

TRANSFORMING GROWTH FACTOR (TGF) β-REGULATED GENES ARE INCREASED SIGNIFICANTLY IN THE HUMAN CERVIX DURING CERVICAL RIPENING

Results from microarray analysis of cervical tissues from women before or after cervical ripening indicate that numerous TGF-β-regulated genes are upregulated during cervical ripening (unpublished results). Thrombospondin-1 (TSP-1) is a classical TGF-β-responsive gene in multiple cell types.[100] Thrombospondins are matricellular proteins that bind simultaneously to extracellular matrix proteins and to cell-surface receptors or other molecules that interact with the cell surface. TSP-1 is intimately involved in processes important to tissue remodeling, including the promotion of monocyte chemotaxis and the induction of monocyte chemoattractant protein (MCP-1) expression. Furthermore, TSP-1 promotes activation of latent TGF-β.

TSP-1 mRNA and protein levels are significantly increased in myometrial tissues from women in labor.[99] In addition, TSP-1 and other TGF-β-responsive genes, such as connective tissue growth factor and plasminogen activator inhibitor-1, are significantly increased in cervical stromal tissues from women in labor, and the expression of TSP-1 mRNA is temporally regulated in cervical tissues from pregnant mice (unpublished results). In mice, TSP-1 mRNA increases in the cervix 1–2 days prior to parturition (approximately two-fold). In labor and 2–4 h postpartum, mRNA levels are increased 6–7-fold relative to the nonpregnant cervix or the cervix during early pregnancy. Thereafter, TSP-1 mRNA decreases to nonpregnant values within 48 h. The data indicate that TSP-1, a TGF-β-induced gene, is increased significantly in both mouse and human pregnancy. The time-course of TSP-1 gene expression during pregnancy in mice is consistent with the idea that TGF-β-induced gene activation precedes the onset of cervical ripening and is amplified during labor.

The mechanism of increased activation of TGF-β-responsive genes in the cervix is not known. Clear-cut increases in TGF-β mRNA, protein, TGF-β receptors, or activation of latent TGF-β, could not be discerned in tissues from pregnant women in labor. It appears that TGF-β1 is highly expressed and relatively constant in myometrial and cervical tissues from pregnant women, and that TGF-β1 levels are greater in the cervix compared with myometrium. It is possible that downstream effector molecules of TGF-β signaling may be regulated in the cervix by progesterone receptors or other transcription repressor complexes (see Figure 2.5). At term, this repression may be relieved, thereby initiating transcription of TGF-β-responsive genes which may further oppose the actions of progesterone in a number of cell types, including cervical stromal cells.

MODEL OF CERVICAL FUNCTION DURING PREGNANCY

Studies described in this chapter and others are in agreement with the overall concept that cervical adaptations during pregnancy involve four phases (Figure 2.6). The initial softening phase involves a slow progressive process of increased turnover of matrix components resulting in reorganization of the collagen fibrillar network. The second phase, termed cervical ripening, precedes uterine contractions of labor, and involves increased synthesis of proteoglycans, glycosaminoglycans, decreased collagen concentrations and increased collagen solubility despite increases in collagen synthesis. The third phase, involving leukocytes and release of proteases into the extracellular matrix, accompanies cervical dilation during labor. Although the term cervical ripening is often used interchangeably to describe changes in the cervix that occur before and during labor, it appears that changes of the cervix during dilation of the cervix in active labor involve different processes to those of cervical ripening before labor. The fourth and final phase of cervical remodeling occurs after parturition (during uterine involution), with a rapid recovery phase involving resolution of inflammation and re-formation of the dense connective tissue and structural integrity of the cervix. No doubt, many of the described biochemical and molecular changes during the active dilation phase of labor occur in preparation for recovery of the cervix from childbirth. A clear definition of terms that describe each phase would clarify much of the discrepancies in the literature. There is little doubt, however, that these processes represent a continuum of cervical function during pregnancy and may not be sharply demarcated in time.

It is proposed that cervical competency during pregnancy in women is an active process that is orchestrated by complex relationships between several tissue-specific transcription factors in cervical stromal and epithelial cells that facilitate and ensure anti-inflammatory effects, progesterone receptor transcriptional activity, and organization of the cervical extracellular matrix to maintain cervical strength and rigidity (Figure 2.5). Conversely, cervical ripening in women may be initiated through a series of cellular events that negatively impact the ability of progesterone receptors to regulate target genes in the cervix. Furthermore, withdrawal of cervical competence during pregnancy may be induced by mechanical factors that initiate biochemical events to overcome the protective influence of progesterone and anti-inflammatory processes.

Collagen degradation and matrix remodeling during the phase of cervical dilation during labor occurs predominantly through release of proteolytic granules from invading inflammatory cells, rather than induction of collagenase or MMP in fibroblasts. Cytokines secreted from activated neutrophils and monocytes [e.g. IL-1 and tumor necrosis factor (TNF) α] act on cell-surface receptors in fibroblast stromal cells to activate NFκB-signaling pathways. NFκB further opposes progesterone receptor-mediated responses, increases production of cytokines in stromal fibroblasts, and amplifies leukocyte invasion, thereby creating a feed-forward loop to ensure complete cervical remodeling during labor. In the immediate postpartum period, rapid increases in repair processes, together with relief of mechanical stretch, shut off the signaling pathways leading to inflammatory responses and dissolution of the extracellular matrix. Although not studied in detail, it is likely that anti-inflammatory pathways (also activated during parturition) facilitate re-formation of the cervix in the puerperium.

Several aspects of the model proposed in Figure 2.5 are well-established, and some are under active investigation in various laboratories. Specifically, cervical ripening in human and rat pregnancy is accompanied by phenotypic alterations in fibroblast cells to activated myofibroblasts,[101,102] cervical dilation is an inflammatory process characterized by the influx of leukocytes,[27,103,104] inflammatory mediators such as IL-1, TNF-α, IL-8 and PGE_2 induce cervical ripening,[23,105,106] and the transcription factor NFκB, activated in response to various cytokines, antagonizes progesterone receptor function.[93,95] Mechanical stretch also activates NFκB signaling in fibroblasts,[107,108] and would further compromise progesterone receptor function. Studies involving the role of leukocyte trafficking, pro-inflammatory cytokines, and matrix proteases in cervical ripening are important in defining the final

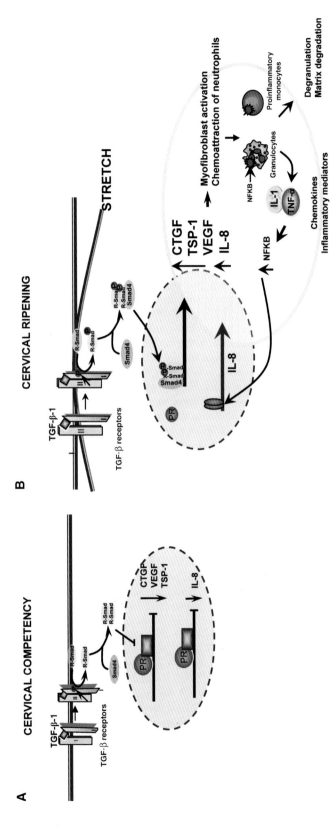

Figure 2.5 Proposed regulation of cervical function during pregnancy and parturition. Cervical competency (A) is maintained by interactions between progesterone receptors (PR) and other transcriptional complexes to induce anti-inflammatory events including suppression of transforming growth factor (TGF) β signaling through the downstream effectors of TGF-β signaling; Smad2 or -3 (R-Smad) are activated and phosphorylated upon TGF-β binding to type I and II receptors. During cervical competency, activation of specific TGF-β target genes may be inhibited by transcriptional repressor complexes thereby facilitating PR function. (B) During cervical ripening, TGF-β signaling occurs through TGF-β receptors that phosphorylate regulatory Smad proteins. Regulatory Smad proteins homo- or heterodimerize with Smad4 and the phosphorylated complex is translocated to the nucleus to induce responsive genes. Connective tissue growth factor (CTGF), an important mediator of fibroblast activation, is induced in stromal cells by TGF-β in the presence of mechanical stretch. Thrombospondin-1 (TSP-1) and plasminogen activator inhibitor-1 (PAI-1) mediate inflammatory responses including recruitment of neutrophils and activation of nuclear factor κB (NFκB) in granulocytes and inflammatory monocytes. Collagen degradation and matrix remodeling occurs predominantly through release of proteolytic granules from invading neutrophils. Cytokines secreted from activated neutrophils and monocytes [e.g. interleukin (IL) 1 and TNF-α] act on cell-surface receptors in fibroblast stromal cells to induce NFκB-signaling pathways. NFκB further opposes PR-mediated responses, increases synthesis of cytokines in stromal fibroblasts, and amplifies leukocyte invasion.

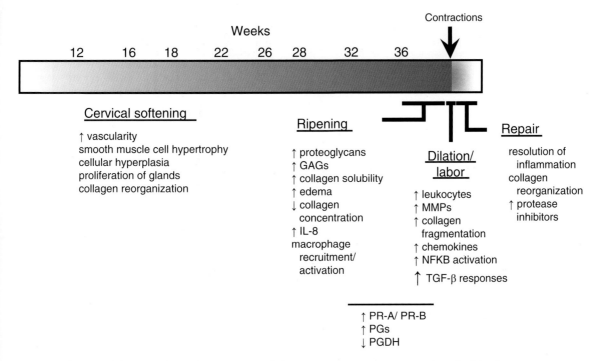

Figure 2.6 Cervical function during pregnancy and the puerperium. Processes are described in the text.

common pathway of cervical ripening, which is dissolution of the cervical extracellular matrix. Nevertheless, there is still a void in our knowledge of the events that initiate this final common pathway which is virtually impossible to reverse once it has begun.

SUMMARY AND PERSPECTIVE

A wealth of literature has established the importance of cervical dilation and effacement in successful parturition at term, and as an independent predictor of preterm birth. Preterm birth is associated with numerous risk factors, including low maternal prepregnancy weight, socioeconomic status, racial and ethnic factors, maternal education, maternal work patterns, physical effort during pregnancy, maternal sexual activity, tobacco use, interval between pregnancies, bacterial vaginosis and other types of bacterial colonization, uterine abnormalities, number of fetuses, and more. Nevertheless, despite these numerous risk factors, results from a number of studies indicate that the single most predictive factor for preterm birth in women with premature labor is the state of the cervix at the time of presentation. Furthermore, cervical length in the second trimester is significantly decreased in women with recurrent preterm birth,[109] and women with increased cervical dilation and effacement are at extreme risk for preterm

delivery within 48 h even in the presence of tocolytic agents. It is therefore important to understand not only the mechanisms of cervical ripening but also the mechanisms by which the cervix normally resists effacement and dilation during pregnancy. The pathophysiology of preterm cervical dilation, which facilitates ascending infection and preterm labor, may involve a dual mechanism whereby failure to maintain cervical competency during pregnancy leads to loss of the protective cervical barrier, and induction of preterm cervical dilation through opportunistic inflammatory mediators.

ACKNOWLEDGMENTS

The authors wish to thank the physicians and staff of Parkland Memorial Hospital, and Ms Sheila Brandon and Ms Valencia Hoffman for their valuable assistance in tissue procurement. We thank the Human Tissue and Biologic Fluid Core Laboratory and the support of NIH HD11149.

REFERENCES

1. Wiggins R, Hicks SJ, Soothill PW et al. Mucinases and sialidases: their role in the pathogenesis of sexually transmitted infections in the female genital tract. Sex Transm Infect 2001; 77(6): 402–8.

2. Owen J. Evaluation of the cervix by ultrasound for the prediction of preterm birth. Clin Perinatol 2003; 30(4): 735–55.

3. Yost NP, Cox SM. Infection and preterm labor. Clin Obstet Gynecol 2000; 43(4): 759–67.

4. Owen J, Iams JD, Hauth JC. Vaginal sonography and cervical incompetence. Am J Obstet Gynecol 2003; 188(2): 586–96.

5. Andrews WW, Copper R, Hauth JC et al. Second-trimester cervical ultrasound: associations with increased risk for recurrent early spontaneous delivery. Obstet Gynecol 2000; 95(2): 222–6.

6. Chegini N, Verala J, Luo X et al. Gene expression profile of leiomyoma and myometrium and the effect of gonadotropin releasing hormone analogue therapy. J Soc Gynecol Invest 2003; 10(3): 161–71.

7. Naim A, Haberman S, Burgess T et al. Changes in cervical length and the risk of preterm labor. Am J Obstet Gynecol 2002; 186(5): 887–9.

8. Havelock JC, Keller P, Muleba N et al. Human myometrial gene expression before and during parturition. Biol Reprod 2005; 72(3): 707–19.

9. Barclay CG, Brennand JE, Kelly RW, Calder AA. Interleukin-8 production by the human cervix. Am J Obstet Gynecol 1993; 169(3): 625–32.

10. Becher N, Hein M, Danielsen CC, Uldbjerg N. Matrix metalloproteinases and their inhibitors in the cervical mucus plug at term of pregnancy. Am J Obstet Gynecol 2004; 191(4): 1232–9.

11. Moriyama A, Shimoya K, Ogata I et al. Secretory leukocyte protease inhibitor (SLPI) concentrations in cervical mucus of women with normal menstrual cycle. Mol Hum Reprod 1999; 5(7): 656–61.

12. Pfundt R, van Ruissen F, van Vlijmen-Willems IMJJ et al. Constitutive and inducible expression of SKALP/elafin provides anti-elastase defense in human epithelia. J Clin Invest 1996; 98(6): 1389–99.

13. Mahendroo MS, Porter A, Russell DW, Word RA. The parturition defect in steroid 5alpha-reductase type 1 knockout mice is due to impaired cervical ripening. Mol Endocrinol 1999; 13(6): 981–92.

14. Minjarez DA, Miller RT, Lindqvist A, Andersson S, Word RA. Regulation of steroid hormone metabolism by 17-hydroxysteroid dehydrogenase type 2 in the human cervix. J Soc Gynecol Invest 2000; 7: 124A.

15. Yoshimatsu K, Sekiya T, Ishihara K et al. Detection of the cervical gland area in threatened preterm labor using transvaginal sonography in the assessment of cervical maturation and the outcome of pregnancy. Gynecol Obstet Invest 2002; 53(3): 149–56.

16. Bishop EH. Pelvic scoring for elective induction. Obstet Gynecol 1964; 24: 266–8.

17. Shi L, Shi SQ, Saade GR, Chwalisz K, Garfield RE. Studies of cervical ripening in pregnant rats: effects of various treatments. Mol Hum Reprod 2000; 6(4): 382–9.

18. Garfield RE, Saade G, Buhimschi C et al. Control and assessment of the uterus and cervix during pregnancy and labour. Hum Reprod Update 1998; 4(5): 673–95.

19. Buhimschi IA, Dussably L, Buhimschi CS, Ahmed A, Weiner CP. Physical and biomechanical characteristics of rat cervical ripening are not consistent with increased collagenase activity. Am J Obstet Gynecol 2004; 191(5): 1695–704.

20. Harkness MLR, Harkness RD. Changes in the physical properties of the uterine cervix of the rat during pregnancy. J Physiol 1959; 148: 524–47.

21. Hollingsworth M, Williams LM. Increases in the creep rate of the rat cervix occurring just prior to parturition. J Physiol 1980; 301: 90–1.

22. Hindson JC, Schofield BM, Turner CB. Some factors affecting dilatation of the ovine cervix. Res Vet Sci 1968; 9(5): 474–80.

23. Chwalisz K. The use of progesterone antagonists for cervical ripening and as an adjunct to labour and delivery. Hum Reprod 1994; 9(Suppl 1): 131–61.

24. Word RA, Landrum CP, Timmons BC, Young SG, Mahendroo MS. Transgene insertion on mouse chromosome 6 impairs function of the uterine cervix and causes Failure of parturition. Biol Reprod 2005; 73(5): 1046–56.

25. Kokenyesi R, Armstrong LC, Agah A, Artal R, Bornstein P. Thrombospondin 2 deficiency in pregnant mice results in premature softening of the uterine cervix. Biol Reprod 2004; 70(2): 385–90.

26. Drzewiecki G, Tozzi C, Yu S, Leppert PC. A dual mechanism of biomechanical change in rat cervix in gestation and postpartum: applied vascular mechanics. Cardiovasc Eng 2005; 5(4): 187–93.

27. Winkler M, Rath W. Changes in the cervical extracellular matrix during pregnancy and parturition. J Perinat Med 1999; 27(1): 45–60.

28. Ludmir J, Schdev HM. Anatomy and physiology of the uterine cervix. Clin Obstet Gynecol 2000; 43(3): 433–9.

29. Westergren-Thorsson G, Norman M, Bjornsson S et al. Differential expressions of mRNA for proteoglycans, collagens and transforming growth factor-[beta] in the human cervix during pregnancy and involution. Biochim Biophys Acta 1998; 1406(2): 203–13.

30. Leppert PC. Anatomy and physiology of cervical ripening. Clin Obstet Gynecol 1995; 38(2): 267–79.

31. Straach KJ, Shelton JM, Richardson JA, Hascall VC, Mahendroo MS. Regulation of hyaluronan expression during cervical ripening. Glycobiology 2005; 15(1): 55–65.

32. Uchiyama T, Matsumoto T, Suzuki Y et al. Endogenous hyaluronan: a cytokine-like factor present in rabbit uterine cervix during pregnancy. Biol Pharm Bull 2004; 27(12): 1907–12.

33. Obara M, Hirano H, Ogawa M et al. Changes in molecular weight of hyaluronan and hyaluronidase activity in uterine cervical mucus in cervical ripening. Acta Obstet Gynecol Scand 2001; 80(6): 492–6.

34. Timmons BC, Mahendroo MS. Timing of neutrophil activation and expression of proinflammatory markers do not support a role for neutrophils in cervical ripening in the mouse. Biol Reprod 2006; 74(2): 236–45.

35. Sakamoto Y, Moran P, Searle RF, Bulmer JN, Robson SC. Interleukin-8 is involved in cervical dilatation but not in prelabour cervical ripening. Clin Exp Immunol 2004; 138(1): 151–7.

36. Sakamoto Y, Moran P, Bulmer JN, Searle RF, Robson SC. Macrophages and not granulocytes are involved in cervical ripening. J Reprod Immunol 2005; 66(2): 161–73.

37. Sennstrom MK, Brauner A, Lu Y et al. Interleukin-8 is a mediator of the final cervical ripening in humans. Eur J Obstet Gynecol Reprod Biol 1997; 74(1): 89–92.

38. Roth J, Vogl T, Sorg C, Sunderkotter C. Phagocyte-specific S100 proteins: a novel group of proinflammatory molecules. Trends Immunol 2003; 24(4): 155–8.

39. Newton RA, Hogg N. The human S100 protein MRP-14 is a novel activator of the {beta}2 integrin Mac-1 on neutrophils. J Immunol 1998; 160(3): 1427–35.

40. Gravett MG, Novy MJ, Rosenfeld RG et al. Diagnosis of intra-amniotic infection by proteomic profiling and identification of novel biomarkers. JAMA 2004; 292(4): 462–9.

41. Buhimschi IA, Christner R, Buhimschi CS. Proteomic biomarker analysis of amniotic fluid for identification of intra-amniotic inflammation. BJOG 2005; 112(2): 173–81.

42. Ruetschi U, Rosen A, Karlsson G et al. Proteomic analysis using protein chips to detect biomarkers in cervical and amniotic fluid in women with intra-amniotic inflammation. J Proteome Res 2005; 4(6): 2236–42.

43. Havelock JC, Keller P, Muleba N et al. Human myometrial gene expression before and during parturition. Biol Reprod 2005; 72(3): 707–19.

44. Uldbjerg N, Ekman G, Malmstrom A, Ulmsten U, Wingerup L. Biochemical changes in human cervical connective tissue after local application of prostaglandin E2. Gynecol Obstet Invest 1983; 15(5): 291–9.

45. Rath W, Osmers R, Adelmann-Grill B et al. Biochemical changes in human cervical connective tissue after intracervical application of prostaglandin E2. Prostaglandins 1993; 45(4): 375–84.

46. Fittkow CT, Maul H, Olson G et al. Light-induced fluorescence of the human cervix decreases after prostaglandin application for induction of labor at term. Eur J Obstet Gynecol Reprod Biol 2005; 123(1): 62–6.

47. Denison FC, Calder AA, Kelly RW. The action of prostaglandin E2 on the human cervix: stimulation of interleukin 8 and inhibition of secretory leukocyte protease inhibitor. Am J Obstet Gynecol 1999; 180(3 Pt 1): 614–20.

48. Kavanagh J, Kelly AJ, Thomas J. Sexual intercourse for cervical ripening and induction of labour. Cochrane Database Syst Rev 20012: CD003093.

49. Platz-Christensen JJ, Pernevi P, Bokstrom H, Wiqvist N. Prostaglandin E and F2 alpha concentration in the cervical mucus and mechanism of cervical ripening. Prostaglandins 1997; 53(4): 253–61.

50. Toth M, Rehnstrom J, Fuchs AR. Prostaglandins E and F in cervical mucus of pregnant women. Am J Perinatol 1989; 6(2): 142–4.

51. Chien EK, Macgregor C. Expression and regulation of the rat prostaglandin E2 receptor type 4 (EP4) in pregnant cervical tissue. Am J Obstet Gynecol 2003; 189(5): 1501–10.

52. Smith GC, Baguma-Nibasheka M, Wu WX, Nathanielsz PW. Regional variations in contractile responses to prostaglandins and prostanoid receptor messenger ribonucleic acid in pregnant baboon uterus. Am J Obstet Gynecol 1998; 179(6 Pt 1): 1545–52.

53. Feltovich H, Ji H, Janowski JW et al. Effects of selective and non-selective PGE2 receptor agonists on cervical tensile strength and collagen organization and microstructure in the pregnant rat at term. Am J Obstet Gynecol 2005; 192(3): 753–60.

54. Smith GC, Wu WX, Nathanielsz PW. Effects of gestational age and labor on the expression of prostanoid receptor genes in pregnant baboon cervix. Prostaglandins Other Lipid Mediat 2001; 63(4): 153–63.

55. Tornblom SA, Patel FA, Bystrom B et al. 15-Hydroxy-prostaglandin dehydrogenase and cyclooxygenase 2 messenger ribonucleic acid expression and immunohistochemical localization in human cervical tissue during term and preterm labor. J Clin Endocrinol Metab 2004; 89(6): 2909–15.

56. Gardner MO, Owen J, Skelly S, Hauth JC. Preterm delivery after indomethacin. A risk factor for neonatal complications? J Reprod Med 1996; 41(12): 903–6.

57. Ruiz RJ, Fullerton J, Dudley DJ. The interrelationship of maternal stress, endocrine factors and inflammation on gestational length. Obstet Gynecol Surv 2003; 58(6): 415–28.

58. Mohan AR, Loudon JA, Bennett PR. Molecular and biochemical mechanisms of preterm labour. Semin Fetal Neonatal Med 2004; 9(6): 437–44.

59. Stjernholm-Vladic Y, Stygar D, Mansson C et al. Factors involved in the inflammatory events of cervical ripening in humans. Reprod Biol Endocrinol 2004; 2(1): 74.

60. Stjernholm Y, Sahlin L, Akerberg S et al. Cervical ripening in humans: potential roles of estrogen, progesterone, and insulin-like growth factor-I. Am J Obstet Gynecol 1996; 174(3): 1065–71.

61. Ekman-Ordeberg G, Stjernholm Y, Wang H, Stygar D, Sahlin L. Endocrine regulation of cervical ripening in humans – potential roles for gonadal steroids and insulin-like growth factor-I. Steroids 2003; 68(10–13): 837–47.

62. Leppert PC. Anatomy and physiology of cervical ripening. Clin Obstet Gynecol 1995; 38(2): 267–79.

63. Sparey C, Robson SC, Bailey J, Lyall F, Nicholas Europe-Finner G. The differential expression of myometrial connexin-43, cyclooxygenase-1 and -2, and Gs{alpha} proteins in the upper and lower segments of the human uterus during pregnancy and labor. J Clin Endocrinol Metab 1999; 84(5): 1705–10.

64. Havelock JC, Keller P, Muleba N et al. Human myometrial gene expression before and during parturition. Biol Reprod 2005; 72(3): 707–19.

65. Cabro LD, Dallot E, Bienkiewicz A et al. Cyclooxygenase and lipoxygenase inhibitors – induced changes in the distribution of glycosaminoglycans in the pregnant rat uterine cervix. Prostaglandins 1990; 39(5): 515–23.

66. Tornblom SA, Patel FA, Bystrom B et al. 15-Hydroxy-prostaglandin dehydrogenase and cyclooxygenase 2 messenger ribonucleic acid expression and immunohistochemical localization in human cervical tissue during term and preterm labor. J Clin Endocrinol Metab 2004; 89(6): 2909–15.

67. Fuchs A-R, Ivell R, Balvers M, Chang S-M, Fields M. Oxytocin receptors in bovine cervix during pregnancy and parturition: gene expression and cellular localization. Am J Obstet Gynecol 1996; 175(6): 1654–60.

68. Blanks AM, Vatish M, Allen MJ et al. Paracrine oxytocin and estradiol demonstrate a spatial increase in human intrauterine tissues with labor. J Clin Endocrinol Metab 2003; 88(7): 3392–400.

69. Nishimori K, Young LJ, Guo Q et al. Oxytocin is required for nursing but is not essential for parturition or reproductive behavior. Proc Natl Acad Sci USA 1996; 93(21): 11 699–704.

70. Shemesh M, Dombrovski L, Gurevich M et al. Regulation of bovine cervical secretion of prostaglandins and synthesis of cyclooxygenase by oxytocin. Reprod Fertil Dev 1997; 9(5): 525–30.

71. Blanks AM, Thornton S. The role of oxytocin in parturition. BJOG 2003; 110 (Suppl 20): 46–51.

72. Alexandrova M, Soloff MS. Oxytocin receptors and parturition. I. Control of oxytocin receptor concentration in the rat myometrium at term. Endocrinology 1980; 106(3): 730–5.

73. Strauss 3rd JF, Sokoloski J, Caploe P et al. On the role of prostaglandins in parturition in the rat. Endocrinology 1975; 96(4): 1040–3.

74. Virgo BB, Bellward GD. Serum progesterone levels in the pregnant and postpartum laboratory mouse. Endocrinology 1974; 95(5): 1486–90.

75. Minjarez D, Konda V, Word RA. Regulation of uterine 5 alpha-reductase type 1 in mice. Biol of Reprod 2001; 65(5): 1378–82.

76. Elliott C, Brennand J, Calder A. The effects of mifepristone on cervical ripening and labor induction in primigravidae. Obstet Gynecol 1998; 92(5): 804–9.

77. Stenlund PM, Ekman G, Aedo AR, Bygdeman M. Induction of labor with mifepristone – a randomized, double-blind study versus placebo. Acta Obstet Gynecol Scand 1999; 78(9): 793–8.

78. Giacalone PL, Daures JP, Faure JM et al. The effects of mifepristone on uterine sensitivity to oxytocin and on fetal heart rate patterns. Eur J Obstet Gynecol Reprod Biol 2001; 97(1): 30–4.

79. Bygdeman M, Gemzell Danielsson K, Marions L, Swahn M. Pregnancy termination. Steroids 2000; 65(10–11): 801–5.

80. Clark K, Ji H, Feltovich H et al. Mifepristone-induced cervical ripening: structural, biomechanical, and molecular events. Am J Obstet Gynecol 2006; 194(5): 1391–8.

81. Hegele-Hartung C, Chwalisz K, Beier HM, Elger W. Ripening of the uterine cervix of the guinea-pig after treatment with the progesterone antagonist onapristone (ZK 98.299): an electron microscopic study. Hum Reprod 1989; 4(4): 369–77.

82. Wolf JP, Sinosich M, Anderson TL et al. Progesterone antagonist (RU 486) for cervical dilation, labor induction, and delivery in monkeys: effectiveness in combination with oxytocin. Am J Obstet Gynecol 1989; 160(1): 45–7.

83. Chwalisz K, Hegele-Hartung C, Schulz R et al. Progesterone control of cervical ripening – experimenal studies with the progesterone antagonists onapristone, lilopristone, and mifepristone. Ithaca: Perinatology Press, 1991.

84. Bukowski R, Scholz P, Hasan SH, Chwalisz K. Induction of preterm parturition with the interleukin-1beta, tumor necrosis factor alpha, and with LPS in guinea pigs. Soc Gynecol Invest 1993: S26.

85. Maul H, Marx S, Baier P, Garfield RE, Saade GR. Platelet-activating factor antagonist WEB-2170 does not inhibit antiprogestin induced preterm cervical ripening. J Soc Gynecol Invest 2003; 10(2): 260.

86. Deng D, Keller PK, Lo J, Word RA. Estrogen and progesterone receptor isoform distribution in cervical stroma during human pregnancy. J Soc Gynecol Invest 2003; 10(2): 256.

87. Stygar D, Wang H, Vladic YS et al. Co-localization of oestrogen receptor {beta} and leukocyte markers in the human cervix. Mol Hum Reprod 2001; 7(9): 881–6.

88. Wang H, Stjernholm Y, Ekman G, Eriksson H, Sahlin L. Different regulation of oestrogen receptors {alpha} and {beta} in the human cervix at term pregnancy. Mol Hum Reprod 2001; 7(3): 293–300.

89. Madsen G, Zakar T, Ku CY et al. Prostaglandins differentially modulate progesterone receptor-A and -B expression in human myometrial cells: evidence for prostaglandin-induced functional progesterone withdrawal. J Clin Endocrinol Metab 2004; 89(2): 1010–13.

90. Chwalisz K, Garfield RE. Role of nitric oxide in the uterus and cervix: implications for the management of labor. J Perinat Med 1998; 26(6): 448–57.

91. Ito A, Imada K, Sato T et al. Suppression of interleukin 8 production by progesterone in rabbit uterine cervix. Biochem J 1994; 301(Pt 1): 183–6.

92. Greenland KJ, Jantke I, Jenatschke S, Bracken KE, Vinson C, Gellersen B. The human NAD+-dependent 15-hydroxy-prostaglandin dehydrogenase gene promoter is controlled by Ets and activating protein-1 transcription factors and progesterone. Endocrinology 2000; 141(2): 581–97.

93. Kalkhoven E, Wissink S, van der Saag PT, van der Burg B. Negative interaction between the RelA(p65) subunit of NF-kappaB and the progesterone receptor. J Biol Chem 1996; 271(11): 6217–24.

94. Allport VC, Pieber D, Slater DM et al. Human labour is associated with nuclear factor-{kappa}}B activity which mediates cyclo-oxygenase-2 expression and is involved with the 'functional progesterone withdrawal'. Mol Hum Reprod 2001; 7(6): 581–6.

95. Davies S, Dai D, Feldman I, Pickett G, Leslie KK. Identification of a novel mechanism of NF-[kappa]B inactivation by progesterone through progesterone receptors in Hec50co poorly differentiated endometrial cancer cells: induction of A20 and ABIN-2. Gynecol Oncol 2004; 94(2): 463–70.

96. Arici A, MacDonald P, Casey M. Modulation of the levels of interleukin-8 messenger ribonucleic acid and interleukin-8 protein synthesis in human endometrial stromal cells by transforming growth factor-beta 1. J Clin Endocrinol Metab 1996; 81(8): 3004–9.

97. Casey ML, MacDonald PC. The endothelin-parathyroid hormone-related protein vasoactive peptide system in human endometrium: modulation by transforming growth factor-beta. Hum Reprod 1996; 2: 62–82.

98. Casey ML, MacDonald PC. Transforming growth factor-beta inhibits progesterone-induced enkephalinase expression in human endometrial stromal cells. J Clin Endocrinol Metab 1996; 81(11): 4022–7.

99. Morimoto T, Head J, MacDonald P, Casey M. Thrombospondin-1 expression in human myometrium before and during pregnancy, before and during labor, and in human myometrial cells in culture. J Clin Endocrinol Metab 1998; 59(4): 862–70.

100. Adams JC, Lawler J. The thrombospondins. Int J Biochem Cell Biol 2004; 36(6): 961–8.

101. Montes GS, Zugaib M, Joazeiro PP et al. Phenotypic modulation of fibroblastic cells in the mucous layer of the human uterine cervix at term. Reproduction 2002; 124(6): 783–90.

102. Varayoud J, Ramos JG, Joazeiro PP et al. Characterization of fibroblastic cell plasticity in the lamina propria of the rat uterine cervix at term. Biol Reprod 2001; 65(2): 375–83.

103. Hunt JS, Petroff MG, Burnett TG. Uterine leukocytes: key players in pregnancy. Semin Cell Dev Biol 2000; 11(2): 127–37.

104. Mackler AM, Iezza G, Akin MR, McMillan P, Yellon SM. Macrophage trafficking in the uterus and cervix precedes parturition in the mouse. Biol Reprod 1999; 61(4): 879–83.

105. Calder AA. Prostaglandins and biological control of cervical function. Aust NZ J Obstet Gynaecol 1994; 34(3): 347–51.

106. Maul H, Shi L, Marx SG, Garfield RE, Saade GR. Local application of platelet-activating factor induces cervical ripening accompanied by infiltration of polymorphonuclear leukocytes in rats. Am J Obstet Gynecol 2002; 187(4): 829–33.

107. Gruden G, Setti G, Hayward A et al. Mechanical stretch induces monocyte chemoattractant activity via an NF-{kappa}B-dependent monocyte chemoattractant protein-1-mediated pathway in human mesangial cells: inhibition by rosiglitazone. J Am Soc Nephrol 2005; 16(3): 688–96.

108. Amma H, Naruse K, Ishiguro N, Sokabe M. Involvement of reactive oxygen species in cyclic stretch-induced NF-[kappa]B activation in human fibroblast cells. Br J Pharmacol 2005; 145(3): 364–73.

109. Mercer BM, Macpherson CA, Goldenberg RL et al. Are women with recurrent spontaneous preterm births different from those without such history? Am J Obstet Gynecol 2006; 194(4): 1176–84.

3

Endocrine and paracrine mechanisms in human placenta and fetal membranes in preterm birth

Michela Torricelli, Alessia Giovannelli, Paolo Boy Torres, Letizia Galleri, Pasquale Florio, Filiberto Severi, Fernando M Reis, and Felice Petraglia

INTRODUCTION

Parturition results from a complex interplay of a variety of different maternal and fetal factors, which act upon the myometrium to trigger molecular pathways involved in the development of coordinated uterine contractility.[1] However, the molecular mechanisms driving the onset of human labor still remain uncertain, although several key players have been identified.

Human placenta and fetal membranes are unique tissues, genetically originated from the fetus and physiologically engaged as mediators of the maternal–fetal dialog. They produce a huge number of signaling substances including cytokines, neuropeptides, steroids and amines. These are released into the amniotic fluid, or act on the adjacent tissues, and thereby are able to modulate myometrial contractility and cervical ripening in a paracrine fashion.[2] As a result, placenta and membranes are putatively involved in both physiological and pathological mechanisms leading to the initiation of labor. The placental and fetal membranes hormones play an important role in human parturition by: (i) endocrine mechanisms, with increasing secretion of placental hormones, and (ii) paracrine mechanisms activation, characterized by local inflammation, myometrial contractility and cervical ripening.

VASOACTIVE PEPTIDES

Neuropeptide Y (NPY)

Expression and localization

Human NPY is a peptide of 36 amino acid residues belonging to a family of regulatory peptides.[3] It is widespread and abundantly expressed in the central and peripheral nervous system. Physiological effects attributed to NPY include the stimulation of food intake, vasoconstriction, and regulation of gut motility. Moreover, there is evidence that NPY is involved in the regulation of luteinizing hormone (LH) secretion from the anterior pituitary.[3]

NPY is produced by human placenta, maternal decidua and fetal membranes.[4,5] Acidic extracts of human placental tissues collected at term pregnancy contain high immunoreactive NPY (irNPY) concentrations, and the extracted irNPY elutes with the same retention time as synthetic NPY. An intense NPY staining is present in the cytoplasm of the epithelial amnion cells, of the cytotrophoblast cells, and the intermediate trophoblast of the chorion.

Receptors and biological effects

Binding sites for NPY are present in all peripheral cells of placental terminal villi.[6] The various NPY receptors mediate their responses through pertussis toxin sensitive G-proteins of the Gi/0 family, resulting in inhibition of adenylate cyclase activity, but they are also able to increase intracellular Ca^{2+} levels.[3] Among the receptor subtypes for NPY, the Y1 and Y3 receptor have been identified within placenta.[6] NPY1R and NPY3R are located on brush-border membranes of syncytiotrophoblastic cells of placental villi and in human myometrium (Figure 3.1).[6] In vitro studies have shown an involvement of NPY in the regulation of uterine blood flow, and of uterine contractility.[7]

Levels in biological fluids

During pregnancy, human placenta secretes NPY in maternal and fetal circulation, and in amniotic fluid. Maternal plasma NPY levels are higher than in nonpregnant

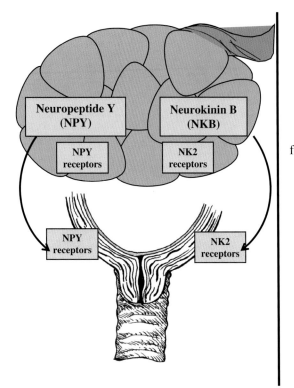

Figure 3.1 Placental expression of neurokinin B (NKB) and neuropeptide Y (NPY) and their actions in intrauterine tissues.

women, without significant changes throughout gestation. During labor, maternal plasma NPY levels progressively increase, matching the highest levels at the most advanced stages of cervical dilatation and at the time of vaginal delivery.[8] NPY levels in amniotic fluid and umbilical cord serum are comparable to those found in the maternal circulation, being highest at term and mainly during the early or late stages of labor. Plasma NPY levels fall immediately after delivery, supporting its placental origin during pregnancy.[8]

Neurokinin B (NKB)

Expression and localization

NKB is a 10 amino acid peptide belonging to the family of tachykinin-related peptides; it also comprises substance P (SP) and neurokinin A. It is expressed in the central nervous system and spinal cord, where it plays a role as an excitatory neurotransmitter, and it modulates blood pressure in mammals.[9] NKB is expressed by the syncytiotrophoblast of the human placenta.[10,11]

Receptors and biological effects

NKB is able to bind to three G-protein-linked receptors – NK1R, NK2R, and NK3R – and it exhibits agonist

activity on each receptor subtype, in which its rank order of potency is NK3R>NK2R>NK1R.[9] In human placenta at term, there is predominant expression of NK1R, some expression of NK2R, and absent expression of NK3R mRNA. NK1R and NK2R, but not NK3R, expression are detectable in the human umbilical vein endothelial cells (HUVEC).[10] The mRNA of NK1R is also expressed by the myometrium from pregnant women.[11]

NKB act as a paracrine regulator of fetal placental vascular tone in the human placenta, predominantly through the tachykinin NK1 receptor. In fact, it causes concentration-dependent relaxation of isolated human placental resistance vessels.[10,12]

NKB is an important modulator of myometrial contractility, since it elicits contractile effects on human myometrium – an effect mediated by NK2R.[13] An excitatory effect of tachykinin on the near-term gravid uterus suggests a possible role for NKB in the initiation of parturition, where the release of tachykinin could contribute to the cascade of events leading to labor (Figure 3.1).

Levels in biological fluids

NKB concentration in maternal blood increases as pregnancy advances, and decreases rapidly after delivery, confirming that NKB is derived mainly from the placenta.[14,15]

GROWTH FACTORS

Activin A

Expression and localization

Activin A is a growth factor belonging to the transforming growth factor β (TGF-β) superfamily; composed of two subunits it is an homodimer of the βA subunit.[16]

During pregnancy, activin A mRNA is localized to placental trophoblast fetal membranes, and decidua.[17,18] In detail, it is localized in the external syncytial layer of placental villi, in the stroma, in maternal decidual cells, in some amnion and chorionic cells, and in some endothelial cells within the placental villi.[17,18]

Receptor binding proteins and biological effects

Activin A signals through a heteromeric complex of receptor serine kinases which include at least two type I (IA and IB) and two type II (IIA and IIB) receptors. These receptors are all transmembrane proteins.[19] First and second trimester placentae express the various receptor proteins in the syncytium, whereas at term the distribution is confined to vascular endothelial cells of villous blood vessels. In the fetal membranes they are localized to some epithelial cells, mesenchyme and chorionic trophoblast.[20]

The activity of activin A is tightly regulated by follistatin, a structurally unrelated protein that binds with high affinity to activin to neutralize its activity.[21] This affinity is similar to that for activin receptors; thus, it plays a major role in regulating activin bioavailability on target tissues and functions. Recently, a new binding protein of 70 amino acids for activin A has been identified, namely follistatin-related gene (FLRG). FLRG is closely related to follistatin which interacts physically with activin A and, preventing binding on activin receptors, regulates activin A functions.[22] Follistatin and FLRG are both present in trophoblast, decidua, and fetal membranes amnion and chorion. But FLRG protein immunolocalization differs from that shown for follistatin, as FLRG is predominantly present in the walls of decidual and placental blood vessels,[23] whilst follistatin is more localized in cyto- and syncytiotrophoblast cells.[21]

The finding of FLRG, activin receptors and activin A distribution in vascular endothelial cells of deciduas and villous blood vessels in term placenta supports the hypothesis that FLRG may act by paracrine/autocrine mechanisms as a modulator of activin A vascular actions, as activin A is known to affect endothelial proliferation and angiogenesis.[24]

In placental tissues, activin A increases the production of the uterotonic agents, prostaglandin E2, and oxytocin.[25-27] Administration of inflammatory cytokines to gestational tissue resulted in increased activin A production, which may be particularly relevant in cases of preterm delivery occurring secondary to intrauterine infection.[28]

Levels in biological fluids

Activin A concentrations significantly increase in maternal serum with advancing gestation, and are significantly higher in women at term who had spontaneous vaginal delivery than in women who had an elective Cesarean delivery.[29,30] Activin A mRNA is upregulated in membranes of preterm delivery, and high amniotic fluid concentrations are detectable in women with preterm labor,[31] since, both spontaneous labor at term and pathological preterm labor are associated with changes in the expression of activin A and activin receptor mRNA in fetal membranes. The activin βA subunit and activin receptor type II mRNA levels in both chorion and amnion in women delivering at term, or after preterm labor, were significantly higher than in women delivering without undergoing labor.[31] Maternal serum activin A levels were higher in women with preterm labor than in a preterm nonlabor group.[32]

NEUROPEPTIDES

Corticotrophin-releasing factor (CRF) and related peptides

Expression and localization

CRF is a 41 amino acid peptide released from the medial eminence of the hypothalamus, acting at the corticotroph cells in the anterior pituitary to stimulate the release of adrenocorticotrophic hormone (ACTH) and related peptides in response to stress events, and to modulate behavioral, vascular and immune response to stress.[33] Urocortin belongs to the family of CRF: it is a 40 amino acid peptide, shares a 45% sequence identity to CRF, and binds to the CRF receptors.[34] Human placenta, decidua, chorion and amnion express and secrete CRF and urocortin.[35,36]

CRF binding protein (CRF-BP) is a 37 KDa protein of 322 amino acids, mainly produced by the human brain and liver.[33] It is able to bind circulating CRF and urocortin. Further sources of CRF-BP during pregnancy are placental trophoblast, decidua and fetal membranes.[37]

Very recently, the newly described urocortin 2 (UCN2; also known as stresscopin-related peptide)[38] and urocortin 3 (UCN3; also known as stresscopin)[39] are also expressed by human trophoblast, fetal membranes and maternal deciduas.[40] Opposed to CRF and urocortin, UCN2 or UCN3 do not stimulate the release of ACTH from explants of placental villi.[35,40]

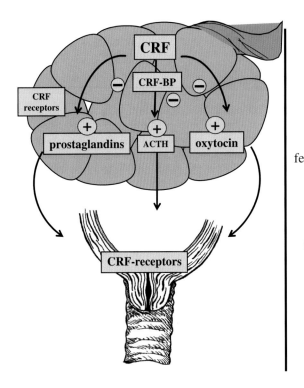

Figure 3.2 Biological effects of corticotrophin-releasing factor (CRF) and corticotrophin-releasing factor binding protein (CRF-BP) on placental hormone secretion and uterine contractility.

Receptors and biological effects

CRF and urocortin interact with two distinct receptors: R1 (R1α, R1β, R1c, and R1d subtypes) and R2 (R2α, R2β, and R2γ subtypes).[41,42] Fluorescent in situ hybridization and immunofluorescence demonstrated that syncytiotrophoblast cells and amniotic epithelium are the cell types expressing CRF-R1α, CRF-Rc, and CRF-R2β mRNA.[43]

CRF-receptors (mRNA and protein) have been also described in human myometrium,[43] and CRF-R1α is also expressed by uterine cervix, suggesting a possible involvement of its ligands in cervical ripening, probably mediated by an effect on metalloproteinases, fibronectin or nitric oxide.[44]

Urocortin binds to CRF receptors types 1 and 2, with a particularly high affinity for type 2 receptor, while UCN2 and UCN3 specifically bind only to CRF-R2.[39] Binding to diverse receptor subtypes, CRF and urocortin may stimulate the local release of uterotonins, i.e. ACTH, oxytocin and prostaglandins (Figure 3.2).[35,45,46]

CRF stimulates uterine contractility when the myometrial intracellular pathways have been already primed by uterotonic agents (oxytocin, prostaglandins).[47,48] Urocortin directly and indirectly triggers myometrial contractility (Figure 3.2).[49]

Levels in biological fluids

During pregnancy, CRF and urocortin are secreted with a different pattern in maternal plasma. CRF levels increase till term (Figure 3.3),[50] while urocortin levels are constant during gestation.[51] Placental mRNA expression of CRF and urocortin parallels the maternal circulating changes. Both CRF and urocortin levels increase at term labor, and women with preterm labor have maternal plasma CRF and urocortin levels significantly higher than those detected in normal pregnancy.[52,53] The levels are higher in the fetal than maternal bloodstream; and placental urocortin mRNA expression does not change depending on labor.[54]

CRF-BP is measurable in maternal plasma, and levels remain stable in nonpregnant women and during gestation until the third trimester of pregnancy.[55] At this time, maternal plasma CRF-BP concentrations significantly and rapidly decrease in the last 4–6 weeks before labor,[50] returning to approximately nonpregnant levels during the first 24 h postpartum. Thus, opposite changes in concentrations of CRF (higher) and CRF-BP (lower) in maternal plasma occur at term, giving an increased availability of bioactive CRF at labor (Figure 3.3). Indeed, women with preterm labor have maternal plasma CRF-BP levels significantly higher than those detected in normal pregnancy (Figure 3.3). Cord blood CRF-BP levels are

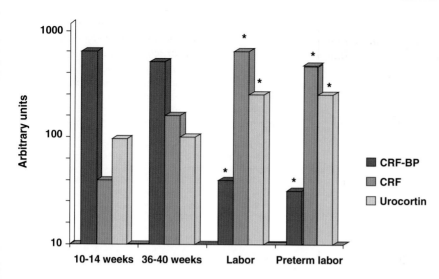

Figure 3.3 Changes of corticotrophin-releasing factor (CRF), corticotrophin-releasing factor binding protein (CRF-BP) and urocortin in maternal circulation throughout pregnancy and at the time of term or preterm labor.

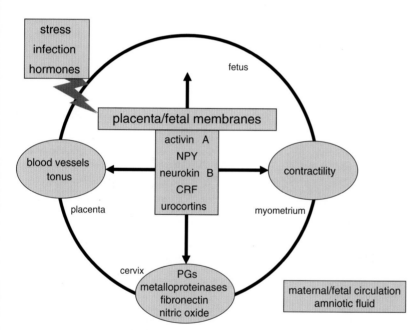

Figure 3.4 Endocrine and paracrine effects of activin A, neuropeptide Y (NPY), neurokinin B (neurokin B), corticotrophin-releasing factor (CRF) and urocortins on the gestational tissues, fetal, and maternal circulation during preterm labor.

higher[56] and amniotic fluid levels are lower than in maternal plasma; they have a similar trend, decreasing until term pregnancy.[57] During spontaneous physiological labor a significant decrease in CRF-BP levels in maternal plasma,[55] cord blood,[56] and amniotic fluid[57] occurs. Furthermore, maternal and fetal plasma CRF-BP levels are low in preterm labor.[54]

CONCLUSIONS

Human placenta and fetal membranes undertake a physiological role of intermediary barriers and active messengers in the maternal–fetal dialog, producing and releasing substances acting as endocrine, paracrine and autocrine factors to control the secretion of other regulatory molecules. In cases when a gestational diseases occurs, such as preterm labor, human placenta and fetal membranes take part in the adaptive response to adverse condition, and change their hormonal secretory ability with the aim to avoid an adverse intrauterine environment. Placental and fetal membranes hormone secretion changes occurring in pathological pregnancies may be monitored and measured in clinically accessible sites (maternal serum, amniotic fluid, saliva, and urine), both for diagnosis and evaluation of the current risk.

In a setting of maternal and/or fetal stress elicited by pathological conditions, these molecules appear to play a role in coordinating the adaptive changes in uterine contractility, triggering uterine cervix, myometrial contractility, blood vessels tonus, and fetal pituitary and adrenal glands (Figure 3.4). A whole body of evidence supports a role for the placenta and fetal membranes in the initiation of labor, and in the mechanisms determining preterm labor.

REFERENCES

1. Challis JRG, Matthews SG, Gibb W, Lye SJ. Endocrine and paracrine regulation of birth at term and preterm. Endocrinol Rev 2000; 21: 514–50.

2. Petraglia F, Florio P, Nappi C, Gennazzani AR. Peptide signaling in human placenta and membranes: autocrine, paracrine, and endocrine mechanisms. Endocrinol Rev 1996; 17: 156–86.

3. Pedrazzini T, Pralong F, Grouzmann E. Neuropeptide Y: the universal soldier. Cell Mol Life Sci 2003; 60: 350–77.

4. Petraglia F, Calzà L, Giardino L et al. Identification of immunoreactive neuropeptide-gamma in human placenta: localization, secretion, and binding sites. Endocrinology 1989; 124: 2016–22.

5. Petraglia F, Calza L, Giardino L et al. Maternal decidua and fetal membranes contain immunoreactive neuropeptide Y. J Endocrinol Invest 1993; 16: 201–5.

6. Robidoux J, Simoneau L, St-Pierre S, Ech-Chadli H, Lafond J. Human syncytiotrophoblast NPY receptors are located on BBM and activate PLC-to-PKC axis. Am J Physiol 1998; 274: E502–9.

7. Fallgren B, Edvinsson L, Ekblad E, Ekman R. Involvement of perivascular neuropeptide Y nerve fibres in uterine arterial vasoconstriction in conjunction with pregnancy. Regul Pept 1989; 24: 119–30.

8. Petraglia F, Coukos G, Battaglia C et al. Plasma and amniotic fluid immunoreactive neuropeptide-Y level changes during pregnancy, labor, and at parturition. J Clin Endocrinol Metab 1989; 69: 324–8.

9. Nussdorfer GG, Malendowicz LK. Role of tachykinins in the regulation of the hypothalamo–pituitary–adrenal axis. Peptides 1998; 19: 949–68.

10. Brownbill P, Bell NJ, Woods RJ et al. Neurokinin B is a paracrine vasodilator in the human fetal placental circulation. J Clin Endocrinol Metab 2003; 88: 2164–70.

11. Patak E, Candenas ML, Pennefather JN et al. Tachykinins and tachykinin receptors in human uterus. Br J Pharmacol 2003; 139: 523–32.

12. Laliberte C, DiMarzo L, Morrish DW, Kaufman S. Neurokinin B causes concentration-dependent relaxation of isolated human placental resistance vessels. Regul Pept 2004; 117: 123–6.

13. Patak EN, Ziccone S, Story ME et al. Activation of neurokinin NK2 receptors by tachinin peptides causes contraction of uterus in pregnant women near term. Mol Hum Reprod 2000; 6: 549–54.

14. Page NM, Woods RJ, Gardiner SM et al. Excessive placental secretion of neurokinin B during the third trimester causes preeclampsia. Nature 2000; 405: 797–800.

15 Sakamoto R, Osada H, Iitsuka Y et al. Profile of neurokinin B concentrations in maternal and cord blood in normal pregnancy. Clin Endocrinol 2003; 58: 597–600.

16. Vale W, Rivier C, Hsueh A et al. Chemical and biological characterization of the inhibin family of protein hormones. Recent Prog Horm Res 1988; 44: 1–34.

17. Petraglia F, Sawchenko P, Lim AT, Rivier J, Vae W. Localization, secretion, and action of inhibin in human placenta. Science 1997; 237: 187–9.

18. Petraglia F, Calza L, Garuti GC et al. Presence and synthesis of inhibin subunits in human decidua. J Clin Endocrinol Metab 1990; 71: 487–92.

19. Petraglia F, Gallinelli A, De Vita D et al. Activin at parturition: changes of maternal serum levels and evidence for binding sites in placenta and fetal membranes. Obstet Gynecol 1994; 41: 95–101.

20. Schneider-Kolsky ME, Manuelpillai U, Waldron K, Dole A, Wallace EM. The distribution of activin and activin receptors in gestational tissues across human pregnancy and during labour. Placenta 2002; 23: 294–302.

21. Petraglia F, Gallinelli A, Grande A et al. Local production and action of follistatin in human placenta. J Clin Endocrinol Metab 1994; 78: 205–10.

22. Ando N, Hirahara F, Fukushima J et al. Differential gene expression of TGF-beta isoforms and TGF-beta receptors during the first trimester of pregnancy at the human maternal-fetal interface. Am J Reprod Immunol 1998; 40: 48–56.

23. Ciarmela P, Florio P, Toti P et al. Human placenta and fetal membranes express follistatin-related gene (FLRG) mRNA and protein. J Endocrinol Invest 2003; 26: 641–5.

24. Kozian DH, Ziche M, Augustin HG. The activin-binding protein follistatin regulates autocrine endothelial cell activity and induces angiogenesis. Lab Invest 1997; 76: 267–76.

25. Petraglia F, Anceschi MM, Calza L et al. Inhibin and activin in human fetal membranes: evidence for a local effect on prostaglandin release. J Clin Endocrinol Metab 1993; 77: 542–8.

26. Florio P, Lombardo M, Gallo R et al. Activin A, corticotrophin-releasing factor, and prostaglandin F2α increase immunoreactive oxytocin release from cultured human placental cells. Placenta 1996; 17: 307–11.

27. Keelan JA, Zhou RL, Mitchell MD. Activin A exerts both pro and anti-inflammatory effects on human term gestational tissues. Placenta 2000; 21: 38–43.

28. Keelan JA, Zhou RL, Evans LW, Groome NP, Mitchell MD. Regulation of activin A, inhibin A, and follistatin production in human amnion and choriodecidual explants by inflammatory mediators. J Soc Gynecol Invest 2000; 7: 291–6.

29. Petraglia F, De Vita D, Gallinelli A et al. Abnormal concentration of maternal serum activin-A in gestational disease. J Clin Endocrinol Metab 1995; 80: 558–61.

30. Florio P, Benedetto C, Luisi S et al. Activin A, inhibin A, inhibin B, and parturition: changes of maternal and cord serum levels according to the mode of delivery. Br J Obstet Gynecol 1999; 106: 1061–5.

31. Petraglia F, Di Blasio AM, Florio P et al. High levels of fetal membrane activin beta A and activin receptor IIB mRNAs and augmented concentration of amniotic fluid activin A in women in term or preterm labor. J Endocrinol 1997; 154: 95–101.

32. Plevyak MP, Lambert-Messerlian GM, Farina A et al. Concentrations of serum total activin A and inhibin A in preterm and term labor patients: a cross-sectional study. J Soc Gynecol Invest 2003; 10(4): 231–6.

33. Bale TL, Vale WW. CRF and CRF receptors: role in stress responsivity and other behaviors. Annu Rev Pharmacol Toxicol 2004; 44: 525–57.

34. Donaldson CJ, Sutton SW, Perrin MH et al. Cloning and characterization of human urocortin. Endocrinology 1996; 137: 2167–70.

35. Petraglia F, Sawchenko PE, Rivier J, Vale W. Evidence for local stimulation of ACTH secretion by corticotropin-releasing factor in human placenta. Nature 1987; 328: 717–19.

36. Petraglia F, Florio P, Gallo R et al. Human placenta and fetal membranes express human urocortin mRNA and peptide. J Endocrinol Metab 1996; 8: 3807–10.

37. Petraglia F, Potter E, Cameron VA et al. Corticotropin-releasing factor-binding protein is produced by human placenta and intrauterine tissues. J Clin Endocrinol Metab 1993; 77: 919–24.

38. Reyes TM, Lewis K, Perrin MH et al. Urocortin II: a member of the corticotropin-releasing factor (CRF) neuropeptide family that is selectively bound by type 2 CRF receptors. Proc Natl Acad Sci USA 2001; 98: 2843–8.

39. Lewis K, Li C, Perrin MH et al. Identification of urocortin III, an additional member of the corticotropin-releasing factor (CRF) family with high affinity for the CRF2 receptor. Proc Natl Acad Sci USA 2001; 98: 7570–5.

40. Imperatore A, Florio P, Torres PB et al. Urocortin 2 and urocortin 3 are expressed by the human placenta, decidua and fetal membranes. Am J Obstet Gynecol 2006; 195: 288–95.

41. Hillhouse EW, Grammatopoulos D, Milton NG, Quartero HW. The identification of a human myometrial corticotropin-releasing hormone receptor that increases in affinity during pregnancy. J Clin Endocrinol Metab 1993; 76: 736–41.

42. Florio P, Franchini A, Reis FM et al. Human placenta, chorion, amnion and decidua express different variants of corticotropin-releasing factor receptor messenger RNA. Placenta 2000; 21: 32–7.

43. Hillhouse EW, Randeva H, Ladds G, Grammatopoulos D. Corticotropin-releasing hormone receptors. Biochem Soc Trans 2002; 30: 428–32.

44. Klimaviciute A, Calciolari J, Bertucci E et al. CRH, CRH-BP, CRH-R1 and CRH-R2 in cervix and corpus uteri in non-pregnant state, during preterm and term labor. Abstract SGI 2005 no. 26.

45. Petraglia F, Florio P, Benedetto C et al. Urocortin stimulates placental adrenocorticotropin and prostaglandin release and myometrial contractility in vitro. J Clin Endocrinol Metab 1999; 84: 1420–3.

46. Reis FM, Luisi S, Florio P, Degrassi A, Petraglia F. Corticotropin-releasing factor, urocortin and endothelin-1 stimulate activin A release from cultured human placental cells. Placenta 2002; 23: 522–5.

47. Benedetto C, Petraglia F, Marozio L et al. Corticotropin-releasing hormone increases prostaglandin F2 alpha activity on human myometrium in vitro. Am J Obstet Gynecol 1994; 171: 126–31.

48. Hillhouse EW, Grammatopoulos DK. Role of stress peptides during human pregnancy and labour. Reproduction 2002; 124: 323–9.

49. Grammatopoulos DK, Chrousos GP. Functional characteristics of CRH receptors and potential clinical applications of CRH-receptor antagonists. Trends Endocrinol Metab 2002; 13: 436–44.

50. Wolfe CD, Patel SP, Linton EA et al. Plasma corticotrophin-releasing factor (CRF) in abnormal pregnancy. Br J Obstet Gynaecol 1988; 95: 1003–6.

51. Glynn BP, Wolton A, Rodriguez-Linares B, Phaneuf S, Linton EA. Urocortin in pregnancy. Am J Obstet Gynecol 1998; 179: 533–9.

52. Florio P, Cobellis L, Woodman J et al. Levels of maternal plasma corticotropin-releasing factor and urocortin during labor. J Soc Gynecol Invest 2002; 9: 233–7.

53. Berkowitz GS, Lapinski RH, Lockwood CJ et al. Corticotropin-releasing factor and its binding protein: maternal serum levels in term and preterm deliveries. Am J Obstet Gynecol 1996; 174: 1477–83.

54. Florio P, Torricelli M, Galleri L et al. High fetal urocortin levels at term and preterm labor. J Clin Endocrinol Metab 2005; 90: 5361–5.

55. Linton EA, Perkins AV, Woods RJ et al. Corticotropin releasing hormone-binding protein (CRH-BP): plasma levels decrease during the third trimester of normal human pregnancy. J Clin Endocrinol Metab 1993; 76: 260–2.

56. Petraglia F, Florio P, Simoncini T et al. Cord plasma corticotropin-releasing factor-binding protein (CRF-BP) in term and preterm labour. Placenta 1997; 18: 115–19.

57. Florio P, Woods RJ, Genazzani AR, Lowry PJ, Petraglia F. Changes in amniotic fluid immunoreactive corticotropin-releasing factor (CRF) and CRF-binding protein levels in pregnant women at term and during labor. J Clin Endocrinol Metab 1997; 82: 835–8.

4

Stress and the pathophysiology of human birth

Roger Smith

LINK BETWEEN THE PLACENTA AND THE STRESS RESPONSE

The human placenta produces many peptide hormones that are similar to those produced by the hypothalamus or pituitary. Such peptides include placental lactogen and placental variant growth hormone, which are similar to pituitary growth hormone, and human chorionic gonadotrophin, which is similar to luteinizing hormone; the placenta also produces gonadotrophin-releasing hormone. Thus, the placenta contains a growth-promoting axis similar to the pituitary, and a gonadal axis with similarities to the hypothalamic–pituitary system.[1] Intriguingly, it also contains elements of the hypothalamic–pituitary adrenal axis. The placenta and membranes express the 11β hydroxysteroid dehydrogenase (11βHSD) enzymes that can either inactivate cortisol (11βHSD type 2) or generate cortisol from cortisone (11βHSD type 1),[2] it also synthesizes the pro-opiomelanocortin precursor of adrenocorticotrophic hormone (ACTH),[2] and the hypothalamic-releasing hormone corticotrophin-releasing hormone (CRH).

CRH was first discovered in the placenta by Shibasaki et al in 1982.[3] Two years later Sasaki et al[4] reported high levels in the blood of pregnant women. The surprise discovery of this hormone at high concentrations in the blood of pregnant women initiated a flurry of research activity. In the USA, Robin Goland,[5] and in the UK, Elizabeth Linton,[6] both found that maternal plasma CRH concentrations were elevated in the blood of women presenting in preterm labor. It was also clearly demonstrated that the maternal plasma CRH was derived from placental production. The placenta released the CRH primarily into the maternal circulation, although smaller amounts were also released into the fetal circulation.

Fetal stress has been linked to increased placental CRH production by several studies. Goland et al[7] examined the cord blood CRH in fetuses that were affected by pre-eclampsia, growth retardation[8] or were acidemic,[9] while Giles et al[10] examined the cord blood CRH in fetuses where Doppler flow studies indicated reduced flow. Both observed increased CRH concentrations in these situations of fetal distress.

A PARADOXICAL RELATIONSHIP BETWEEN PLACENTAL CORTICOTROPHIN-RELEASING HORMONE (CRH) PRODUCTION AND CORTISOL

Robinson et al,[11] working in Joe Majzoub's laboratory in Boston, were studying the production of CRH mRNA in the placenta. They identified that cortisol stimulated placental CRH expression, which is the opposite to the inhibitory effects of cortisol in the hypothalamus.[11] Further work in Newcastle, Australia, has determined that glucocorticoids stimulate CRH production through an interaction with the promoter of the CRH gene.[12,13] Intriguingly, this interaction does not occur through a classical glucocorticoid response element but via the cyclic adenosine monophosphate (cAMP) response element. The positive interaction between cortisol and CRH allows cortisol to stimulate CRH production, while CRH, through its effect on the maternal and fetal pituitary, can stimulate ACTH production, which in turn stimulates cortisol production.[14] The net result is an exponential increase in CRH. The exponential increase in CRH predicted by these endocrine interactions is exactly what is observed in pregnant women followed through pregnancy.[15]

CHANGING CONCENTRATIONS OF MATERNAL PLASMA CORTICOTROPHIN-RELEASING HORMONE (CRH) AND THE TIMING OF BIRTH

In longitudinal studies of maternal plasma CRH, an exponential rise in concentrations is observed which is consistent with mathematical modeling of a feed-forward system. In women who are destined to deliver preterm, the exponential rise is more rapid; in those who will deliver post dates, the rise is slower.[16,17] Thus, the rate of rise of maternal plasma CRH is predictive of the timing of birth.[18] More recently this has been related to elevated maternal concentrations of cortisol.[19] A potential further interaction involves the fetal, and perhaps the maternal, adrenal. CRH receptors exist on the fetal adrenal and in vitro CRH have been shown to directly stimulate both cortisol and dehydroepiandrosterone (DHEAS) production from fetal adrenal tissue.[20] It seems likely that fetal stress initiates increased cortisol production, which increases placental CRH production, which leads in turn to a more rapid increase in placental CRH production and preterm birth.

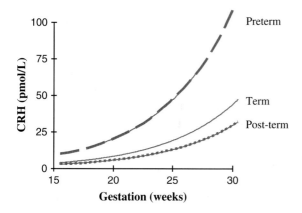

Figure 4.1 Maternal plasma corticotrophin-releasing hormone (CRH) versus gestation. (From McLean et al, Nat Med 1995; 1: 460–3.)

CONTROVERSIES IN THE CORTICOTROPHIN-RELEASING HORMONE (CRH) LITERATURE

While the majority of studies relating maternal plasma CRH to the timing of birth have found high plasma CRH in those who will deliver preterm, several notable exceptions exist. A large study by Berkowitz et al[21] reported a weak trend, and more recently a second moderate-sized study failed to find an association between increased CRH levels and preterm birth.[22] Two factors appear to be important in this conflict in the literature. Firstly, the exponential increase in plasma CRH means that CRH levels in late pregnancy are extremely high, but the corollary is that levels in early pregnancy are low or undetectable. Therefore, samples taken early in pregnancy are the most challenging from an assay methodological point of view, and many assays will not have the required sensitivity to separate normal from elevated levels at this stage of pregnancy. A second issue is that CRH production appears to be different in different racial groups; most notably, in African Americans CRH concentrations are lower than in Caucasian individuals. However, in African Americans CRH is still elevated in those who deliver prematurely compared to race-matched controls.[23] The studies that have failed to identify an elevation in the rate of rise of maternal plasma CRH in those giving birth prematurely have used a cohort with a mixture of African Americans and other racial groups, with blood sampling relatively early in gestation. African Americans have a high rate of preterm birth and it will be interesting to learn what polymorphisms in the regulation of CRH determine the altered dynamics in African Americans, and to determine if this is pathophysiologically linked to the high rate of preterm birth. It seems likely that a relationship between genes and environment exists in this area, with African Americans living in disadvantaged circumstances being predisposed by particular haplotypes to be more at risk for preterm birth than other racial groups experiencing similar disadvantage.

EVOLUTION OF CORTICOTROPHIN-RELEASING HORMONE (CRH) INVOLVEMENT IN THE TIMING OF BIRTH

Amphibians were the first vertebrates to leave the oceans and adapt to life on land. To achieve this transition a process of metamorphosis was required. Amphibian metamorphosis allows the development of a number of physiological changes which make life on land possible. Key changes include the development of lungs for breathing, and limbs for locomotion. It has been known for many decades that metamorphosis is regulated by increasing production of thyroid hormone. Tadpoles in which the thyroid gland has been removed do not undergo metamorphosis while administration of thyroid hormone can force tadpoles into an early metamorphic change. Recently, work by Denver[24] has indicated an important link between CRH and metamorphosis. In tadpoles, the thyroid-stimulating hormone (TSH) produced by the pituitary gland is regulated by CRH release from the hypothalamus. Consequently, when the tadpole is stressed by environmental factors in its pond, CRH production is increased and metamorphosis occurs earlier than usual (see Figure 4.2). This developmental plasticity in the rate of maturation in amphibians confers a survival advantage, and allows the developing individual to control the period of time that is spent in an aquatic environment. It seems this role for CRH evolved roughly 300 million years ago. There are obvious parallels in mammalian biology where the development of the embryo and fetus occurs in the watery environment contained within the amniotic cavity. The event of birth for mammals requires a transition to air breathing and terrestrial locomotion similar to that provided by metamorphosis in the amphibian.

In mammals there is evidence linking CRH to the timing of birth, and the transition to a terrestrial environment. In the mouse, knockout of the CRH gene leads to death at birth from respiratory failure[25] – i.e. the mouse requires CRH-stimulated cortisol production to adapt to air breathing. If glucocorticoids are administered to mature the fetal lungs then the mouse is subsequently normally viable, indicating that birth is the only time in the life of a mouse when CRH is essential. Recently, in studies on mice, Condon et al[26] linked maturation of the lungs to the onset of labor mediated by the lung production of surfactant protein A, which stimulates inflammatory processes in the myometrium; lung maturation is modulated by fetal cortisol production, probably under CRH control. In the sheep, infusion of a CRH antagonist is able to delay delivery, indicating that CRH is linked to the timing of birth in this species.[27] Again in the sheep, cortisol production is part of the linkage, and administration of glucocorticoids to the pregnant sheep can precipitate delivery and concurrent maturation of the fetal lungs (see Figure 4.3).

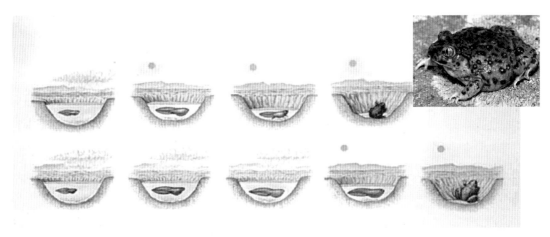

Figure 4.2 Environmental stress regulates metamorphosis in amphibians – the American spadefoot toad. (Reproduced from Smith R. The timing of birth. Sci Am 1999; 280(3): 68–75.)

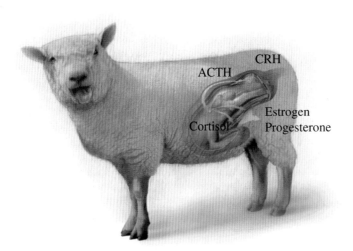

Figure 4.3 Corticotrophin-releasing hormone production and labor in the sheep. In the sheep the fetal hypothalamus produces CRH, which drives ACTH and cortisol production. Cortisol promotes lung maturation and changes in placental steroid metabolism leading to a fall in progesterone and arise in estrogen that directly stimulates the onset of labor. (Reproduced from Smith R. The timing of birth. Sci Am 1999; 280(3): 68–75.)

While fetal production of CRH in the hypothalamus appears central to birth in sheep the situation is more complicated in primates. Robinson et al[28] examined placental CRH gene expression in primates and other mammals, but CRH was only detected in primates. More recent studies of CRH protein expression have also only identified CRH within the placentae of primates.

Within the order of primates, placental CRH production does not occur in lemurs but has been identified in the maternal blood of all New and Old World monkeys that have been examined, and also in the blood of chimpanzees and gorillas.[29,30] In both New and Old World monkeys, a peak in CRH concentration occurs at mid-gestation (see Figure 4.4). In gorillas and chimpanzees

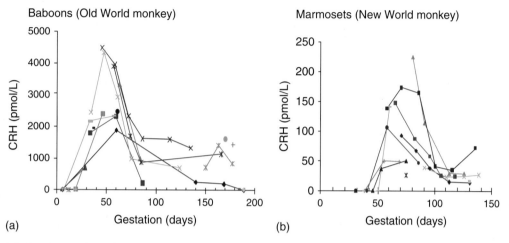

Figure 4.4 Corticotrophin-releasing hormone (CRH) in pregnant (a) Old and (b) New World monkeys. [(a) From Bowman et al, Am J Primatol 2001; 53: 123–30. (b) from Power et al, Am J Primatol 2006; 68: 181–8.]

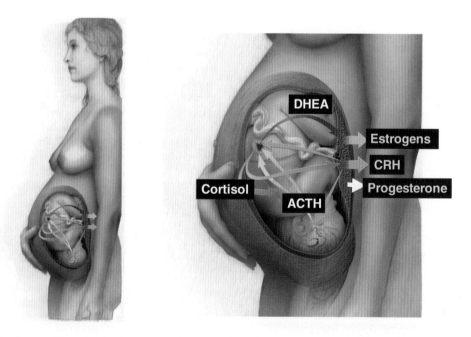

Figure 4.5 Corticotrophin-releasing hormone (CRH) is released into maternal and fetal circulations. ACTH, adrenocorticotrophic hormone; DHEAS, dehydroepiandrostesterone. (From Smith, Sci Am 1999; 250: 68–75.) In the mother the CRH may have direct actions on the myometrium. In the fetus CRH may promote fetal adrenal production of DHEAS that is converted to estrogens in the placenta.

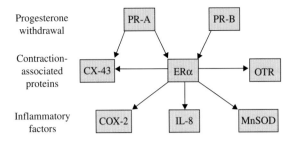

LISREL: $P = 0.499$ $df = 22$ $Chi^2 = 21.35$ MXC2: $P = 0.859 \pm 0.007$
DGraph: $P = 0.280$ $df = 40$ $Chi^2 = 44.72$

Figure 4.6 Identifying pathways leading to uterine activation. COX-2, cyclooxygenase-2; CX-43, connexin43; Erα, estrogen receptor alpha; IL-8, interleukin 8; MnSOD, manganese superoxide dismutase; OTR, oxytocin receptor; PR-A and PR-B, isoforms of progesterone receptor. (From Bisits et al, PLoS Comput Biol 2005; 1: 132–6.)

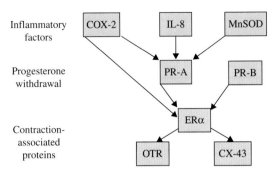

LISREL: $P = 0.925$ $df = 23$ $Chi^2 = 14.08$ MXC2: $P = 0.990 \pm 0.002$
DGraph: $P = 0.684$ $df = 40$ $Chi^2 = 35.24$

Figure 4.7 Identifying pathways leading to uterine activation. COX-2, cyclooxygenase-2; CX-43, connexin43; Erα, estrogen receptor alpha; IL-8, interleukin 8; MnSOD, manganese superoxide dismutase; OTR, oxytocin receptor; PR-A and PR-B, isoforms of progesterone receptor. (From Bisits et al, PloS Comput Biol 2005; 1: 132–6.)

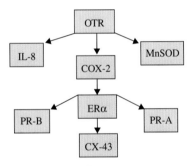

LISREL: $P = 0.091$ $df = 22$ $Chi^2 = 31.25$ MXC2: $P = 0.470 \pm 0.009$
DGraph: $P = 0.04$ $df = 42$ $Chi^2 = 59.28$

Figure 4.8 Identifying pathways leading to uterine activation. COX-2, cyclooxygenase-2; CX-43, connexin43; Erα, estrogen receptor alpha; IL-8, interleukin 8; MnSOD, manganese superoxide dismutase; OTR, oxytocin receptor; PR-A and PR-B, isoforms of progesterone receptor. (From Bisits et al, PloS Comput Biol 2005; 1: 132–6.)

an exponential rise in maternal plasma concentrations occurs, similar to that observed in humans.[31]

POTENTIAL PATHWAYS BY WHICH CORTICOTROPHIN-RELEASING HORMONE (CRH) MAY MEDIATE PARTURITION

While the association between placental CRH production and parturition appears robust, the link between CRH and the onset of myometrial contractions in humans remains unclear. CRH receptors have been identified on the myometrial cells,[32] the pituitary cells of the mother and fetus, and the adrenal cells of the fetus.[33] CRH may act on the pituitary of the fetus to drive production of ACTH, and therefore cortisol, which matures fetal lung tissue. The maturation of fetal lungs may promote the onset of parturition through the production of surfactant protein A or other phospholipids. Indeed, Laatikinen et al[34] reported that amniotic fluid phospholipid concentrations are correlated with amniotic fluid CRH concentrations. Fetal adrenal zone tissue responds to CRH with preferential synthesis of DHEAS, which is converted in the placenta into estrogens; estrogens increase the production of contraction-associated proteins such as oxytocin receptors in many systems (see Figure 4.5). CRH also stimulates fetal adrenal cortisol synthesis and, as previously mentioned, cortisol may act to stimulate lung maturation and labor onset. CRH may also act via the CRH receptors expressed on myometrial cells. Early reports suggested that CRH may potentiate the action of uterotonics such as oxytocin or prostaglandins;[35] however, more recent studies have suggested that CRH may promote relaxation. CRH receptors are usually linked via Gas proteins to increased cAMP synthesis, as cAMP promotes relaxation a role for CRH in maintaining uterine quiescence has been proposed.[36] However, late in pregnancy multiple forms of CRH receptor are expressed in myometrial cells, some of which appear to be linked to the phospholipase C pathway, which when activated promotes Ca entry into cells and increased contractility. Therefore it may be possible

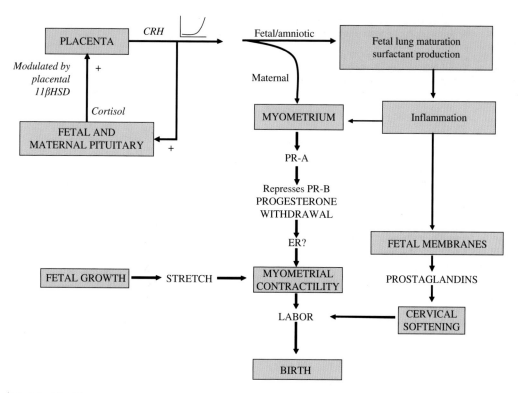

Figure 4.9 Model of human parturition.

that CRH is bifunctional, promoting relaxation early in gestation and contraction in the final stages of parturition. Resolving these uncertainties may require novel experimental approaches to determine cause and effect relationships between the variables thought to play a role in labor.

DETERMINING CAUSE AND EFFECT RELATIONSHIPS IN HUMAN LABOR

Several features of human pregnancy are unique to primates and some appear specific to the great apes. For this reason, experiments on processes of parturition in common laboratory animals are difficult to extrapolate to humans. Yet it is not possible to perform experiments on pregnant women. This situation has restricted progress in understanding the process of labor in humans. Recently, novel mathematical approaches have been developed that allow conclusions to be drawn on the likely causal relationships between variables without conducting experimental interventions. This approach has been applied to the expression of different genes in myometrial samples obtained from women in labor and prior to labor. Using 'directed graphs' the likelihood of different potential pathways linking the variables can be statistically tested.

With this approach, strong support for an inflammatory pathway has been produced (see Figures 4.6, 4.7 and 4.8).[37] In the future it may be possible to expand this pathway to include other variables such as those involved in the stress axis, and thereby resolve the nature of the link between stress and human preterm birth (See Figure 4.9).

REFERENCES

1. Reis FM, Florio P, Cobellis L et al. Human placenta as a source of neuroendocrine factors. Biol Neonate 2001; 79: 150–6.
2. Challis JR, Sloboda D, Matthews SG et al. The fetal placental hypothalamic–pituitary–adrenal (HPA) axis, parturition and post natal health. Mol Cell Endocrinol 2001; 185: 135–44.
3. Shibasaki T, Odagiri E, Shizume K, Ling N. corticotropin-releasing factor-like activity in human placental extracts. J Clin Endocrinol Metab 1982; 55(2): 384–6.
4. Sasaki A, Liotta AS, Luckey MM et al. Immunoreactive corticotropin-releasing factor is present in human maternal plasma during the third trimester of pregnancy. J Clin Endocrinol Metab 1984; 59: 812–14.
5. Goland RS, Wardlaw SL, Stark RI et al. High levels of Corticotrophin-releasing hormone immunoactivity in maternal and fetal plasma during pregnancy. J Clin Endocrinol Metab 1986; 63: 1199–203.
6. Wolfe C, Poston L, Jones M. Digoxin-like immunoreactive factor, corticotropin releasing factor, and pregnancy. Lancet 1987; 1: 335–6

7. Goland RS, Conwell IM, Jozak S. The effect of pre-eclampsia on human placental corticotrophin-releasing hormone content and processing. Placenta 1995; 16: 375–82.

8. Goland RS, Jozak S, Warren WB et al. Elevated levels of umbilical cord plasma corticotropin-releasing hormone in growth-retarded fetuses. J Clin Endocrinol Metab 1993; 77: 1174–9.

9. Goland RS, Tropper PJ, Warren WB et al. Concentrations of corticotrophin-releasing hormone in the umbilical-cord blood of pregnancies complicated by pre-eclampsia. Reprod Fertil Dev 1995; 7: 1227–30.

10. Giles WB, McLean M, Davies JJ, Smith R. Abnormal umbilical artery Doppler waveforms and cord blood corticotropin-releasing hormone. Obstet Gynecol 1996; 87: 107–11.

11. Robinson BG, Emanuel RL, Frim DM, Majzoub JA. Glucocorticoid stimulates expression of corticotropin-releasing hormone gene in human placenta. Proc Natl Acad Sci USA 1988; 85: 5244–8.

12. Cheng YH, Nicholson RC, King B et al. Glucocorticoid stimulation of corticotropin-releasing hormone gene expression requires a cyclic adenosine 3',5'-monophosphate regulatory element in human primary placental cytotrophoblast cells. J Clin Endocrinol Metab 2000; 85: 1937–45.

13. Cheng YH, Nicholson RC, King B et al. Corticotropin-releasing hormone gene expression in primary placental cells is modulated by cyclic adenosine 3',5'-monophosphate. J Clin Endocrinol Metab 2000; 85: 1239–44.

14. Thomson M, Smith R. The action of hypothalamic and placental corticotropin releasing factor on the corticotrope. Mol Cell Endocrinol 1989; 62: 1–12.

15. Emanuel RL, Robinson BG, Seely EW et al. Corticotrophin releasing hormone levels in human plasma and amniotic fluid during gestation. Clin Endocrinol (Oxf) 1994; 40: 257–62.

16. McLean M, Bisits A, Davies J et al. A placental clock controlling the length of human pregnancy. Nat Med 1995; 1: 460–3.

17. Inder WJ, Prickett TC, Ellis MJ et al. The utility of plasma CRH as a predictor of preterm delivery. J Clin Endocrinol Metab 2001; 86: 5706–10.

18. Leung TN, Chung TK, Madsen G et al. Analysis of mid-trimester corticotrophin-releasing hormone and alpha-fetoprotein concentrations for predicting pre-eclampsia. Hum Reprod 2000; 15: 1813–18.

19. Sandman CA, Glynn L, Schetter CD et al. Elevated maternal cortisol early in pregnancy predicts third trimester levels of placental corticotropin releasing hormone (CRH): priming the placental clock. Peptides 2006; 27(6): 1457–63.

20. Mesiano S, Chan EC, Fitter JT et al. Progesterone withdrawal and estrogen activation in human parturition are coordinated by progesterone receptor A expression in the myometrium. J Clin Endocrinol Metab 2002; 87: 2924–30.

21. Berkowitz GS, Lapinski RH, Lockwood CJ et al. Corticotropin-releasing factor and its binding protein: maternal serum levels in term and preterm deliveries. Am J Obstet Gynecol 1996; 174: 1477–83.

22. Sibai B, Meis PJ, Klebanoff M et al. Plasma CRH measurement at 16 to 20 weeks' gestation does not predict preterm delivery in women at high-risk for preterm delivery. Am J Obstet Gynecol 2005; 193: 1181–6.

23. Holzman C, Jetton J, Siler-Khodr T, Fisher R, Rip T. Second trimester corticotropin-releasing hormone levels in relation to preterm delivery and ethnicity. Obstet Gynecol 2001; 97: 657–63.

24. Denver RJ. Hormonal correlates of environmentally induced metamorphosis in the Western spadefoot toad, Scaphiopus hammondii. Gen Comp Endocrinol 1998; 110: 326–36.

25. Muglia LJ, Bae DS, Brown TT et al. Proliferation and differentiation defects during lung development in corticotropin-releasing hormone-deficient mice. Am J Respir Cell Mol Biol 1999; 20: 181–8.

26. Condon JC, Jeyasuria P, Faust JM, Mendelson CR. Surfactant protein secreted by the maturing mouse fetal lung acts as a hormone that signals the initiation of parturition. Proc Natl Acad Sci USA 2004; 101: 4978–83.

27. Chan EC, Falconer J, Madsen G et al. A corticotropin-releasing hormone type I receptor antagonist delays parturition in sheep. Endocrinology 1998; 139: 3357–60.

28. Robinson BG, Arbiser JL, Emanuel RL, Majzoub JA. Species-specific placental corticotropin releasing hormone messenger RNA and peptide expression. Mol Cell Endocrinol 1989; 62: 337–41.

29. Bowman ME, Lopata A, Jaffe RB et al. Corticotropin-releasing hormone-binding protein in primates. Am J Primatol 2001; 53: 123–30.

30. Power ML, Bowman ME, Smith R et al. Pattern of maternal serum corticotropin-releasing hormone concentration during pregnancy in the common marmoset (Callithrix jacchus). Am J Primatol 2006; 68: 181–8.

31. Smith R, Wickings EJ, Bowman ME et al. Corticotropin-releasing hormone in chimpanzee and gorilla pregnancies. J Clin Endocrinol Metab 1999; 84: 2820–5.

32. Grammatopoulos D, Thompson S, Hillhouse EW. The human myometrium expresses multiple isoforms of the corticotropin-releasing hormone receptor. J Clin Endocrinol Metab 1995; 80: 2388–93.

33. Smith R, Mesiano S, Chan EC, Brown S, Jaffe RB. Corticotropin-releasing hormone directly and preferentially stimulates dehydroepiandrosterone sulfate secretion by human fetal adrenal cortical cells. J Clin Endocrinol Metab 1998; 83: 2916–20.

34. Laatikainen TJ, Raisanen IJ, Salminen KR. Corticotropin-releasing hormone in amniotic fluid during gestation and labor and in relation to fetal lung maturation. Am J Obstet Gynecol 1988; 159: 891–5.

35. Quartero HW, Fry CH. Placental corticotrophin releasing factor may modulate human parturition. Placenta 1989; 10: 439–43.

36. Grammatopoulos DK, Hillhouse EW. Role of corticotropin-releasing hormone in onset of labour. Lancet 1999; 354: 1546–9.

37. Bisits AM, Smith R, Mesiano S et al. Inflammatory aetiology of human myometrial activation tested using directed graphs. PLoS Comput Biol 2005; 1: 132–6.

SECTION II

MEDIATORS

5

Undernutrition, preterm birth, and the prostaglandin pathway

John RG Challis

INTRODUCTION

It is clear from studies in many species that the onset of birth at term is initiated by the fetus. In sheep, the influence of the fetal genome is expressed through two independent but interrelating pathways, a fetal growth pathway and a fetal endocrine pathway. During pregnancy, the growing fetus provides a stretch stimulus to the development of the uterus, under the influence of progesterone. At term, as the influence of progesterone wanes, this stretch influence results in upregulation of a cassette of genes responsible for myometrial activation and the potential for myometrial contractility. The fetal endocrine pathway involves maturation of the fetal hypothalamic–pituitary–adrenal (HPA) axis, increased output of cortisol, which provides not only the stimulation to maturation of those organ systems required for extrauterine survival but also the stimulus to an altered pattern of placental steroidogenesis. In this species, as in many others, there is a clear decrease in the concentration of progesterone in maternal plasma before the onset of parturition. This change is followed by a terminal increase in maternal estrogen concentrations, and increased output of prostaglandin $F_{2\alpha}$ ($PGF_{2\alpha}$) from the maternal endometrium. The mechanism by which cortisol effects these changes is thought to be associated with upregulation of prostaglandin synthase ($PGHS_2$) activity in the placenta, in a manner which is dependent on cortisol but independent of changes in estrogen. In turn, this leads to an increase in the concentration of prostaglandin E_2 (PGE_2) in the fetal circulation which occurs with a time-course coincident with the prepartum increase in fetal cortisol. The observation that PGE_2 increases expression, in fetal trophoblast cells, of P450C17 lyase suggests that this may be the mechanism by which fetal endocrine events are translated into altered placental steroid output. Maternal increases in

$PGF_{2\alpha}$ from induced $PGHS_2$ in endometrium require the prepartum increase in estrogen. Changes in maternal uterotonins, such as $PGF_{2\alpha}$, then interact with the stretch pathway to stimulate the activated myometrium.[1]

It is also clear that the overall sequence of events associated with human labor may have remarkable similarities to that described in the sheep model. Key differences are the absence of a maternal progesterone withdrawal, lack of P450C17 lyase induction in the human placenta at term, and the possibility that in human pregnancy increased output of placental corticotrophin-releasing hormone (CRH) subserves the functions effected by rising PGE_2 in ovine pregnancy.

Human preterm labor is a syndrome that may arise from different causes. Before 30 weeks of gestation, infection appears to predominate amongst these. In later gestation, premature activation of the fetal HPA axis in response to an adverse intrauterine environment, e.g. hypoxemia, undernutrition (UN) or even infection, may underlie the stimulus to prematurity. A third pathway clearly involves vascular thrombotic processes. It would seem that these different pathways may occur separately, or be activated to different degrees in the same patient.

PRETERM BIRTH AND PROGRAMMING

Although dismissed in the early observations,[2] it is now apparent that there is an obvious link between preterm birth, growth restriction, and programming later-life disease. We have discussed elsewhere the likelihood that in normal pregnancy the prepartum increase in fetal cortisol occurs at an appropriate developmental time, leading to the maturation of organ systems required for postnatal health after term birth.[3] We have suggested that preterm birth may be associated with an inappropriate increase in fetal HPA activation and a rise in fetal cortisol at an inappropriate developmental window. Fetal hypercortisolemia predisposes to cessation of tissue proliferation and overall fetal growth restriction. Thus, these babies, born prematurely, may be exposed in utero to inappropriate levels of glucocorticoids, known to precipitate programming of the cardiovascular and metabolic axes. The coincidence of growth restriction and preterm birth is an outcome of these pregnancies.

Many workers have shown that UN during pregnancy leads to growth restriction of the fetuses, the postnatal development of hypertension, and characteristics of the metabolic syndrome.[2,4] In rats, restriction of maternal casein during the second half of pregnancy led to growth-restricted pups at birth, and a significant reduction in expression of the enzyme 11β hydroxysteroid dehydrogenase type 2 (11βHSD-2) in the placenta. The reduced expression of this enzyme in the placenta would diminish the capacity to metabolize maternal corticosterone and restrict its transfer to the fetuses. Hence, the developing pups would be exposed to inappropriately high levels of glucocorticoids. Reduction of placental 11βHSD-2 may explain the interrelationship between UN and elevations of glucorticoids, and subserve later-life programming. In this context, the recent observation showing that similar dietary restriction during pregnancy in mice also leads to a reduction in placental 11βHSD-2 and preterm birth is further evidence linking growth restriction, premature birth and programming.[5]

UNDERNUTRITION (UN) AND PRETERM BIRTH

We examined the relationship between periconceptional UN, fetal development and preterm birth in sheep. Ewes were subject to a modest degree of UN for 60 days before the start of pregnancy and for the 30 days of gestation. The degree of UN was 'titrated' to produce a 15% decrease in maternal body weight; this weight loss corrected after re-feeding. We were surprised to find that fetuses in about one-half of the undernourished mothers delivered prematurely.[6] This significant change was associated with precocious increases in adrenocorticotrophic hormone (ACTH) and cortisol in the fetal circulation, and increased levels of mRNA encoding proopiomelanocortin (POMC) and prohormone convertase-1 (PC-1) in the pars intermedia of the fetal pituitary.[7]

At day 130 of gestation there were also significant increases in the critical enzyme for cortisol biosynthesis – P450C17 – in the adrenal, attesting to the bioactivity of the raised immunoreactive ACTH in the fetal circulation. Furthermore, expression of PGHS$_2$ was also elevated at day 130 of gestation in pregnancies where the mothers were undernourished during the periconceptional period. Thus, in sheep, periconceptional UN results, 100 days later in pregnancy, in precocious activation of fetal HPA function and preterm birth in a significant proportion of the animals. We are currently exploring the mechanisms underlying this process. Our hypothesis is that it may be associated with altered gene expression and/or with methylation in an epigenetic manner of a key gene or genes in the fetal HPA activation pathway. It is clear, however, that there may be other mechanisms involved. For example, maternal plasma progesterone levels are lower in early pregnancy after periconceptional UN and placental 11βHSD-2 activity is reduced at day 50 of gestation in these animals.

Next, it was of obvious concern to examine whether there were human correlates of these observations. Outcome from pregnancies during the Dutch famine of the Second World War suggested that the preterm labor rate was increased in those women pregnant in the first trimester during the period of famine, although it is impossible to separate the effects of UN from the overriding stressful circumstances prevailing at that time. We collaborated with Professor Keith Godfrey and colleagues at the University of Southampton, UK, to study pregnancies that were monitored closely as part of the Southampton Women's Survey. We asked the simple question of women before pregnancy whether they were dieting in order to lose weight. We recognize of course that this question does not inform the duration or magnitude of diet, although the effects seen are independent of the maternal BMI, ethnicity, parity and socioeconomic status. In preliminary observations of the first 600 women, about 25% acknowledged dieting deliberately before the start of their pregnancy.[8] Many of these went to term, but in a subset, studied in detail, their placentae had lowered expression of 11βHSD-2 and increased expression of PGHS$_2$, just as we had seen and others had reported in the earlier animal studies referred to above. Of particular interest was the preliminary observation that the incidence of preterm birth was approximately three-fold higher in women who acknowledged dieting to lose weight before the start of pregnancy compared to those who did not. These results need substantiating in a larger cohort recruited through the Southampton Women's Study. They are, however, consistent with observations across species linking modest UN with altered expression of placental 11βHSD-2, increased prostaglandin synthesis, and preterm birth. The implications for public health policy in potentially reducing the incidence of preterm birth might be quite important.

ROLE OF PROSTAGLANDINS

All of the pathways discussed above, which may be associated with an increased incidence of preterm birth, appear to do so through increased potential for the generation of bioactive prostaglandins within the intrauterine tissues. Studies conducted using human placental tissue and fetal membranes in tissue culture have shown an increased output of prostaglandin and increased expression of $PGHS_2$ in response to glucocorticoids, and in response to proinflammatory cytokines (see ref 1). Cytokines such as tumor necrosis factor-α (TNF-α) or interleukin-1 (IL-1β) produce coordinate increases in inducible $PGHS_2$ and membrane-associated PGE synthase (mPGES). We were able to co-localize these enzymes in cultures of primary trophoblasts and in the choriocarcinoma JEG-3 cell line, and showed increased expression of both enzymes in some, although not all, placental trophoblast cells maintained in culture in the presence of IL-1β.[9] We and others have demonstrated that IL-1β also decreases expression and activity of the key prostaglandin metabolizing enzyme, type 1 prostaglandin dehydrogenase (PGDH). Moreover, in JEG-3 cells, and in primary trophoblasts, IL-1β increases expression of EP1 and EP3 receptors for PGE_2, an effect that is attenuated in the presence of the anti-inflammatory cytokine IL-10. Thus, as postulated in the classical studies of Romero, Mitchell and colleagues (see ref 1), in the presence of infection, increases in proinflammatory cytokine act through nuclear factor κB (NFκB) pathway to increase expression, coordinately, of prostaglandin synthesizing enzymes while decreasing the metabolism of prostaglandins and increasing tissue-receptor responses by upregulating key receptor species. Clinically, it may be quite relevant that several of these activities can be blocked or reduced in the presence of IL-10.

Many years ago, several groups of investigators [including those of Gibb et al (see ref 1)] made the surprising observation that, in human amnion, glucocorticoids increased expression of $PGHS_2$ and increased output of PGE_2. In amnion, the predominant responsive cell type appears to be the fibroblast-like cells within the mesenchymal layer. In vivo, these cells might respond to cortisol derived from the amniotic fluid, or, because they express 11βHSD-1 they, and amniotic epithelial cells, have the capacity to metabolize cortisone, also derived from amniotic fluid into biologically active cortisol. We have found that the chorion trophoblast cells also exhibit increased $PGHS_2$ expression in response to addition of cortisol. These cells also express 11βHSD-1 and have the capacity to produce cortisol locally from cortisone, and this activity is increased further by $PGF_{2\alpha}$ and PGE_2 in a dose-dependent manner.[10] Thus, there exist between and within amnion and chorion novel, locally effective cascades between glucocorticoids and prostaglandins which enhance prostaglandin output. For much of pregnancy, however, the potential effect of these stimuli is balanced by the abundant expression of PGDH in chorion trophoblast. Our group has shown that, during pregnancy, expression and activity of this enzyme is sustained in a local tonic fashion by progesterone. However, the effect of progesterone on PGDH can be countered by cortisol. Of even greater interest is the observation that when chorion trophoblast cells are cultured in the presence of trilostane, an inhibitor of the enzyme 3β hydroxysteroid dehydrogenase (3βHSD), PGDH expression and activity is reduced. Addition of progesterone to trilostane-treated cells restores PGDH activity. This effect of progesterone can be partially attenuated by antagonists of the progesterone receptor but, most importantly, are also antagonized by a specific inhibitor of the glucocorticoids receptor (see ref 1).[11] Thus, it seems possible that part of the action of progesterone in maintaining pregnancy is through tonically upregulating PGDH as a means of controlling levels of bioactive prostaglandins. It appears that this effect may be mediated, at least in part, through the glucocorticoid receptor, and that this activity could be blocked by rising glucocorticoids either through their endogenous production at term, or through the increased local synthesis within the chorion as a result of prostaglandin-induced increases in chorionic 11βHSD-1. If PGDH is considered as a progesterone-dependent enzyme contributing to pregnancy maintenance, then we have has described a mechanism by which the local intrauterine withdrawal of progesterone action might be effected.[12]

PROGESTERONE WITHDRAWAL AND HUMAN LABOR

The withdrawal of the progesterone block to the myometrium is central to the dogma surrounding the process of parturition in virtually all animal species. The failure to detect a decrease in maternal progesterone in association with human labor continues to confound our understanding of this process.

It is now generally accepted that in human pregnancy there may well be 'progesterone withdrawal', but this occurs through a number of different potential mechanisms, and in a 'local' manner within the tissues of the pregnant uterus. It remains possible that progesterone withdrawal could occur through the formation of a specific metabolite of this steroid in late gestation, or indeed that the action of progesterone through pregnancy is effected not by progesterone but by an alternative metabolite, and the generation of this candidate steroid might decrease at term (see ref 1).

The action of progesterone is effected through the progesterone receptor, of which there are at least three isoforms – PR-A, PR-B and PR-C. We used Syrian hamster myocytes (SHM) cells, transfected with different progesterone receptor isoforms, and with a PRE or mouse mammary tumor virus (MMTV)-luciferase reporter system to show that PR-B was far more effective in transducing progesterone responses than PR-A.[13] However, increasing amounts of PR-A were able to attenuate progesterone-mediated transactivation of PR-B. It has been reported that levels of mRNA encoding PR-A increase during late gestation, potentially stimulated by estrogen, and this interaction between PR-A and PR-B might account for progesterone withdrawal by reducing progesterone receptor activity. Further clarification of this concept is required, however, as not all studies measuring PR-A and PR-B protein levels have replicated the findings based on changes in mRNA.

Recently, in an elegant series of studies from Carol Mendelson's laboratory, it has been shown that progesterone receptor activation depends on the presence of particular co-activator proteins such as steroid receptor co-activator (SRC)-1, -2 and -3.[14] In mouse and human tissues, SRC activity is reduced in association with labor. Moreover, these changes can be induced by administration into the amniotic fluid of the surfactant protein A (SP-A), and would appear to involve a cytokine-mediated NFκB pathway.

Recently, Dong et al[15] identified a novel co-repressor of progesterone receptor activation. This material, PSF, decreased the activation of PR-B that follows addition of progesterone to SHM cells. It appears that PSF not only blocks progesterone receptor transactivation but also increases progesterone receptor degradation. In the rat, spontaneous parturition is associated with increased levels of intrauterine PSF and a simultaneous decrease in PR-B expression. Further studies on the regulation and action of PSF in human labor at term and preterm are eagerly awaited.

MATRIX METALLOPROTEINASES (MMP)

Birth at term and preterm is associated with detachment of the placenta, and with weakening and rupture of the fetal membranes. Preterm, premature rupture of the membranes (PPROM) is commonly associated with infection-driven preterm birth. MMP-2 and MMP-9 are key enzymes expressed in the placenta and fetal membranes. MMP-9 is expressed exclusively in amnion epithelium, and expressed with MMP-2 in chorion trophoblasts.[16] The activity of MMP enzymes is regulated, in part, by tissue inhibitors of matrix metalloproteinase (TIMP family). Thus, a balance between MMP-2, MMP-9 and TIMP is important in determining the basis of local collagenolytic activity.

We found that lipopolysaccharide (LPS) increases MMP-9 expression and protein activity by chorion trophoblasts. This occurred in the absence of changes in MMP-2, and without change in TIMP-1. The activity of LPS could be blocked by meloxicam, a specific inhibitor of $PGHS_2$, and restored by the addition of increasing amounts of PGE_2 and $PGF_{2\alpha}$.[17] Thus prostaglandins, in addition to their other activities at the time of labor, appear also to regulate MMP expression. Recently, we showed that this activity could be reproduced by IL-1β, in a dose-dependent manner, an action that was blocked by the anti-inflammatory IL-10. These actions appear to be associated with altered phosphorylation of intermediates on the mitogen activated protein kinase (MAPK) pathway.

CRH also increases MMP-9. This is of obvious interest given the findings that maternal plasma levels of CRH are precociously elevated in women at risk of preterm labor. We have presumed that rises in maternal CRH reflect stimulation in the placenta and membranes of CRH gene expression by glucocorticoids of either maternal or fetal adrenal origin (see ref 1). However, proinflammatory cytokines also stimulate CRH expression in trophoblasts, suggesting a common pathway in infection or in the presence of a low-grade inflammatory process. The effect of CRH on uterine contractility is confusing. It is apparently inhibitory for much of pregnancy, but stimulatory at term either through altered receptor coupling or through CRH-induced increases in prostaglandin biosynthesis. An effect on MMP offers the possibility of other locally important actions of CRH. We found that these actions could be reproduced by addition of the related peptide urocortin, and were countered in chorion, but not amnion, by CRH-2 receptor antagonists.[18] In amnion, only the CRH-1 receptor antagonist was effective, consistent with early reports that in this tissue only corticotropin releasing hormone receptor 1 (CRHR-1) is expressed.[19]

These studies – in addition to emphasizing potentially novel roles for CRH and related neuropeptides in the mechanisms of human labor – have emphasized further the reliance of this process on multiple, interconnecting feed-forward pathways. The experimental evidence, of course, for such pathways is based predominantly on in vitro experimentation. For many studies there are appropriate animal models: for others, including those on CRH, studies have to be conducted using human tissues. New approaches, perhaps using small inhibitory RNA, may be required to determine the relative importance of individual feed-forward cascades. Finally, it is apparent that there is no normal homeostatic regulator of these feed-forward loops. They act to exaggerate and accelerate each other. The point at which they are broken, and the outcome of their interaction, is birth.

ACKNOWLEDGMENTS

I am indebted to many colleagues, without whose contributions this chapter, and the work described in it, would not have been possible. In particular, studies on undernutrition in sheep have involved Drs Frank Bloomfield, Jane Harding and Peter Gluckman, and Ms Kristin Connor. Studies with the Southampton Women's Survey would not have been possible without Professor Keith Godfrey, and involved Mr Jim Johnstone. Students and postdocs in my own laboratory have included Drs Elif Unlugedik, Marina Premyslova, Wei Li, Fal Patel, and Nadia Alfaidy. Collaboration with Professors Steve Lye, Bill Gibb and Alan Bocking (Toronto), John Newnham and Tim Moss (Perth, Australia), and more recently with Professor Felice Petraglia and Alberto Imperatore (Siena, Italy), have provided a consistent source of provocative and productive discussion. Work in my laboratory has been supported principally through operating grants from the Canadian Institutes of Health Research, and from the CIHR Group Grant in Fetal and Neonatal Health and Development.

REFERENCES

1. Challis JRG, Matthews SG, Gibb W, Lye SJ. Endocrine and paracrine regulation of birth at term, and preterm. Endocr Rev 2000; 21: 514–50.
2. Barker DJP. Mothers, babies and Health in Later Life, 2nd edn. Edinburgh: Churchill Livingstone, 1998.
3. Challis JRG, Bloomfield FH, Bocking AD et al. Fetal signals and parturition. J Obstet Gynecol Res 2005; 6: 492–9.
4. Gluckman P, Hanson M. The Fetal Matrix. Evolution, Development and Disease. Cambridge, UK: Cambridge University Press, 2005.
5. Knight BS, Pennel CE, Adamson L, Lye SJ. Strain differences in the impact of dietary restriction on fetal growth and pregnancy in mice. Annual Meeting of the Society for Gynecologic Investigation, Abstract No. 102, Toronto, February 2005.
6. Bloomfield F, Oliver M, Hawkins P et al. A periconceptional nutritional origin for non-infectious preterm birth. Science 2003; 300: 606.
7. Bloomfield FH, Oliver MH, Giannoulias CD et al. Brief undernutrition in late-gestation sheep programmes the HPA axis in adult offspring. Endocrinology 2003; 144: 2933–40.
8. Johnstone JF, Lewis RM, Crozier S et al. Maternal dieting behaviour before pregnancy and its relation to the incidence of preterm delivery. J Soc Gynecol Investig 2006; 13(Suppl): 176A, 340.
9. Premyslova M, Chisaka H, Okamura K, Challis JRG. 1L-1 β treatment does not co-ordinately up-regulate mPGES-1 and COX-2 mRNA expression, but results in higher degree of cellular and intracellular co-localization of their immunoreactive proteins in human placenta trophoblast cells. Placenta 2006; 27: 576–86.
10. Alfaidy N, Li W, MacIntosh T, Yang K, Challis JRG. Late gestation increase in 11β-HSD1 expression in human fetal membranes: a novel intrauterine source of cortisol. J Clin Endocrinol Metab 2003; 88: 5033–8.
11. Patel FA, Funder JW, Challis JRG. Mechanism of cortisol/progesterone antagonism in the regulation of 15-hydroxyprostaglandin dehydrogenase activity and mRNA levels in human chorion and placental trophoblast cells at term. J Clin Endocrinol Metab 2003; 88: 2922–33.
12. Gibb W, Lye SJ, Challis JRG. Parturition. In: Knobil E, Neill JD, eds. Knobil and Neill's Physiology of Reproduction, 3rd edn. Boston, MA: Elsevier 2006: 2925–73.
13. Dong X, Challis JRG, Lye SJ. Intramolecular interactions between the AF3 domain and the C-terminus of the human progesterone receptor are mediated through two LXXLL motifs. J Mol Endocrinol 2004; 32: 843–57.
14. Condon JC, Jeyasuria P, Faust JM, Wilson JW, Mendelson CR. A decline in the levels of progesterone receptor coactivators in the pregnant uterus at term may antagonize progesterone receptor function and contribute to the initiation of parturition. Proc Natl Acad Sci USA 2003; 100: 9518–23.
15. Dong X, Shylnova O, Challis JRG, Lye SJ. Identification and characterization of PSF as a negative coregulator of progesterone receptor. J Biol Chem 2005; 280: 13 329–40.
16. Xu P, Alfaidy N, Challis JRG. Expression of matrix metalloproteinase (MMP)-2 and MMP-9 in human placenta and fetal membranes in relation to preterm and term labor. J Clin Endocrinol Metab 2002; 87: 1353–61.
17. Li W, Unlugedik E, Bocking AD, Challis JRG. The role of postglandins in the mechanism of lipopolysaccharide-induced proMMP-9 secretion from human placental and fetal membrane cells. AM J Ob Gyn (submitted).
18. Li W, Challis JRG. Corticotrophin-releasing hormone and urocortin induce secretion of matrix metalloproteinase-9 (MMP-9) without change in tissue inhibitors of MMP-1 by cultured cells from human placenta and fetal membranes. J Clin Endocrinol Metab 2005; 90: 6569–74.
19. Florio P, Vale W, Petraglia F. Urocortins in human reproduction. Science 2004; 25: 1751–7.

6

Gene redundancy in parturition: lessons for tocolysis?

Andrew M Blanks and Steven Thornton

INTRODUCTION

The purpose of this chapter is to review recent observations about parturition in transgenic mice. We focus on the demonstration of redundant mechanisms in the oxytocin/prostaglandin (OT/PG) pathways and extrapolate, with support from pharmacological experiments, the potential lessons to be learned about the parturition process as a whole and for the treatment of preterm labor by tocolysis.

WHAT IS REDUNDANCY?

Ever since scientists have had the ability to transgenically modify organisms by the targeted deletion of genetic loci the phenomenon of gene redundancy has been described. Redundancy can be attributed to a number of mechanisms, both at the gene level and at the physiological level. At the gene level, redundancy is largely understood to have arisen from the evolutionary multiplication of alleles from a common ancestor to which they share some remaining function. In complex genomes, genes may have a number of paralogs that are capable of maintaining a given function in the presence of the chosen deletion, particularly if the deletion is made congenitally. This process alludes to two very important principles. Firstly, in the creation of a complex system, evolution has maintained a certain degree of redundancy within genomes to allow for adaptability and robustness. Secondly, a property of the complex system is that it can adapt to perturbations at points within it (be they human-made or environmental) by sensing deficits and re-establishing equilibrium near to preset values.

Subtleties of gene redundancy have only become apparent since the large-scale sequencing of genomes where the relatedness of gene families can really be appreciated on a broad scale. Perhaps a good example of this subtlety is that of the calmodulin family of proteins. The calmodulin protein is essential to the function of all cell types, where its expression is tightly regulated both at a transcriptional and post-transcriptional level. The protein itself is surprisingly encoded by a family of non-allelic genes, raising questions as to the necessity to conserve diverse alleles encoding the same protein. One explanation for the conservation of this diversity might lie in the complexity of the specific control of the expression, translation, post-translational modification, and cellular trafficking of the protein for its many functions.[1] Thus, out of diversity and complexity, gene redundancy is almost inevitable – and although its consequence is advantageous in itself, in terms of adaptability, this adaptability is not necessarily the reason for its conservation. Whatever the reason for the existence of redundancy, the implications for any treatment of a disease, or perturbation of a physiological system, must be considered when interpreting data sets.

In addition to redundancy at the gene level, where evolutionarily related genes may replace the function of a perturbed protein, a similar replacement may occur by an unrelated protein or proteins which perform a common physiological function. Similar arguments for the existence of gene network complexity apply at the level of physiological networks, although the nature of evolutionary conservation of such mechanisms is perhaps more difficult to determine. There are now described mechanisms of redundancy in one of the most important physiological processes of all, that of parturition. We propose here that the complexity of the parturition process, both at a gene and physiological level, has given rise to partly redundant systems that are robust in the face of environmental challenges. We further propose that, scientifically and clinically, the implications of redundancy must be considered when interpreting data or designing perturbations to arrest the parturition cascade.

TRANSGENIC MICE, PROSTAGLANDINS, AND OXYTOCIN

A host of transgenic studies in mice have illustrated previously unknown physiological interrelationships and function for some the main protagonists of parturition. Some of these studies involving PG and OT intimate redundancy in the physiology of parturition, and, further, suggest physiological co-regulation of networks and compensation.

Oxytocin

In 1996, the century-old thesis that OT was required for parturition was falsified by the surprisingly normal delivery of OT (–/–) null mice.[2,3] Although homozygote OT null mice die postpartum, due to the inability of the mother to lactate, delivery of viable pups occurs unhindered on the normal day of parturition. Thus, in mice, OT is critical for the milk ejection reflex but not parturition. Although difficult to reconcile with the wealth of data supporting a role for OT in the timing of parturition, subsequent analysis of the OT null mouse in conjunction with other transgenic mice has revealed far more about the role of OT in mouse parturition than was previously described. Perhaps the most important implication of the OT null mouse is the interrelationship of OT with PG.

Prostaglandins

In mice, a late gestation rise in systemic prostaglandin $F_{2\alpha}$ ($PGF_{2\alpha}$) originating from the uterine epithelium, is critical for inducing luteolysis, and the subsequent progesterone withdrawal necessary for labor. This conclusion is established from failed labor in mice null for cytosolic phospholipase A_2 ($cPLA_2$),[4,5] the $PGF_{2\alpha}$ receptor[6] and cyclooxygenase-1 (COX-1).[7,8] All of these manipulations prevent $PGF_{2\alpha}$ formation or activity at the corpus luteum, luteolysis and labor. Surgical or pharmacological luteolysis can rescue these phenotypes and restore progesterone withdrawal and normal labor. Thus, removal of neither OT nor PG is sufficient to generate a noncontractile phenotype once progesterone withdrawal has been initiated, which leads to the question of what is the key uterotonin in these mice? To answer this question it is necessary to discuss the knockout phenotypes further.

In mice there is a surge of prepartum $PGF_{2\alpha}$ in maternal plasma leading to luteolysis that occurs around day 18.5 of gestation,[9] but events leading to $PGF_{2\alpha}$ synthesis occur from day 15.5. During this time, uterine epithelial prostaglandin F synthase (PGF-S) protein and COX-1 mRNA increase, whilst the PG degrading enzyme 15-hydroxyprostaglandin dehydrogenase (PGDH) begins to decrease.[9] Following the increase in COX-1 mRNA there is a gradual increase in COX-1 protein which peaks on the day of delivery, while $cPLA_2$ protein and activity remain unchanged throughout gestation. Therefore, arachidonic acid and PGF-S are increased, and PGDH decreased by the day of the $PGF_{2\alpha}$ surge, when a maximal increase in COX-1 enzyme provides the PGH_2 substrate for PGF-S.

Oxytocin, prostaglandins, and redundancy

The extent to which OT interacts with this pathway was revealed when mating COX-1 null mice with OT null mice. Surprisingly, the COX-1/OT null mouse initiates labor on the normal day of delivery by luteolysis, but labor is prolonged in some mice over a number of days.[8] Since COX-1 null mice do not labor due to failed luteolysis, this suggests that OT has luteotrophic actions which are only unmasked in the double knockout genotype. Perhaps more importantly, since only the double knockout genotype experiences labor difficulties, significant compensation must occur between $PGF_{2\alpha}$ and OT in generating the uterotonic phenotype of the single knockouts. With the exception of the overexpression of the small conductance calcium-sensitive potassium channel SK3,[10] the double knockout is the only phenotype in the literature where the myometrium cannot contract properly once labor has been initiated. Thus, the double knockout uncovers redundancy between the main uterotonic hormones of parturition. And although this is not at the gene level, it is likely to be at the physiological level of a common signal transduction pathway stimulating the myometrium. It is interesting to speculate that compensation occurs at the post-receptor level, since both $PGF_{2\alpha}$ and OT activate receptors in the myometrium that couple to the α-G_q G-protein, thus stimulating phospholipase C, inositol phosphate, and calcium release.

The precise regulation of the opposing luteotrophic and uterotonic actions of OT in the mouse were determined in an elegant set of experiments in the OT null mouse.[11] Infusion of OT on day 15.5 into the OT null and wild-type mouse elicits dose-dependent inhibitory and stimulatory effects. Although the precise mechanism of action is unknown at lower concentrations, gestation is prolonged by maintenance of the corpus luteum in both mice. However, at higher concentrations both mice initiate premature labor within 24 h. Interestingly, the responses in both mice are dose dependent, but the OT null mouse is more sensitive to the effects of OT. The initiation of premature labor in both mice is not associated with luteolysis and progesterone withdrawal, and is not prevented by co-administration of indomethacin. The induction of premature labor in this model is therefore independent of PG and mediated by the uterotonic actions of OT, and illustrates a further property of a complex physiological system. That is, despite OT being a redundant agonist in the normal physiology of labor, overactivation of its physiological pathway results in labor distinct from normal physiology. This point is vital when understanding the multiple etiologies of preterm labor.

Detailed analysis of the OT receptor mRNA, and protein levels in the ovary and uterus, indicate a reciprocal relationship whereby ovarian OT receptor levels decrease on day 19 whilst increasing dramatically after progesterone withdrawal in the uterus. Therefore, although the absence of OT does not significantly affect the timing of term labor in mice, abnormal modulation of OT action – either by peptide or receptor – does influence the onset of labor. Taken together these studies suggest that the role of the OT/ oxytocin receptor (OTR) system in mice is to focus the timing of the onset of labor. The OT null mice also illustrate the importance of the tissue-specific control of OT receptor expression in modulating the OT receptor system.

Co-regulation of parturition networks and compensation

The congenital lack of OT in the OT knockout mouse clearly makes the animal more sensitive to exogenous doses of OT. The origins of this heightened sensitivity are almost certainly due to upregulation of receptor in a naïve system. However, a picture of a greater degree of intercommunication between contraction-associated proteins is beginning to appear. A recent study using a knockdown strategy has given some insight into how perturbation of the equilibrium of myometrial activation may be resisted by compensation.[12] In this model the targeted insertion of a neomycin cassette in the tenth intron of the COX-1 gene results in a substantial decrease in COX-1 transcription, and subsequent uterine production of only 8% $PGF_{2\alpha}$, and 3.3% PGE_2 and 3.2% PGD_2 when compared to wild-type values. This substantial decrease in PG production is sufficient to affect platelet aggregation, prevent thrombosis and depress macrophage PGE_2 production, but was insufficient to affect parturition. Interestingly, the levels of $PGF_{2\alpha}$, PGE_2 and PGD_2 are not much greater than those values observed in the full COX-1 knockout of

1.1% $PGF_{2\alpha}$, 1.1% PGE_2 and 0.4% PGD_2 where parturition is impaired. Although the levels of PG were very low in the COX-1 hypomorphic mice, the expression of the OTR in the myometrium of these mice was by contrast upregulated by 50%. Thus, by some yet-to-be-described mechanism, the network equilibrium in these mice responds to, and compensates for, the low amount of PG being produced by increasing the expression of the receptor for another key agonist. Although not described in this study, it would be interesting to know whether this effect was limited to the OTR or whether other contraction-associated proteins were similarly regulated.

The fact that there appears to be a common link between two physiologically redundant arms of a similar physiological pathway is in itself intriguing, since, in theory at least, such a link may be a better target for perturbing the system rather than having to block two pathways simultaneously. That notwithstanding, a greater understanding in the future of the intercommunication between the different pathways of the cascade of parturition will prove to be very interesting.

PHARMACOLOGICAL MANIPULATIONS

As illustrated perfectly in the hypomorphic COX-1 mice, different physiological processes rely to a greater or lesser extent on differing amounts of key proteins. This principle is exploited by many drug treatments in that an appropriate dose can be found to achieve a relatively high level of therapeutic effect whist maintaining an appropriate level of selectivity. However, given the previously described work utilizing selective knockouts and knockdowns in mice, can we postulate that to achieve effective tocolysis by targeting the key stimulatory contraction proteins we must target two pathways simultaneously? The answer to this question may already have been partially answered in pharmacological experiments undertaken in sheep. In the study of Grigsby et al,[13] co-administration of the COX-2 antagonist nimesulide and atosiban into dexamethasone-infused sheep prevented mean labor onset over a 98 h treatment period in all animals, at which time the study was terminated. This was in contrast to labor onset at a mean 72 h in nimesulide treatment alone and 51 h in vehicle-treated ewes. The authors concluded that co-administration of OT and COX-2 antagonists offers significantly greater tocolytic potential. This principle was further demonstrated by a follow-up study to assess the potential of co-administration in preventing established preterm labor. In this study, co-administration successfully inhibited established labor for a 48 h study period in four of six ewes.[14] Thus, the principle of redundancy between OT and PG as described from transgenic studies in mice appears to be strongly supported by pharmacological manipulations in a different species (sheep). It may therefore be possible to postulate that any intervention, however efficacious, targeted at a single pathway of either OT or PG will be ineffective (in the long term) as a treatment for tocolysis because of physiological redundancy. Of course, ultimately this proof must come from studies in humans, although careful consideration needs to be given to possible adverse effects of dual use of compounds.

ROBUSTNESS AND PERTURBATION OF THE SYSTEM

During this discussion, we have only given detailed consideration to the stimulation phase of parturition and concentrated on the physiological redundancy of two key players, and their interrelationships in maintaining an active contractile phenotype. It is beyond the remit of this text to extrapolate in detail to other processes of parturition, although the ripening of the cervix is of course another critical process. Equally, we cannot discuss the important issues of defining the different etiologies of the preterm labor syndrome before the informed decision to use tocolysis can be made. We can however summarize lessons to be learned for devising effective tocolysis to perturb parturition effectively.

The principles established in this discussion, in terms of physiological redundancy, are particularly pertinent to parturition since the process appears to be able to be activated in a number of different ways. Our general thesis states that the reason parturition is so complex, involving so many apparently parallel processes, is that it gives the system robustness. That is, given changes in physiological circumstance, by unfavorable or favorable conditions either to the mother or fetus, the equilibrium of the process can attempt to create the best outcome. We must appreciate this robustness and, as biologists and clinicians wishing to understand a complex process, we must understand this fact particularly when considering ways in which to perturb the network. We must design tocolytic strategies that inhibit network breakpoints or simultaneously inhibit parallel pathways such that the network cannot compensate. Only then will

effective tocolysis be achieved and only with accurate diagnosis of the etiology of the labor will it be effectively used.

REFERENCES

1. Toutenhoofd SL, Strehler EE. The calmodulin multigene family as a unique case of genetic redundancy: multiple levels of regulation to provide spatial and temporal control of calmodulin pools? Cell Calcium 2000; 28(2): 83–96.
2. Nishimori K, Young LJ, Guo Q et al. Oxytocin is required for nursing but is not essential for parturition or reproductive behaviour. Proc Natl Acad Sci USA 1996; 93: 11 699–704.
3. Young WS, Shepard E, Amico J et al. Deficiency in mouse oxytocin prevents milk ejection, but not fertility or parturition. J Neuroendocrinol 1996; 8: 847–53.
4. Uozumi N, Kume K, Nagase T et al. Role of cytosolic phospholipase A2 in allergic response and parturition. Nature 1997; 390: 618–22.
5. Bonventre JV, Huang Z, Taheri MR et al. Reduced fertility and postischaemic brain injury in mice deficient in cytosolic phospholipase A2. Nature 1997; 390: 622–5.
6. Sugimoto Y, Yamasaki A, Segi E et al. Failure of parturition in mice lacking the prostaglandin F receptor. Science 1997; 277: 681–3.
7. Langenbach R, Morham SG, Tiano HF et al. Prostaglandin synthase 1 gene disruption in mice reduces arachadonic-acid induced inflammation and indomethacin-induced gastric ulceration. Cell 1995; 83: 483–92.
8. Gross GA, Imamura T, Luedke CE et al. Opposing actions of prostaglandins and oxytocin determine the onset of murine labor. Proc Natl Acad Sci USA 1998; 95: 11 875–9.
9. Winchester SK, Imamura T, Gross GA et al. Coordinate regulation of prostaglandin metabolism for induction of parturition in mice. Endocrinology 2002; 143: 2593–8.
10. Bond CT, Sprengel R, Bissonnette JM et al. Respiration and parturition affected by conditional over expression of the Ca^{2+}-activated K^+ channel subunit, SK3. Science 2000; 289(5486): 1942–6.
11. Imamura T, Leudke CE, Vogt SK, Muglia LJ. Oxytocin modulates the onset of murine parturition by competing ovarian and uterine effects. Am J Physiol Regul Integr Comp Physiol 2000; 279: R1061–R1067.
12. Yu Y, Cheng Y, Fan J et al. Differential impact of prostaglandin H synthase 1 knockdown on platelets and parturition. J Clin Invest 2005; 115(4): 986–95 (Epub 2005, Mar 1).
13. Grigsby PL, Poore KR, Hirst JJ, Jenkins G. Inhibition of premature labor in sheep by a combined treatment of nimesulide, a prostaglandin synthase type 2 inhibitor, and atosiban, an oxytocin antagonist. Am J Obstet Gynecol 2000; 183(3): 649–57.
14. Scott JE, Grigsby PL, Hirst JJ, Jenkin G. Inhibition of prostaglandin synthesis and its effect on uterine activity during established premature labour in sheep. J Soc Gynecol Invest 2001; 8: 266–76.

7

Regulation of inflammatory response pathways during pregnancy and labor

Carole R Mendelson, Jennifer C Condon, and Daniel B Hardy

LABOR AND THE INFLAMMATORY RESPONSE

There is considerable evidence that the initiation of labor, both preterm and at term, is associated with an inflammatory response. Up to 30% of pregnancies ending in preterm labor (with intact membranes) are associated with infection.[1] Furthermore, it has been suggested that even in those cases of preterm labor in which there are no clinical symptoms, there is a 'silent' infection.[2] Interleukin (IL) 1β has been detected in amniotic fluid samples from around 30% of pregnancies ending in preterm labor, and in a comparable proportion of amniotic fluid samples from women in spontaneous labor at term.[3,4] In studies with pregnant rhesus monkeys, intra-amniotic infusion of IL-1β caused a rapid increase in amniotic fluid levels of tumor necrosis factor (TNF) α, prostaglandin E_2 (PGE_2) and prostaglandin $F_2α$ ($PGF_2α$),followed by preterm uterine contractions.[5] The potential role of IL-1 in the initiation of human labor, both preterm and at term, is emphasized by the finding that IL-1β is undetectable in amniotic fluids from pregnancies with intact membranes before the onset of labor at any stage of gestation.[4] Concentrations of IL-1α, IL-1β and TNF-α also were found to be increased in cervicovaginal secretions of women at normal term labor in the absence of infection, as compared to women at term who were not in labor.[6] It is likely that the inflammatory cytokines present in amniotic fluid are produced by macrophages, monocytes and neutrophils which are recruited into the amniotic space.[7] The mechanism whereby activated inflammatory cells within the amniotic cavity traverse fetal membranes and decidua to enter the myometrium is uncertain. However, neutrophils and macrophages were observed to densely infiltrate both upper and lower uterine segments of the human myometrium during spontaneous labor at term, whereas few inflammatory cells were detected in the myometrium of non-laboring women.[8] IL-1α and IL-1β mRNA levels were also observed to increase markedly in rat[9] and mouse[7] myometrium towards term.

PROGESTERONE MAINTAINS UTERINE QUIESCENCE THROUGHOUT PREGNANCY

Uterine quiescence throughout pregnancy is maintained by progesterone acting via its nuclear receptor (PR). We have proposed that progesterone/PR prevents uterine contractility by suppressing inflammatory response pathways,[10] and consequently blocking expression of 'contractile genes', including cyclooxygenase 2 (COX-2),[10] the oxytocin receptor[11] and the gap junction protein connexin 43.[12] The decline in circulating levels of progesterone which accompanies the onset of labor in most mammalian species suggests that progesterone withdrawal is critical for the increase in uterine contractility leading to labor,[13] although in some species (e.g. the mouse) the levels of progesterone at term still exceed equilibrium dissociation constant (K_d) for its binding to the PR. Paradoxically, in humans and other primates, levels of circulating progesterone and of myometrial PR remain elevated throughout pregnancy and into labor.[14–17] However, in women at term, treatment with the PR antagonist mifepristone (RU486) caused increased cervical ripening and spontaneous labor, or increased sensitivity to labor induction by oxytocin.[18–21] In term pregnant guinea pigs – a species that also fails to manifest spontaneous progesterone withdrawal – the PR antagonists RU486 and onapristone caused increased myometrial responsiveness to prostaglandins and oxytocin, increased formation of myometrial gap junctions and cervical ripening.[22] Collectively, these findings suggest that PR serves an important role in the maintenance of uterine quiescence during pregnancy in all species.

The maintenance of elevated circulating progesterone levels throughout the end of pregnancy, together with the observation that levels of PR in the human uterus and cervix also remain elevated, has led us to postulate that parturition is caused by a series of molecular events that impair PR function.[10] We propose that PR function near term may be compromised by changes at several levels. These include changes in: expression of co-activators and co-repressors;[23,24] increased metabolism of progesterone within the cervix[25] and myometrium;[26] upregulation of inflammatory response pathways leading to activation of nuclear factor κB (NF-κB), an inflammatory transcription factor that antagonizes PR function;[27] and alterations in the relative levels of PR isoforms which are expressed.[28] Conversely, we also suggest that PR mediates uterine quiescence throughout most of pregnancy by antagonizing the activation of NFκB and that it does so via ligand-dependent and ligand-independent mechanisms.[10]

In this chapter, we will briefly review our findings to suggest that augmented surfactant production by the maturing fetal lung, and the subsequent secretion of surfactant lipids and proteins into amniotic fluid, provide a key signal for the uterine inflammatory response that leads to parturition at term. The mechanisms whereby PR and NFκB exert antagonistic roles in the regulation of myometrial quiescence versus contractility also will be considered.

FETAL LUNG SECRETES A SIGNAL FOR THE INITIATION OF LABOR

It has been suggested that the fetus may provide a signal for parturition. Mitchell et al[29] reported that a substance(s) in human amniotic fluid caused a marked increase in PGE_2 production by cultured human amnion cells. They suggested that this substance was secreted by the fetal kidney.[29] Lopez et al[30] postulated that a stimulus may emanate from the maturing fetal lung. They found that pulmonary surfactant isolated from human amniotic fluid stimulated PGE synthesis by discs of human amnion, and suggested that surfactant phospholipids secreted into amniotic fluid provide a source of arachidonic acid precursor for prostaglandin synthesis by the avascular amnion. Toyoshima et al[31] proposed that platelet-activating factor – an alkyl ether phospholipid component of the fetal lung surfactant lipids secreted into amniotic fluid at term – may play an important role in activation of myometrial contractility. In recent studies, we obtained evidence that the surfactant-associated

protein – surfactant protein A (SP-A), which is secreted by the fetal lung into amniotic fluid in association with surfactant glycerophospholipids – provides an important signal for the initiation of parturition in the mouse.[7]

Synthesis of the glycerophospholipid-rich lipoprotein surfactant by fetal lung type II cells is initiated during the third trimester of gestation. Inadequate surfactant production by the lungs of premature infants can result in respiratory distress syndrome,[32] the primary cause of neonatal morbidity and mortality in developed countries. In addition to SP-A, there are three other proteins associated with lung surfactant: SP-B, SP-C and SP-D. Whereas SP-B and SP-C are lipophilic proteins that reduce alveolar surface tension,[33] SP-A and SP-D are C-type lectins that act within the lung alveolus as part of the innate immune response to microbial pathogens.[34] SP-A enhances immune function within the lung alveolus by activating alveolar macrophages, increasing cytokine production and NF-κB DNA-binding activity.[34–36] In studies using primary cultures of human fetal lung type II cells, we observed that *SP-A* gene expression was increased by IL-1 through activation of NF-κB,[37] and by hormones and factors that increase cyclic adenosine monophosfate (cAMP).[37,38] Furthermore, intra-amniotic administration of IL-1 in pregnant rabbits was observed to increase SP-A expression in fetal lung[39] and caused preterm birth.[40] These and other studies suggest that the type II cell and the alveolar macrophage exist in a positive feedback loop, whereby SP-A secreted by type II cells stimulates cytokine production by alveolar macrophages, which acts back on type II cells to enhance SP-A expression.

SP-A synthesis by the fetal lung is initiated after around 80% of gestation is complete in association with enhanced surfactant glycerophospholipid synthesis, and reaches maximal levels prior to term.[41] In this regard, SP-A serves as an excellent marker of fetal lung maturity. SP-A mRNA, which was barely detectable in fetal mouse lung at 16 days post-coitum (dpc), was evident at 17 dpc, and increased markedly to term.[42,43] Similarly, SP-A protein in amniotic fluid, which was absent on day 16 of gestation, was readily detectable on day 17 and increased to extremely high levels on day 19 (term).[7] This gestational increase in SP-A secretion by the fetal lung was associated with a parallel increase in IL-1β protein expression in macrophages isolated from amniotic fluid,[7] with migration of activated macrophages to the pregnant mouse uterus and with activation of uterine NF-κB.[7] Using a transgenic mouse model in which fetal macrophages stained positively for β-galactosidase, we obtained evidence that a major proportion of the macrophages present within the maternal uterus near term are derived from the fetus.[7]

Furthermore, treatment of amniotic fluid macrophages from fetal mice at 15, 17 and 19 dpc with SP-A for 30 min stimulated IL-1β expression.[7]

These findings suggested that SP-A secreted into amniotic fluid near term activates fetal macrophages, causing them to migrate to the maternal uterus where they produce cytokines, resulting in activation of NF-κB within the myometrium. To directly assess the capacity of SP-A to initiate labor in vivo, parallel groups of mice were injected with the purified SP-A protein preparation or with a control preparation that was depleted of SP-A on a mannose D column.[7] Of 17 mice injected with SP-A on 15 dpc, 14 delivered premature fetuses that were surrounded by intact amniotic membranes from the injected uterine horn on day 16–17 of gestation. Fetuses in the uninjected horn were not delivered

and were ultimately resorbed. Mice injected intra-amniotically with mannose D-extracted, SP-A-depleted preparation delivered normally at term.[7] To further evaluate the role of endogenous SP-A in the initiation of labor, another series of 15 dpc pregnant mice were intra-amniotically injected with an antibody raised against human SP-A to deplete endogenous levels of the surfactant protein in amniotic fluid. Interestingly, all of the mice in this group delivered viable pups 24h late (day 20).[7]

Based on these collective findings, we suggest that augmented production of SP-A by the maturing fetal lung near term provides a hormonal stimulus for activation of a cascade of inflammatory signals within the maternal uterus that culminate in the enhanced myometrial contractility leading to parturition (Figure 7.1).[44]

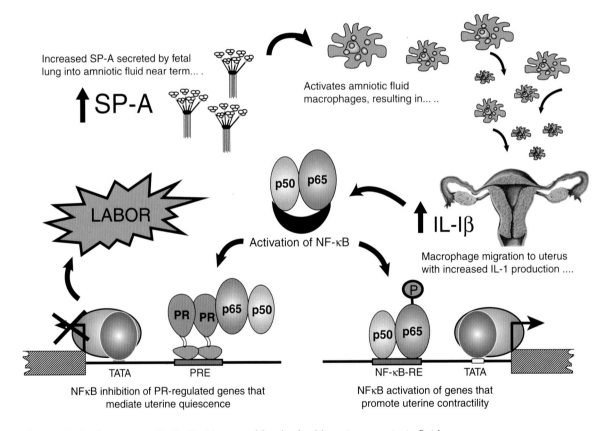

Figure 7.1 Surfactant protein A (SP-A) secreted by the fetal lung into amniotic fluid near term may serve as a hormone of parturition. SP-A, the major surfactant protein, is secreted by the fetal lung into amniotic fluid at high concentrations near term. SP-A activates amniotic fluid macrophages, causing them to migrate to the maternal uterus where they produce cytokines resulting in activation of nuclear factor κB (NF-κB). We propose that the activated NF-κB promotes increased uterine contractility resulting in parturition by two mechanisms: (i) direct binding and increased transcription of genes encoding proteins that promote increased smooth muscle contraction; (ii) inhibition of progesterone receptor (PR) target genes that maintain uterine quiescence via functional antagonism of PR-mediated transcription. (From Mendelson CR, Condon JC. J Steroid Biochem Mol Biol 2005; 93: 113–19.)

This hormonal stimulus, which is transmitted to the uterus by fetal amniotic macrophages, reveals that the fetal lungs are sufficiently developed to withstand the critical transition from an aqueous to an aerobic environment. Our findings further suggest that NF-κB serves as a key transcriptional mediator of the inflammatory response leading to labor. We propose that activated NF-κB promotes increased uterine contractility by direct and indirect mechanisms. On the one hand, NF-κB can bind directly to the promoters of genes that mediate increased uterine contractility, including the $PGF_{2\alpha}$ receptor,[45] the gap junction protein connexin 43,[46] the oxytocin receptor[47] and COX-2.[48] Alternatively, NF-κB can block the capacity of the PR to activate genes that control uterine quiescence (Figure 7.1). Mutual transcriptional repression between PR and NF-κB p65 has previously been described in COS-1 and HeLa cells, and was attributed to direct physical interaction of these proteins.[27] However, to date, the PR-responsive genes that prevent uterine contractility remain to be identified, as are the mechanisms that compromise PR function at term.

CYCLOOXYGENASE 2 (COX-2) EXPRESSION IN MYOMETRIUM IS INCREASED BY INFLAMMATORY CYTOKINES THROUGH NUCLEAR FACTOR κB (NF-κB) AND INHIBITED BY PROGESTERONE ACTING THROUGH ITS NUCLEAR RECEPTOR

In studies in our laboratory[10] and others,[49] COX-2 mRNA was found to be upregulated in fundal myometrium of women during labor. Using matched biopsies of lower uterine segment (LUS) and fundal myometrium from women in labor (n = 8) and not in labor (n = 8), we observed a seven-fold increase in the expression of COX-2 mRNA in fundal myometrium of laboring women as compared to fundal myometrium from women not in labor (Figure 7.2). By contrast, no labor-associated differences were observed in myometrium from the LUS (Figure 7.2). The finding of a fundus-specific induction of COX-2 mRNA is significant, since during labor increased contractility occurs within the fundus, while the LUS myometrium relaxes to allow expulsion of the fetus.[50] This is of great interest with regard to our recent finding that NF-κB activation occurs specifically in the fundus during labor.[28] This would likely mediate the spatial induction of COX-2 and other contractile genes within the uterus during labor. On the other hand, COX-1 mRNA levels remained unchanged during labor.[51] This is not surprising, since the *COX-1* gene is constitutively regulated and lacks functional NF-κB response elements.[52] In pregnant

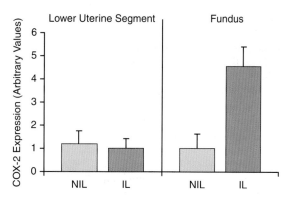

Figure 7.2 Cyclooxygenase 2 (COX-2) mRNA levels are selectively increased in fundal myometrium of women in labor. RNA was isolated from paired fundal and lower uterine segment (LUS) myometrial tissues from eight women not in labor (NIL) and eight women in labor (IL) near term. The RNA was analyzed for COX-2 mRNA transcripts and normalized against ribosomal RNA using real-time quantitative reverse transcriptase polymerase chain reaction (Q-PCR).

mouse uterus, we and others have observed that COX-2 mRNA levels remain low through gestational day 18 and then increase dramatically during labor on day 19.[10,53]

To elucidate the mechanisms for the regulation of uterine *COX-2* during pregnancy and labor, immortalized human fundal myometrial cells (hTERT) were treated with IL-1β ± progesterone. IL-1β alone caused a pronounced upregulation of COX-2 mRNA, while treatment with progesterone markedly suppressed this induction (Figure 7.3). The human *COX-2* gene contains two well-characterized NF-κB response elements in its promoter.[48,54,55] Using chromatin immunoprecipitation (ChIP) with primers, which amplified the genomic region surrounding each of these response elements, we[10] and others[48] observed that the IL-1β stimulated rapid recruitment of NF-κB p65 to both proximal and distal NF-κB elements of the *COX-2* promoter. Importantly, we found that this was markedly diminished by co-incubation with progesterone.[10] These findings indicate that progesterone acting through PR antagonizes NF-κB induction of *COX-2* gene transcription. Recently, we found that siRNA-induced ablation of PR-A and PR-B isoforms in breast cancer cells resulted in a marked increase in NF-κB activity and in *COX-2* expression. This induction was observed in the absence of cytokines or progesterone, suggesting that PR exerts a ligand-independent inhibitory effect on NF-κB activity.[10] Thus, the progesterone/PR-mediated decrease in p65 binding to the *COX-2* promoter might be caused, in part, by a direct physical interaction of PR with p65,

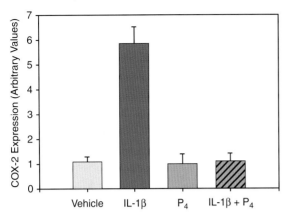

Figure 7.3 Progesterone impairs interleukin (IL) 1β induction of cyclooxygenase-2 (COX-2) expression. Immortalized human fundal myometrial cells (hTERT) were cultured for 12 h in the absence or presence of IL-1β (10 ng/ml) with or without progesterone (10^{-7} M). RNA was isolated and the expression of COX-2 was analyzed by real-time quantitative reverse transcriptase polymerase chain reaction (Q-PCR). Data are the mean ±SEM of values from four independent experiments and are expressed as fold-induction over the control.

as was previously observed in vitro,[27] resulting in a repression of NF-κB DNA-binding and transcriptional activity.

We also have obtained convincing evidence that the anti-inflammatory effect of progesterone within the myometrium is mediated, in part, by increased expression of inhibitor of κB (IκB)α, a crucial inhibitor of NF-κB transactivation.[10] Progesterone caused rapid induction of IκBα mRNA and protein expression in the immortalized myometrial cells, which preceded its effect to inhibit IL-1β-induced COX-2 expression. Moreover, co-treatment with progesterone prevented the IL-1β-mediated decline in IκBα protein levels,[10] suggesting an effect of progesterone/PR to block IκBα degradation via the proteasome pathway.[56] Progesterone action to inhibit NF-κB activation by induction of IκBα was previously reported in macrophage cell lines[57] and in T47D cells.[58]

PROGESTERONE RECEPTOR (PR) FUNCTION IN FUNDAL MYOMETRIUM AT TERM IS COMPROMISED BY UPREGULATION OF THE TRUNCATED PR-C ISOFORM

PR is expressed as three isoforms – PR-A, PR-B and PR-C – which are generated from a single gene by utilization of different promoters[59,60] and translation initiation sites.[61] PR-B has been shown to function as a strong transactivator of progesterone-regulated genes; when PR-A and PR-B are co-expressed, the A-isoform can repress the action of PR-B.[62,63] The inhibitory action of PR-A protein was suggested to be due to its inability to efficiently recruit co-activators and its increased interaction with co-repressors, as compared to PR-B.[62] It should be noted that although PR-A has been proposed to serve as an antagonist of PR-B function in a cell- and promoter-specific manner,[63] and was found to inhibit PR-B transcriptional activity in cultured human LUS myometrial cells,[64] mice with a selective knockout of the PR-B isoform are fertile and apparently deliver normally,[65] suggesting that PR-A has the capacity to mediate the action of progesterone to maintain myometrial quiescence. The third PR isoform, PR-C (60 kDa), which is truncated at the amino terminus and lacks the DNA binding domain, is primarily localized in the cytosolic fraction.[66] PR-C cannot bind DNA, but is able to bind progesterone.[67] Thus, PR-C may inhibit PR function by sequestering available progesterone away from the PR-B isoform. PR-C has also been found to bind to PR-B, thereby reducing the capacity of PR-B to bind to PR response elements (PRE).[68]

Recently, we have obtained compelling evidence to suggest that PR-C isoform expression increases dramatically both in human fundal myometrium and in pregnant mouse uterus at term as a result of increased NF-κB activation and binding to the *PR* gene promoter.[28] In those studies, expression of PR-A, PR-B and PR-C isoforms were analyzed in matched fundal and lower uterine segment myometrium of pregnant women in labor and not in labor. PR-B mRNA levels increased dramatically in the fundal and LUS myometrial tissues of women in labor (Figure 7.4A). On the other hand, a pronounced increase in PR-B protein levels was observed specifically in the laboring fundal myometrium. Labor-associated changes in PR-C mRNA and protein levels in fundal myometrium were even more striking than those of PR-B. PR-C mRNA, which was undetectable in the non-laboring myometrium isolated from the LUS, increased to clearly detectable levels in LUS during labor (Figure 7.4B). By contrast, around a 200-fold increase in PR-C mRNA levels was observed in the fundal myometrium of women in labor. PR-C protein, which was evident only in cytoplasmic fractions, was undetectable in LUS but was markedly induced in fundal myometrium of women in labor (Figure 7.4B). PR-A protein was not detected in human LUS or fundal myometrium before or after the initiation of labor.[28] Interestingly, this fundal-specific increase in PR-B and PR-C protein with labor was associated with similar spatial and temporal increases in myometrial NF-κB activation.[28] Expression of PR isoforms in the LUS myometrium of women in labor versus not in labor has previously been investigated.[64,69,70]

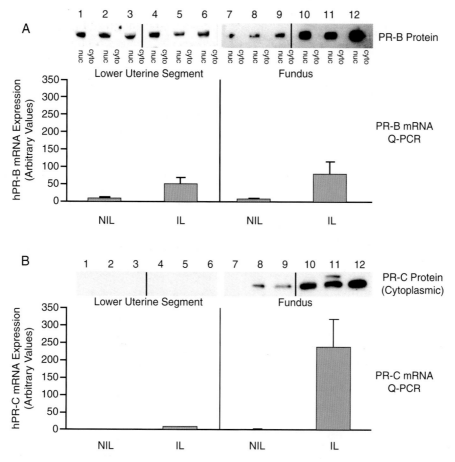

Figure 7.4 Progesterone receptor (PR) isoforms PR-B and PR-C are upregulated in the fundal myometrium of women in labor. (A) Nuclear (nuc) and cytoplasmic (cyto) extracts (11 µg) isolated from lower uterine segment (LUS) (1–6) and fundal (7–12) myometrium of three women in labor (IL) (4–6, 10–12) and three women not in labor (NIL) (1–3, 7–9) (n = 3 for each group) were analyzed for PR-A, PR-B and PR-C expression by immunoblotting (top panel). The relative abundance of PR-B mRNA in the myometrium of six women not in labor and six women in labor was assessed by Q-PCR (bottom panel). (B) Cytoplasmic extracts (20 µg) isolated from LUS (1–6) and fundal (7–12) myometrium of three women in labor (IL) (4–6, 10–12) and not in labor (NIL) (1–3, 7–9) (n = 3 for each group) were analyzed for PR-A, PR-B and PR-C expression by immunoblotting (top panel). The relative abundance of PR-C mRNA in the myometrium of sixwomen not in labor and six women in labor was assessed by Q-PCR (bottom panel). (From Condon JC, Hardy DB, Kovaric K et al. Mol Endocrinol 2006; 20: 764–75. © 2006 The Endocrine Society.)

In one study, the ratio of PR-A to PR-B mRNA was found to be increased ten-fold in term LUS myometrium from women in labor.[70] However, the primers used for quantitative reverse transcriptase polymerase chain reaction (Q-PCR) also would have amplified PR-C mRNA.

Similar changes in PR isoform expression were observed in the pregnant mouse during late gestation and into labor. As can be seen in Figure 7.5A, nuclear PR-B protein levels increased modestly in the pregnant mouse uterus towards term, while PR-C levels increased in the cytoplasm between days 15 and 16 of gestation,

and then translocated to the nucleus where they continued to increase between 17 and 19 dpc. PR-A, which was undetectable in cytoplasmic or nuclear fractions through 18 dpc, was only evident in the nucleus on 19 dpc. The increased levels of PR-A, PR-B and PR-C proteins toward term were associated with pronounced increases in the levels of mRNA for all three isoforms (Figure 7.5B–D), and with increased nuclear localization NF-κB p50 and p65.[7] We also found that intra-amniotic injection of SP-A into 15 dpc mice – which as noted above promotes amniotic fluid macrophage migration to

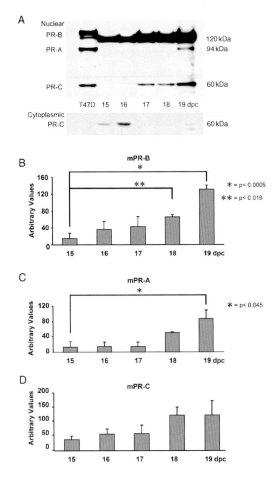

Figure 7.5 The inhibitory progesterone receptor (PR) isoforms PR-C and PR-A are upregulated in the pregnant mouse uterus in late gestation. (A) Nuclear and cytoplasmic extracts from pregnant mouse uterus at 15–19 days post-coitum (dpc) were analyzed for PR-A, PR-B and PR-C expression by immunoblotting. PR-B levels increased between 15 and 19 dpc. The immunoblot shown is representative of findings obtained using uteri from three different gestational series of mice. (B)–(D) RNA isolated from uteri of three series of pregnant mice at 15–19 dpc were analyzed for PR-B, PR-A + PR-B and PR-A + PR-B + PR-C mRNA by real-time quantitative reverse transcriptase polymerase chain reaction (Q-PCR) using oligonucleotides that primed with equivalent efficiency. Levels of PR-B, PR-A and PR-C mRNA were ascertained by subtraction. Data are the mean ±SEM of values from three gestational series of pregnant mice. Expression levels of all three PR isoforms increased toward term. (From Condon JC, Hardy DB, Kovaric K et al. Mol Endocrinol 2006; 20: 764–75. © 2006 The Endocrine Society.)

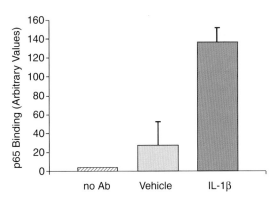

Figure 7.6 Interleukin (IL) 1β enhances recruitment of nuclear factor κB (NF-κB) p65 to the human progesterone receptor (hPR) gene promoter. Immortalized human myometrial (hTERT) fundal cells were cultured for 12h in serum-free medium with (black bar) or without (white bar) IL-1β (10 ng/ml). The cells were then treated with 1% formaldehyde, followed by lysis and sonication to shear and solubilize the crosslinked chromatin, which was immunoprecipitated using an antibody specific for NF-κB p65. A no-antibody immunoprecipitation was used as a control (no Ab) (hatched bar). DNA was purified and the relative abundance of a 100 base pairs (bp) region surrounding the NF-κB response element was quantified by a real-time polymerase chain reaction. Shown is a representation of three independent experiments with comparable results. The data are expressed as arbitrary units. The bars represent the mean ± SEM of values from three sets of culture dishes. (From Condon JC, Hardy DB, Kovaric K et al. Mol Endocrinol 2006; 20: 764–75. © 2006 The Endocrine Society.)

the maternal uterus with increased cytokine production, uterine NF-κB activation, and preterm labor[17] – caused a rapid increase in uterine levels of PR-B and PR-C proteins.[28] In contrast, inhibition of uterine NF-κB activation by intra-amniotic injection of SN50[7] caused a decrease in the uterine levels of both PR-B and PR-C.[28] Notably, using ChIP we observed that IL-1β treatment of human myometrial cells enhanced in vivo p65 binding to a putative NF-κB response element at −1330 base pairs (bp) upstream of the human *PR* gene (Figure 7.6). Thus, *PR* gene expression may be increased by the inflammatory mediators that activate NF-κB. We suggest that the paradoxical increase in PR-B expression in both mouse and human uterus at term may also be a consequence of a decline in PR function, caused, in part, by decreased levels of cAMP response element binding protein (CBP) and steroid receptor coactivator (SRC) coactivators, and of histone acetylation.[23] This decrease in PR function may reduce the capacity of progesterone to negatively regulate PR expression,[71] resulting in the upregulation of a relatively inactive receptor.

Based on our findings, we suggest that in the human uterus at term, there is fundus-specific upregulation of NF-κB activation.[28] This likely results in the increased COX-2 expression (Figure 7.2), a decline in PR coactivator expression[23,72] and histone acetylation,[23] and an upregulation of PR-C isoform expression (Figure 7.4)[28] with an associated decline in PR function within the fundal myometrium. These spatial changes may lead to a further increase in COX-2 expression, prostaglandin production and in uterine contractility leading to labor. A labor-associated increase in oxytocin receptors also has been spatially observed in the fundal myometrium.[47] This regionalization of the pregnant uterus is highlighted by studies using superfused human myometrial strips, in which PGE_2 and $PGF_2\alpha$ were found to stimulate contractility in the fundal myometrium but not in the LUS.[50] These observations are consistent with findings of Myatt and Lye,[73] who reported increased expression of 'relaxant' PGE_2 receptors (EP_4) and decreased expression of 'contractile' $PGF_2\alpha$ receptors (FP) in LUS myometrium with the onset of labor.

CONCLUSIONS

We suggest that uterine quiescence throughout most of pregnancy is mediated, in part, by progesterone/PR inhibition of genes involved in the inflammatory response. This may occur via direct PR interaction with NF-κB proteins and upregulation of IκBα. Near term, we propose that the augmented secretion of surfactant lipids and SP-A into amniotic fluid activates amniotic fluid macrophages (which also are of fetal origin), causing them to migrate to the myometrium where they produce cytokines resulting in the activation of NF-κB. The activated NF-κB can then directly interact with PR and block its ability to activate 'relaxant' genes, such as *IκBα*. NF-κB also may directly bind to the *PR* gene promoter, resulting in increased expression of inhibitory PR isoforms. This likely would result in further activation of NF-κB, which binds to the promoters of 'contractile' genes, such as *COX-2*, resulting in increased prostaglandin production and enhanced uterine contractility.

ACKNOWLEDGMENTS

Our research was supported by the March of Dimes Birth Defects Foundation (research grant no. 21-FY04-174), the National Institutes of Health (NIH grant 5 P01 HD011149).

REFERENCES

1. Romero R, Mazor M, Wu YK et al. Infection in the pathogenesis of preterm labor. Semin Perinatol 1988; 12: 262–79.
2. Iams JD, Clapp DH, Contos DA et al. Does extra-amniotic infection cause preterm labor? Gas-liquid chromatography studies of amniotic fluid in amnionitis, preterm labor, and normal controls. Obstet Gynecol 1987; 70: 365–8.
3. Romero R, Parvizi ST, Oyarzun E et al. Amniotic fluid interleukin-1 in spontaneous labor at term. J Reprod Med 1990; 35: 235–8.
4. Cox SM, Casey ML, MacDonald PC. Accumulation of interleukin-1β and interleukin-6 in amniotic fluid: a sequela of labour at term and preterm. Hum Reprod Update 1997; 3: 517–27.
5. Baggia S, Gravett MG, Witkin SS et al. Interleukin-1β intra-amniotic infusion induces tumor necrosis factor-α, prostaglandin production, and preterm contractions in pregnant rhesus monkeys. J Soc Gynecol Invest 1996; 3: 121–6.
6. Steinborn A, Kuhnert M, Halberstadt E. Immunmodulating cytokines induce term and preterm parturition. J Perinat Med 1996; 24: 381–90.
7. Condon JC, Jeyasuria P, Faust JM et al. Surfactant protein secreted by the maturing mouse fetal lung acts as a hormone that signals the initiation of parturition. Proc Natl Acad Sci USA 2004; 101: 4978–83.
8. Thomson AJ, Telfer JF, Young A et al. Leukocytes infiltrate the myometrium during human parturition: further evidence that labour is an inflammatory process. Hum Reprod 1999; 14: 229–36.
9. Melendez JA, Vinci JM, Jeffrey JJ et al. Localization and regulation of IL-1α in rat myometrium during late pregnancy and the postpartum period. Am J Physiol Regul Integr Comp Physiol 2001; 280: R879–R888.
10. Hardy DB, Janowski BA, Corey DR et al. Progesterone inhibition of cyclooxygenase-2 (COX-2) expression in human myometrium is mediated by progesterone receptor (PR) antagonism of nuclear factor-κB (NF-κB) activity. J Soc Gynecol Invest 2005; 12: 173A.
11. Ou CW, Chen ZQ, Qi S et al. Increased expression of the rat myometrial oxytocin receptor messenger ribonucleic acid during labor requires both mechanical and hormonal signals. Biol Reprod 1998; 59: 1055–61.
12. Petrocelli T, Lye SJ. Regulation of transcripts encoding the myometrial gap junction protein, connexin-43, by estrogen and progesterone. Endocrinology 1993; 133: 284–90.
13. Virgo BB, Bellward GD. Serum progesterone levels in the pregnant and postpartum laboratory mouse. Endocrinology 1974; 95: 1486–90.
14. Giannopoulos G, Tulchinsky D. Cytoplasmic and nuclear progestin receptors in human myometrium during the menstrual cycle and in pregnancy at term. J Clin Endocrinol Metab 1979; 49: 100–6.
15. Challis JRG, Matthews SG, Gibb W et al. Endocrine and paracrine regulation of birth at term and preterm. Endocr Rev 2000 2000; 21: 514–50.
16. Haluska GJ, Wells TR, Hirst JJ et al. Progesterone receptor localization and isoforms in myometrium, decidua, and fetal membranes from rhesus macaques: evidence for functional progesterone withdrawal at parturition. J Soc Gynecol Invest 2002; 9: 125–36.
17. Bernard A, Duffek L, Torok I et al. Progesterone and oestradiol levels and cytoplasmic receptor concentrations in the human myometrium at term, before labour and during labour. Acta Physiol Hungarica 1988; 71: 507–10.

18. Frydman R, Lelaidier C, Baton-Saint-Mleux C et al. Labor induction in women at term with mifepristone (RU 486): a double-blind, randomized, placebo-controlled study. Obstet Gynecol 1992; 80: 972–5.

19. Elliott CL, Brennand JE, Calder AA. The effects of mifepristone on cervical ripening and labor induction in primigravidae. Obstet Gynecol 1998; 92: 804–9.

20. Stenlund PM, Ekman G, Aedo AR et al. Induction of labor with mifepristone – a randomized, double-blind study versus placebo. Acta Obstet Gynecol Scand 1999; 78: 793–8.

21. Herrmann W, Wyss R, Riondel A et al. The effects of an antiprogesterone steroid in women: interruption of the menstrual cycle and of early pregnancy. C R Seances Acad Sci III 1982; 294: 933–8.

22. Chwalisz K. The use of progesterone antagonists for cervical ripening and as an adjunct to labour and delivery. Hum Reprod 1994; 9 (Suppl-61): 131–61.

23. Condon JC, Jeyasuria P, Faust JM et al. A decline in progesterone receptor coactivators in the pregnant uterus at term may antagonize progesterone receptor function and contribute to the initiation of labor. Proc Natl Acad Sci USA 2003; 100: 9518–23.

24. Dong X, Shylnova O, Challis JR et al. Identification and characterization of the protein-associated splicing factor as a negative co-regulator of the progesterone receptor. J Biol Chem 2005; 280: 13 329–40.

25. Mahendroo MS, Porter A, Russell DW et al. The parturition defect in steroid 5α-reductase type 1 knockout mice is due to impaired cervical ripening. Mol Endocrinol 1999; 13: 981–92.

26. Condon JC, and Mendelson CR. Fetal macrophages, which contain elevated 20α-hydroxysteroid dehydrogenase (20α-HSD) activity and invade the pregnant uterus near term, may contribute to the onset of labor by causing local progesterone withdrawal. J Soc Gynecol Invest 2004; 11(2), 224A.

27. Kalkhoven E, Wissink S, van der Saag PT et al. Negative interaction between the RelA(p65) subunit of NF-κB and the progesterone receptor. J Biol Chem 1996; 271: 6217–24.

28. Condon JC, Hardy DB, Kovaric K et al. Upregulation of the progesterone receptor (PR)-C isoform in laboring myometrium by activation of NF-κB may contribute to the onset of labor through inhibition of PR function. Mol Endocrinol 2006; 20: 764–75.

29. Mitchell MD, MacDonald PC, Casey ML. Stimulation of prostaglandin E2 synthesis in human amnion cells maintained in monolayer culture by a substance(s) in amniotic fluid. Prostaglandins Leukot Med 1984; 15: 399–407.

30. Lopez BA, Newman GE, Phizackerley PJ et al. Surfactant stimulates prostaglandin E production in human amnion. Br J Obstet Gynaecol 1988; 95: 1013–17.

31. Toyoshima K, Narahara H, Furukawa M et al. Platelet-activating factor. Role in fetal lung development and relationship to normal and premature labor. Clin Perinatol 1995; 22: 263–80.

32. Avery ME, Mead J. Surface properties in relation to atelectasis and hyaline membrane disease. AMA J Dis Child 1959; 97: 517–23.

33. Hawgood S, Shiffer K. Structures and properties of the surfactant-associated proteins. Annu Rev Physiol 1991; 53: 375–94.

34. Crouch E, Wright JR. Surfactant proteins A and D and pulmonary host defense. Annu Rev Physiol 2001; 63: 521–54.

35. Kremlev SG, Phelps DS. Surfactant protein A stimulation of inflammatory cytokine and immunoglobulin production. Am J Physiol Lung Cell Mol Physiol 1994; 267: L712–L719.

36. Phelps DS. Surfactant regulation of host defense function in the lung: a question of balance. Pediatr Pathol Mol Med 2001; 20: 269–92.

37. Islam KN, Mendelson CR. Potential role of nuclear factor κB and reactive oxygen species in cAMP and cytokine regulation of surfactant protein-A gene expression in lung type II cells. Mol Endocrinol 2002; 16: 1428–40.

38. Odom MJ, Snyder JM, Mendelson CR. Adenosine 3′,5′-monophosphate analogs and β-adrenergic agonists induce the synthesis of the major surfactant apoprotein in human fetal lung in vitro. Endocrinology 1987; 121: 1155–63.

39. Bry K, Lappalainen U, Hallman M. Intraamniotic interleukin-1 accelerates surfactant protein synthesis in fetal rabbits and improves lung stability after premature birth. J Clin Invest 1997; 99: 2992–9.

40. Bry K, Hallman M. Transforming growth factor-β2 prevents preterm delivery induced by interleukin-1α and tumor necrosis factor-α in the rabbit. Am J Obstet Gynecol 1993; 168: 1318–22.

41. Mendelson CR, Boggaram V. Hormonal and developmental regulation of pulmonary surfactant synthesis in fetal lung. Baillières Clin Endocrinol Metab 1990; 4: 351–78.

42. Korfhagen TR, Bruno MD, Glasser SW et al. Murine pulmonary surfactant SP-A gene: cloning, sequence, and transcriptional activity. Am J Physiol Lung Cell Mol Physiol 1992; 263: L546–L554.

43. Alcorn JL, Hammer RE, Graves KR et al. Analysis of genomic regions involved in regulation of the rabbit surfactant protein A gene in transgenic mice. Am J Physiol Lung Cell Mol Physiol 1999; 277: L349–L361.

44. Mendelson CR, Condon JC. New insights into the molecular endocrinology of parturition. J Steroid Biochem Mol Biol 2005; 93: 113–19.

45. Olson DM. The role of prostaglandins in the initiation of parturition. Best Pract Res Clin Obstet Gynaecol 2003; 17: 717–30.

46. Chow L, Lye SJ. Expression of the gap junction protein connexin-43 is increased in the human myometrium toward term and with the onset of labor. Am J Obstet Gynecol 1994; 170: 788–95.

47. Fuchs AR, Fuchs F, Husslein P et al. Oxytocin receptors in the human uterus during pregnancy and parturition. Am J Obstet Gynecol 1984; 150: 734–41.

48. Soloff MS, Cook Jr DL, Jeng YJ et al. In situ analysis of interleukin-1-induced transcription of COX-2 and IL-8 in cultured human myometrial cells. Endocrinology 2004; 145: 1248–54.

49. Havelock JC, Keller P, Muleba N et al. Human myometrial gene expression before and during parturition. Biol Reprod 2005; 72: 707–19.

50. Wiqvist N, Bryman I, Lindblom B et al. The role of prostaglandins for the coordination of myometrial forces during labour. Acta Physiol Hung 1985; 65: 313–22.

51. Bethin KE, Nagai Y, Sladek R et al. Microarray analysis of uterine gene expression in mouse and human pregnancy. Mol Endocrinol 2003; 17: 1454–69.

52. Wang LH, Hajibeigi A, Xu XM et al. Characterization of the promoter of human prostaglandin H synthase-1 gene. Biochem Biophys Res Commun 1993; 190: 406–11.

53. Tsuboi K, Iwane A, Nakazawa S et al. Role of prostaglandin H2 synthase 2 in murine parturition: study on ovariectomy-induced parturition in prostaglandin F receptor-deficient mice. Biol Reprod 2003; 69: 195–201.

54. Tazawa R, Xu XM, Wu KK et al. Characterization of the genomic structure, chromosomal location and promoter of human prostaglandin H synthase-2 gene. Biochem Biophys Res Commun 1994; 203: 190–9.

55. Newton R, Kuitert LM, Bergmann M et al. Evidence for involvement of NF-κB in the transcriptional control of COX-2 gene expression by IL-1β. Biochem Biophys Res Commun 1997; 237: 28–32.

56. Baldwin ASJ. The NF-κB and IκB proteins: new discoveries and insights. Annu Rev Immunol 1996; 14: 649–83.

57. Miller L, Hunt JS. Regulation of TNF-alpha production in activated mouse macrophages by progesterone. J Immunol 1998; 160: 5098–104.

58. Deroo BJ, Archer TK. Differential activation of the IκBα and mouse mammary tumor virus promoters by progesterone and

glucocorticoid receptors. J Steroid Biochem Mol Biol 2002; 81: 309–17.

59. Kastner P, Bocquel MT, Turcotte B et al. Transient expression of human and chicken progesterone receptors does not support alternative translational initiation from a single mRNA as the mechanism generating two receptor isoforms. J Biol Chem 1990; 265: 12 163–7.

60. Giangrande PH, McDonnell DP. The A and B isoforms of the human progesterone receptor: two functionally different transcription factors encoded by a single gene. Recent Prog Horm Res 1999; 54: 291–313.

61. Conneely OM, Maxwell BL, Toft DO et al. The A and B forms of the chicken progesterone receptor arise by alternate initiation of translation of a unique mRNA. Biochem Biophys Res Commun 1987; 149: 493–501.

62. Giangrande PH, Kimbrel EA, Edwards DP et al. The opposing transcriptional activities of the two isoforms of the human progesterone receptor are due to differential cofactor binding. Mol Cell Biol 2000; 20: 3102–15.

63. Vegeto E, Shahbaz MM, Wen DX et al. Human progesterone receptor A form is a cell- and promoter-specific repressor of human progesterone receptor B function. Mol Endocrinol 1993; 7: 1244–55.

64. Pieber D, Allport VC, Hills F et al. Interactions between progesterone receptor isoforms in myometrial cells in human labour. Mol Hum Reprod 2001; 7: 875–9.

65. Mulac-Jericevic B, Lydon JP, DeMayo FJ et al. Defective mammary gland morphogenesis in mice lacking the progesterone receptor B isoform. Proc Natl Acad Sci USA 2003; 100: 9744–9.

66. Wei LL, Gonzalez-Aller C, Wood WM et al. 5'-Heterogeneity in human progesterone receptor transcripts predicts a new amino-terminal truncated "C"-receptor and unique A-receptor messages. Mol Endocrinol 1990; 4: 1833–40.

67. Wei LL, Hawkins P, Baker C et al. An amino-terminal truncated progesterone receptor isoform, PRc, enhances progestin-induced transcriptional activity. Mol Endocrinol 1996; 10: 1379–87.

68. Wei LL, Norris BM, Baker CJ. An N-terminally truncated third progesterone receptor protein, PR(C), forms heterodimers with PR(B) but interferes in PR(B)-DNA binding. J Steroid Biochem Mol Biol 1997; 62: 287–97.

69. How H, Huang ZH, Zuo J et al. Myometrial estradiol and progesterone receptor changes in preterm and term pregnancies. Obstet Gynecol 1995; 86: 936–40.

70. Mesiano S, Chan EC, Fitter JT et al. Progesterone withdrawal and estrogen activation in human parturition are coordinated by progesterone receptor A expression in the myometrium. J Clin Endocrinol Metab 2002; 87: 2924–30.

71. Nardulli AM, Katzenellenbogen BS. Progesterone receptor regulation in T47D human breast cancer cells: analysis by density labeling of progesterone receptor synthesis and degradation and their modulation by progestin. Endocrinology 1988; 122: 1532–40.

72. Leite RS, Brown AG, Strauss III, JF. Tumor necrosis factor-alpha suppresses the expression of steroid receptor coactivator-1 and -2: a possible mechanism contributing to changes in steroid hormone responsiveness. FASEB J 2004; 18: 1418–20.

73. Myatt L, Lye SJ. Expression, localization and function of prostaglandin receptors in myometrium. Prostaglandins Leukot Essent Fatty Acids 2004; 70: 137–48.

8

Matrix biology and preterm birth

Brian R Heaps, Michael House, Simona Socrate, Phyllis Leppert, and Jerome F Strauss III

EXTRACELLULAR MATRIX (ECM) COMPOSITION

An ECM is found in all mammalian tissues. It is comprised of structural proteins consisting of the numerous and ubiquitous collagen family (over 28 different types of α chains) and elastin. The adhesive proteins, laminin, fibronectin, and tenascin, and the matricellular proteins, including thrombospondin and the proteoglycans are also components of the ECM. The fibrillar collagens, type I, II, III, V and XI, provide structure and form, and are major components of skin and bones, while other collagens function in other ways such as assisting with fibril formation, linkage of fibrils or formation of networks in basement membranes.[1] The predominant collagens of the human cervix are type I and III, and some type IV and V.[2,3] These are also the predominant collagens in the fetal membranes (Figure 8.1). Elastin is responsible for the resilience of tissues. This protein is usually in a recoiled state but is capable of being stretched to double its length. Elastin in tissue is physiologically functional in even small amounts. For example, it is present in the cervix of rodents and non-human primates, and in human cervix is 1–2% of the total ECM and is arranged as a thin membrane.[4] The proteoglycans serve as a gel-like substance that stabilizes the ECM in the aqueous environment of the body.[1] These molecules also play important roles in the remodeling of the ECM. The mammalian cervix contains large quantities of proteoglycans, including hyaluronan (hyaluronic acid) and dermatan sulfate, which increase during pregnancy. Other ECM proteins – laminin, fibronectin, and tenascin – provide adhesive properties to the ECM, while thrombospondins function in wound healing and tissue remodeling.[1,5]

The current understanding of the dynamic interaction of cells and ECM, including the role that the ECM plays in cellular metabolism, has greatly altered our appreciation of the physiology of the cervix and the fetal membranes. Several decades ago it was accepted that the ECM was extremely stable and that once it was laid down in tissue it was rarely altered. One concept from this era that is still present in today's clinical literature is that the ECM changes only by degradation by highly specific proteases. However, current evidence indicates that the ECM is a very dynamic and complex substance, and that its remodeling is highly controlled. That the ECM itself is a body-wide signaling network has been proposed.[6] Thus, there is more complexity to tissue remodeling than mere tissue degradation.

The critical issue in appreciating the roles of the cervix and fetal membranes in preterm birth is to understand how the normal steps in tissue remodeling of the ECM are circumvented or, alternatively, prematurely promoted in premature parturition.[7]

EXTRACELLULAR MATRIX (ECM) BIOLOGY

Collagens

The fibrillar collagens are long, rigid, and primarily nonextensible proteins in their native triple helical state. There are three individual collagen polypeptide chains that make up these helices. Mature collagen consists of a triple helix, which is proline and glycine rich. Every third residue is a glycine that promotes a tight packing of the triple helix.[8] Various combinations of the collagen chains produce the different collagen types. These collagens undergo extensive co- and posttranslational modifications which both stabilize the triple helix and allow the formation of fibrils. Each individual collagen chain is synthesized on ribosomes and then secreted into the endoplasmic reticulum (ER) lumen as a large precursor, pro-α chain. This large precursor chain has

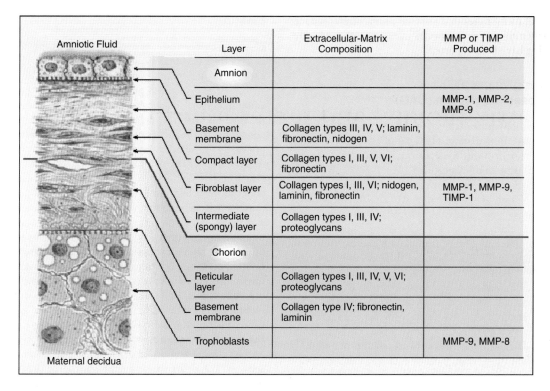

Amniotic Fluid	Layer	Extracellular-Matrix Composition	MMP or TIMP Produced
	Amnion		
	Epithelium		MMP-1, MMP-2, MMP-9
	Basement membrane	Collagen types III, IV, V; laminin, fibronectin, nidogen	
	Compact layer	Collagen types I, III, V, VI; fibronectin	
	Fibroblast layer	Collagen types I, III, VI; nidogen, laminin, fibronectin	MMP-1, MMP-9, TIMP-1
	Intermediate (spongy) layer	Collagen types I, III, IV; proteoglycans	
	Chorion		
	Reticular layer	Collagen types I, III, IV, V, VI; proteoglycans	
	Basement membrane	Collagen type IV; fibronectin, laminin	
	Trophoblasts		MMP-9, MMP-8
Maternal decidua			

Figure 8.1 Schematic drawing of the human fetal membranes and component proteins. MMP, matrix metalloproteinase; TMP, tissue inhibitor of metalloproteinase. Modified from Parry S, Strauss JF 3rd. Premature rupture of the fetal membranes. N Engl J Med 1998; 338(10): 663–70.

nonhelical extensions, propeptides at the amino- and carboxyl-terminal ends, and a signal peptide directs the pro-α chain to the ER. In the ER lumen, selected prolines and lysines are hydroxylated to form hydroxyproline and hydroxylysine, and some of the hydroxylysines are glycolsylated. Pro-α chains then self-assemble and three chains form a procollagen triple-helix. These procollagen molecules are then secreted from the cell into the extracellular matrix where the propeptides are cleaved forming the collagen molecule. At this juncture the collagen molecule self-assembles into a collagen fibril. Fibrils visualized by electron microscopy have a characteristic cross-striated appearance every 67 nm due to the staggered array of the individual collagen molecules.[1] Collagen fibrils are typically 10–300 nm in diameter.

The cytoskeleton of the cells influences the sites, rates and orientation of collagen fibril assembly. Given the complexity of this synthesis process it is easy to understand how the process might be altered in abnormal parturition.[9] After the fibrils are formed, covalent cross-linking occurs between the lysines of the adjacent collagen molecules. These types of cross-links are found only in collagen and elastin. The extent of these cross-links varies from tissue to tissue, and the amount of cross-linking determines the tensile strength of the tissue. For instance, if cross-linking is inhibited the tissue becomes fragile, while highly cross-linked collagen provides tensile strength. During gestation in the rat there is continuous synthesis of new collagen.[10] Newly synthesized collagen is more readily extracted from tissue than older and highly cross-linked collagen.[2] Due to the fact that there is an increase in the amount of water and an increase in proteoglycans in the cervix from conception to parturition, the concentration of collagen is decreased. Thus, many clinicians and some investigators have misunderstood the fact that collagen synthesis is increased because the increase in water and proteoglycan content resulted in a decrease in collagen concentration. This has been a confusing fact and the misunderstanding of the increasing collagen synthesis but decreased concentration has contributed to the idea that collagen degradation is a large component of cervical remodeling. Collagen is altered in cervical insufficiency, further strengthening the point that interstitial collagen has a role in maintaining cervical integrity in gestation.[11]

In fetal membranes that rupture prematurely, reduced collagen content and regionally reduced collagen cross-linking have been reported.

Proteoglycans (PG) and glycosaminoglycans (GAG)

The carbohydrate chains of GAG encode information. There are four distinct GAG families: heparin sulfate (HS), chondroitin(CS)/dermatan sulfate (DS), keratin sulfate (KS) and hyaluronan (HA). GAG are linear carbohydrates of repeating disaccharides of amino sugars, either N-acetyl-D-glucosamine (D-GlcNAc) or N-acetyl-D-galatosamine (GalNAc), as well as an uronic acid; either D-glucuronic acid (D-GlacA) or L-iduronic acid (L-Ido). HS and CS/DS are linked by serine to protein cores that make PG. There are differences in the basic sugars of individual GAG chains. However, it is the sulfation, deacetylation and epimerization of GAG that distinguish the individual chains from one and other. The formation of GAG chains provides great diversity and no two chains are exactly alike. GlcNAc or N-acetyl-D-galactosamine (GalNAc) residues are added to the chains, and modifications occur to GAG on PG in the Golgi by mechanisms that are not completely understood.[12] HA is not the usual GAG as it has a galactose in place of uronic acids, and it is not linked by serine to a protein core. Also, it is not modified by sulfation, deacetylation or epimerization but by two HA synthases. The monosaccharides are added at the reducing end of the HA chain inside the cell membrane, while the growing polysaccharide chain is pushed out into the extracellular space. Thus, HA can be extremely long.[13]

GAG have functional roles in a variety of processes, including activation of cytokines, enzymes and growth factors as well as numerous cell–matrix interactions. They activate various inflammatory cells such as macrophages through CD44-dependent signaling. Recent findings suggest that GAG are able to function as molecular signals of injury in the absence of microbial insult. In some instances, such as scleroderma and inflammatory bowel disease, specific GAG are elevated. However, in other situations it has been suggested that increased levels of GAG may lead to a decrease in the inflammatory response. Small GAG such as decorin (a small DS) are essential to fibrillogenesis of collagen.[14] Decorin is increased in the cervix in late gestation, and contributes to collagen rearrangement and fibril separation.[15–17] HA increases in the cervix as gestation advances, and it is postulated that hyaluronan and water accumulation in ECM may allow dispersion of collagen fibrils, or prevent their aggregation, leading to decreased tensile strength.[18,19]

Elastin

Elastin provides resiliency to tissue and is the component of the ECM that assists in the creation and maintenance of tissue architecture. It is capable of rubber-like stretching to five times greater than a rubber band of equal diameter.[1] Elastic fibers are usually laid down in tissue along with the inelastic collagen fibrils, and thus contribute to the prevention of tissue tearing. Elastin is not easily degraded by enzymes, including many MMP. Although elastin is extremely hydrophobic, when stretched the hydrophobic interactions are disrupted and water is absorbed onto nonpolar groups,[20] indicating that the hydration of tissue is essential for elastin extension. The precursor protein – tropoelastin, a soluble monomer – is secreted by the cell, followed by elastin assembly in the extracellular space. There are two components in mature elastin, amorphous elastin and microfibrils. Recent work suggests that elastic fibers first organize as globules of elastin on the cell surface. These globules then aggregate to form a fiber, a process called microassembly.[21] Cells play a direct role in the shaping of the final fiber through the mechanical forces of the cytoskeleton of the cell and the movement of the cells, as well deformation of the matrix. In the cervix, elastin plays a role in maintaining the shape and architecture of the cervix, where it is organized into very thin sheets which are capable of stretching in all directions. It is laid down in the tissue so that when the cervix is fully effaced the force of the uterine contractions pushing the vertex, or other presenting part, against the cervical tissue will allow maximum stretching.[4] When the presenting part is well applied to the cervix it would appear that the elastic fibers do not recoil or close.[22] The amount of elastin is reduced in cervical insufficiency,[23] supporting the notion of a key role for this ECM component in cervical function.

Post-translational modifications of collagens and elastin

Cross-linking of collagen by lysyl oxidase, a secreted copper-containing enzyme, increases tensile strength and resistance to degradation by matrix-metabolizing enzymes. Elastin is also cross-linked by lysyl oxidases. The lysyl oxidase family of enzymes cross-link proteins by the oxidative deamination of lysine or hydroxylysine residues. There are five members of the family: lysyl oxidase (LOX) and four lysyl oxidase-like enzymes (LOXL-1–4).[74] LOX expression is highest in the amnion mesenchymal cells that lay down the interstitial collagen. However, LOX, and LOXL-1 and LOXL-2, are also expressed in extraembryonic tissues. The phenotype of the Loxl-1 knockout mouse includes postpartum uterine prolapse, which is most likely the result of aberrant elastin cross-linking.

Fibronectins, thrombospondins (TSP), and tenascins

Fibronectins are large molecules consisting of dimers made up of large subunits with multiple binding domains. These subunits are folded into functionally distinct domains which are separated by polypeptide chains. In general, the fibronectins have one domain that binds to collagen, one to heparin and others that bind to certain specific cells. The amino acid sequence, Arg-Gly-Asp, called the RGD sequence, is found on type III fibronectin and binds to integrin. However, tight binding requires more than the RGD sequence. Fibronectins assemble into fibrils only on the surface of specific cells and therefore do not self-assemble. Interestingly, the fibronectin fibrils form on the surface or near the surface of cells in alignment with intracellular actin stress fibers. The actin and myosin of the cytoskeleton pulls the fibronectin, and thus elongates the fibronectin molecule and exposes binding sites which were hidden. Fibronectins function to organize the ECM and to help cells attach to it.[1]

TSP play important roles in wound healing as well as other cell functions.[25] They are part of the matricellular family and act as mediators of cell function as well as modulating the activity of growth factors, proteases and other ECM proteins.[26] They also may either promote or inhibit ECM cell adhesion. In the murine cervix, TSP-2 expression is induced and detected on day 14, and is extracted with noncross-linked collagen. However, on day 18 the expression of TSP increased, where it was observed in noncross-linked and irreversibly cross-linked collagen fractions.[5] Interestingly, TSP-2 appears to modulate matrix metalloproteinase 2 (MMP-2), as this enzyme is observed (on immunohistochemistry) to be more widespread and have a more intense staining in TSP-2 null mice on days 14 and 18 but not on day 10 compared to wild-type animals. Tenascin is also involved in ECM cell adhesion. The roles of these molecules, especially TSP, in cervical remodeling deserve further study.

Matrix metalloproteinases (MMP)

MMP, also called matrixins, degrade both matrix and nonmatrix proteins, including proteolycans within the extracellular space.[27] Humans have 23 MMP.[14] All MMP use a Zn^{2+} ion linked to their catalytic sites to hydrolyse peptide substrates. Human MMP are subdivided into four groups; collagenases, which include MMP-1, MMP-8, (secreted by neutrophils), and (MMP-13; gelatinases, which include MMP-2 and MMP-1; stromelysins, which include MMP-3, MMP-10, and MMP-11; and membrane MMP type 1 (MT1-MMP).[27] They play major roles in tissue repair and remodeling, in wound healing in response to injury, and in morphogenesis. Their function is not limited to ECM degradation as they have important roles in cell-surface and ECM protein activation.[28] MMP break down cell-surface or ECM molecules that alter cell–matrix or cell–cell interactions, and release growth factors. MMP play roles in cell migration, cell differentiation, growth, apoptosis and inflammatory responses not related to the degradation of collagen or other matrix molecules.[29] The various MMP have substrate specificity (Table 8.1). Their synthesis and breakdown in tissue is tightly controlled by protein kinases, cell-type specific and tissue-specific, and inducible and constitutive cell-stage-specific gene expression.[29] Expression is usually low in normal physiological conditions and MMP activity is often not detected.[28] Pro-MMP are secreted by uterine fibroblasts and smooth muscle cells.[30,31] Cytokines, growth factors, hormones, and cell–cell and cell–matrix interactions all control their gene expression.[27] Extracellular matrix metalloproteinase inducer (EMMPRIN) stimulates expression of some MMP (MMP-1, MMP-2, MMP-3 and membrane type 1)[32] by an unclear mechanism. MMP are synthesized in latent forms by a number of cells, including fibroblasts and leukocytes, secreted into the ECM in an inactive form and which require proteolytic cleavage for enzymatic activity. They must be activated by

Table 8.1 Selected matrix metalloproteinases (MMP) and their substrates	
MMP	**Substrate**
MMP-1	Collagen type I, II, III, VII, and X, gelatin, entactin, aggrecan
MMP-2	Gelatin, collagen type I, IV, V, VII, and X, fibronectin, lamin, aggrecan, tenascin-C, vitronectin
MMP-3	Gelatin, fibronectin, lamin, collagen type III, IV, IX, and X, pro-MMP-1, tenascin-C, vitronectin
MMP-8	Collagen type I, II, and III, aggrecan
MMP-9	Gelatin, collagen type IV, V, and XVI, aggrecan, elastin
MMP-12	Elastin
MMP-15	Pro-MMP-2, lamin, fibronectin

protein cleavage after secretion into the ECM, although a few MMP are activated intracellularly by a furin-like mechanism and are thus fully activated when secreted.[33] MMP-1 cleaves the collagen molecule into 1/3–2/3 fragments. Pro-MMP-1 is activated by cleavage of its propeptide by MMP-3.[34] MMP-1 has a narrow binding site that does not accommodate the collagen triple helix. Thus, MMP-1 binds to, and locally unwinds, the triple helix before the peptide bond is hydrolyzed.[35] MMP-9 exhibits activity against type IV collagens and elastic fibers and thus is thought to have elastolytic properties.[36] MMP-9 and MMP-2 are related to the inflammatory response. Pro-MMP-2 is a 72 kDa protein which is secreted and then processed to a 64 kDa (intermediate form) before it is activated in a 62 kDa from. It is regulated by tissue inhibitor of metalloproteinases (TIMP) 2, which can either promote activation of pro-MMP-2 or it can inhibit enzyme activity depend-ing on tissue levels.[37] Finally, MMP are inhibited by α_2-macroglobulin and TIMP, of which there are four types. MMP have a zinc-binding motif in the catalytic domain and a propeptide 'cysteine switch'. Three histidines in the zinc-binding motif, and the cysteine in the propeptide, coordinate with the catalytic zinc atom. This cysteine-zinc coordination also promotes MMP inactivation by preventing a water molecule, needed for catalysis, from binding to the zinc atom.[27] Therefore, the regulation of MMP is extremely complex because the equilibrium between activation and inhibition is delicate.[38] In some situations a signal that regulates one MMP in a coordinated way may have no effect, or even the exact opposite effect, in another situation. A particular signal may regulate one MMP in one direction (activation), but regulate another MMP in the opposite direction (inhibition). Often the regulation by a TIMP depends on the presence (or absence) of hormones in addition to the usual pathways of MMP activation and inhibition.[38]

In summary, there are three levels of regulation of MMP: (i) induction of gene expression (ii) activation of latent proenzymes; and (iii) inhibition of MMP enzymatic activity by α_2-macroglobulin and TIMP. Therefore, in assessing the role of MMP in the initiation of parturition, it is necessary to know if the MMP is activated in the tissue being studied.[39] However, demonstration of the presence of mRNA or protein in a particular tissue is not sufficient to prove the role of an MMP in that tissue.[27,38]

UTERINE CERVIX

In women the cervix is approximately 85%–90% ECM with a 10%–15% cellular component of smooth muscle cells and fibroblasts.[39,40] During pregnancy increased collagen and proteoglycan synthesis,[10,41] cellular turnover (a process which includes proliferation and programmed cell death or apoptosis),[42–45] and increased water content contribute to an expansion of cervical volume.[46] Interstitial collagens are prominent[47] and therefore the most fundamental change throughout gestation is the remodeling of the collagen. Other ECM components of the cervix undergo change as well.[2,48] Interstitial collagens are resistant to stretching and extension.[1] The prevailing view is that cervical collagen is degraded by MMPs released by infiltrating leukocytes.[49] However, there is accumulating evidence that the remodeling of the uterine cervix is not due solely to collagen degradation but to an alteration of the collagen helices by proteoglycans.[5,50] The contribution of the uterine cells to remodeling is unclear. While cellular turnover is a component of cervical change, the individual cells do not proliferate and die simultaneously, and thus the phenomenon of apoptosis in individual cells is fleeting. The only definitive measure of apoptosis is demonstration of DNA degradation fragments revealed by a typical ladder on gel electrophoresis.[42,44] A careful reading of published studies demonstrates that at any one point in time the majority of cervical cells are quiescent.[44,51] Furthermore, even though programmed cell death is increased during a particular stage of pregnancy, cell proliferation occurs at that stage as well, and thus cell populations are not depleted.[43] In rat mid-gestation, apoptotic cells were surrounded by altered collagen fibrils. Postpartum uterine involution is associated with pro-MMP-13 production in rat smooth muscle cells. Apoptotic features and decreased collagen birefringence under polarized light microscopy suggest that these dying cells mediate local pro-MMP production.[52] Apoptosis undoubtedly plays some role in cervical remodeling as it plays an important role in homeostasis by regulation of normal cell populations.[53]

The two essential functions of the cervix are to maintain the fetus in the uterus until biological maturity and to dilate at the time of parturition to allow a normal birth. The biochemical and biomechanical mechanisms that drive these two functions are programmed at the inception of pregnancy and occur throughout gestation. In most mammals, except humans, the timing of parturition is consistent among individuals within a species. Only humans are confronted with rather widespread alterations in the timing of birth. A tissue remodeling cascade of the cervix commences in early gestation, and culminates in the effacement and dilatation at parturition. In human gestation this remodeling is noted by clinicians as consistency, effacement, dilatation, and position of the cervix in relationship to the vagina and pelvis. Abnormalities in the remodeling cascade lead to both preterm birth and postdate pregnancy.

While the length of normal gestation is species specific, the structures and functions of the proteins and glycoproteins of the ECM are highly conserved.[54,55] In mammals, the synthesis, degradation and tissue remodeling processes of the ECM are strikingly similar. Cervical remodeling cascades resemble the inflammatory response, as hormones, cytokines and degradative enzymes, and immune cells are all respected players in the processes. However, these cascades are not a typical inflammatory response.[50] Because of the conserved nature of ECM, animal models of changes in the uterine cervix are instructive for human gestation and parturition cervical remodeling.

The challenge facing scientists studying the complexities of cervical remodeling is to develop a theoretical model which accomodates findings of clinical studies and accepted biomechanics and matrix biology. This theoretical model must also take into consideration the role of various individual genotypes on the process of cervical remodeling. In the genomic era it is essential that physicians/scientists develop careful phenotypes of preterm birth, as numerous perturbations of the remodeling cascades that contribute to this pregnancy outcome are likely.

In this discussion, the focus is on the nature, function and remodeling of ECM proteins, and it highlights recent evidence of how this remodeling may occur. Hormonal regulation will not be discussed in detail, although the reader should appreciate the fact that cervical remodeling is under hormonal, especially prostaglandin, control.

CLINICAL CORRELATES

Very early in human pregnancy, the uterine cervix undergoes a change in consistency. This softening of the cervix is palpable from the tenth week of gestation onwards, and prior to modern diagnostic tests was considered a probable sign of pregnancy. The palpable cervical consistency is similar to the lips of the face, while the nonpregnant cervix feels like the tip of the nose.[56] This change in consistency is thought to be due to increased vascularity of the cervix, as well as to a proliferation of cervical glands and the production of mucus; although the ECM composition of the human cervix in the first ten weeks of human gestation is unclear. While studies of the matrix biology of the human cervix obtained from an individual at various time points throughout gestation has not been conducted for ethical reasons, comparisons of several individuals demonstrate a change in cervical softening from the nonpregnant state to that at 22 weeks of gestation

and then at term.[57] These observations indicate that the changes in cervical consistency (palpated as softness) occur prior to the last month of pregnancy. As pregnancy progresses, the clinical changes in the cervix become more apparent. This remodeling is initiated in the first trimester in women and in early pregnancy in rodents, and constitutes the first phase of cervical remodeling.[58]

Several weeks prior to the onset of labor in women, additional changes in the consistency are noted as 'cervical ripening', the second phase of remodeling.[58] The cervix becomes much softer to palpation, and effaces or shortens. It also may dilate somewhat. Clinicians have long noted that these changes seem to occur earlier in the third trimester in multiparous women. These two phases prepare the cervix for parturition. The final phase of remodeling occurs in labor.[59,60]

In the mid-twentieth century obstetricians/gynecologists began to document cervical changes and develop cervical scoring systems that provided a semi-quantitative means for determining 'ripening' for the purpose of predicting the onset of labor.[61-64] The changes in this third phase of remodeling are cervical effacement and dilatation in conjunction with the descent of the fetal head or vertex or other presenting part. An analysis of cervical changes in labor was a landmark in obstetrics and ushered in a new era in practice based on the widespread use of the 'Friedman Curve'.[64] The utilization of this curve provided clinicians with a means to monitor the rate of cervical change, and to diagnose abnormalities in labor and delivery by plotting the findings against normal standards.

During the same time period, investigators demonstrated that the uterine cervix is composed of ECM.[2,3,47] It became apparent that the cervix does not function as a muscular sphincter opening and shutting like a door, and that dynamic complex changes are necessary for cervical dilatation in parturition.[9,65]

In women, the normal progression of cervical remodeling is altered in two general situations. First, the inability of the cervix to undergo the appropriate biochemical and biomechanical changes near to and at term leads to dysfunctional parturition, including arrest of labor. Post-dates pregnancy constitutes the most severe form of failure of cervical tissue remodeling. Current therapies for this clinical syndrome are not always satisfactory, and the treatment of this condition is challenging.[66] The focus of this text, however, is on the second serious abnormality of cervical remodeling, in which the changes are either accelerated in time or the cascade is dysynchronous, both of which lead to preterm birth.

The term 'cervical incompetency' has been used for over a century to describe a situation in which the cervix dilates without contractions or symptoms in the late second or early third trimester. Some authors suggest the term 'cervical insufficiency' for this syndrome.[67] In this condition a gradual funneling of the endocervical canal is observed, ending in spontaneous loss of the fetus. The condition is usually treated with the placement of a suture around the cervical canal to keep it closed until term. Clinical definitions of this condition are often varied and the criteria for the placement of a closing suture are being examined.[67] The prevention of cervical insufficiency remains a challenge, and investigators strive to find factors in the remodeling cascade which will lead to a diagnostic test, or combination of tests, which will truly allow preventive treatment.[67] It is clear that remodeling cascades are capable of a variable progression, as this syndrome may occur any time from late mid-trimester to early late trimester.

Cervical insufficiency does not account for all preterm births. However, all cases of spontaneous preterm birth are preceded by cervical dilation. Sonography of the cervix has become a reliable method to determine cervical length, a measurement that approximates cervical effacement. A short length in mid-trimester indicates a greater risk of spontaneous preterm birth. Unfortunately, there is no agreement on the actual cervical length that is defined as 'short'. One clinical investigator suggests a definition of 26 mm or shorter at 24 weeks would predict spontaneous preterm birth at 35 weeks or less.[68] With this stringent definition, however, most women will not deliver a preterm infant since only 4.3% of births were preterm in the reported study. Others propose 15 mm or shorter since this length is associated with a 50% risk of spontaneous preterm birth at 32 weeks of gestation or less.[69]

Cervicitis could lead to a pathological acceleration of remodeling and subsequent preterm birth. There is a doubling of preterm births of infants conceived as a result of assisted reproductive technologies (ART). (The role of relaxin, which increases certain MMP, in ART pregnancies is discussed in another section of this book.) The increase of MMP in this instance could contribute to protease activation of cell–matrix interactions as opposed to simply a degradation of interstitial collagen.

The challenge to both clinical and other scientists in determining the etiologies of cervical 'ripening', or acceleration of the remodeling cascade, is to elucidate the particular pathway or pathways which are altered in an individual case. There could be the failure of multiple cascades or a lack of one critical gene. In clinical and translational research it is essential to appreciate that the time in gestation or labor of the specimen collection is important to an understanding of the findings of the study. The expression of various molecules, or the observation of migration of different types of leukocytes at a particular point in gestation or parturition, may not correlate with their activity or their role in remodeling. Investigators must be aware of the temporal relationships to activation of enzymes and leukocytes to actual tissue remodeling. It is not appropriate to equate the immediate post-delivery tissue as reflective of the molecular profile of the cervix at any stage of labor. For example, the immune cell trafficking that is seen in the cervix near the end of parturition is in preparation for the involution remodeling of the cervix in the postpartum period.[50] The determination of whether tissue obtained at the time of Cesarean section is cervical tissue or lower uterine segment (LUS) tissue is difficult. Where does the cervix end and the lower segment of the uterus begin? Is the tissue obtained during low transverse Cesarean section LUS or cervical tissue that has been pushed up during effacement and decent of the fetus? Are there important clinical differences in these two tissues? The existing literature is murky with respect to these issues. Finally, tissues, especially in rodent models, may be contaminated by endometrium.[70] In vitro studies may not provide a complete picture of ECM remodeling since MMP may be secreted in greater abundance from cells in culture than in vivo, as culture conditions can alter the delicate balance between MMP and their inhibitors.[38]

Biomechanics of the cervix

With regard to spontaneous preterm birth, pregnancy outcomes are described within the conceptual framework of solid mechanics: health is associated with a static cervix and disease is associated with cervical deformation. Although cervical dilation is often associated with uterine contractions, clinicians know that a direct correlation between contractions and cervical dilation does not always hold. Many women experience contractions without associated cervical dilation. Other women experience cervical dilation without contractions. Our ability to predict who, among those at risk for preterm delivery, will go on to deliver is limited because it is difficult to predict the specific contractions that will cause cervical dilation. Part of the difficulty is that the biomechanics of cervical deformation is not well defined.

Cervical deformation, whether it is described as funneling, effacement or dilation, is a special case of a general problem – the problem of solid-body deformation. At a simple level, the likelihood of solid deformation involves the balance between two factors: material strength and external loading. The load-bearing tissue within the cervix is assumed to be the cervical stroma. Hence, when the cervical load exceeds the inherent strength of the stroma, the cervix will deform. Like any solid body, the pattern of deformation reflects the stress distribution within the body of the cervix. It is clear to see why cervical biomechanics is complex and a challenge to investigate. Cervical loading depends on three factors: the inherent material properties of the stroma, anatomic geometry and pelvic forces. Each of these factors is associated with wide patient variability, and each factor can change over the course of pregnancy.

Engineers investigate the mechanical behavior of materials through the use of constitutive models. A constitutive model is a mathematical model that shows how the macroscopic behavior of a solid is explained by the mechanical behavior of its constituent parts. Only two notable models have been developed to relate structural features of cervical tissue to mechanical properties. In the first model, the theory of fiber-reinforced composites was applied to cervical tissue in an attempt to explain the reduction of the stiffness of the tissue during the course of pregnancy.[71,72] The model was based on the assumption that the tissue can be considered mechanically equivalent to a fibrous network (corresponding to the collagen fibers) embedded in a ground substance (mainly composed of hydrated glycosaminoglycans). The model achieved its objective in a semi-quantitative way by showing decreased collagen concentration, decreased collagen alignment and changes in collagen – ground substance reinforcement combined to reduce tissue stiffness by a factor of ten. However, the model was limited by its underlying assumptions of linearity and small deformations. Moreover, the model only considered equilibrium properties and did not give insight in transient phenomena such as interstitial fluid flow, which are crucial in the short time range response of the cervix to various loading conditions.

More recently, a three-dimensional constitutive model for the large-strain, time-dependent mechanical behavior of the cervical stroma in pregnancy was presented by Fabvay et al.[73] The model captured the global tissue response, which was controlled by the cooperative contributions of the major constituents. In terms of mechanical behavior, the dominant constituents were the collagen fibers and the hydrated network of glycosaminoglycans. Stiffness in tension was provided by the collagen network. The glycosaminoglycans (proteoglycans and HA), due to their high negative fixed charge density, drew water into the tissue and created a high osmotic pressure responsible for the compressive stiffness of the tissue. Free interstitial fluid flowed in the tissue according to pressure gradients within the porous network, and was a major contributor to the time-dependent properties of the tissue. The effects of the smooth muscle,[74] vessels and cellular components on the passive biomechanical properties were neglected. The contributions of the elastic fibers were integrated within the model used to represent the collagen response.

The mechanical behavior of the cervix depends not only on the mechanical properties of the stroma but also on anatomic geometry and pelvic loading. A robust constitutive model can predict mechanical behavior as long as the loads are well characterized and the boundary conditions are realistic. Computational techniques are often used when complex loading is involved because an analytic solution is not practical. Figures 8.2 and 8.3 show the potential of a using a computational, solid mechanics approach to the study of the cervix.[75] In this simulation, the constitutive model of Fabvey et al[73] was implemented within a finite element framework. Figure 8.2 illustrates an idealized anatomic geometry that was used in the simulation. Anatomic dimensions were derived from magnetic resonance imaging (MRI) scans performed during pregnancy.[76] Pelvic loading (gravity and hydrostatic pressure) was applied using finite element methodology. The simulation in Figure 8.3 demonstrates a TYVU pattern of cervical deformation. TYVU deformation reflects the underlying stress distribution within the cervical stroma. At the outset, the stress is concentrated at the internal os. As the cervix deforms, the stress distribution moves down the cervical canal, which causes progressive funneling. Hence, the pattern of deformation observed clinically is a function of both cervical material properties and pelvic loading. This methodology can also be used to examine, in an

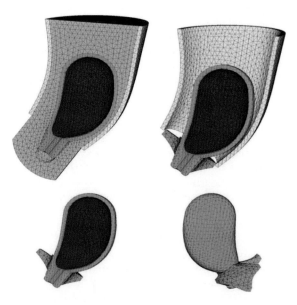

Figure 8.2 The anatomic geometry used for the simulation of cervical funneling. Red, the amniotic cavity, green, the uterus and cervix; orange, the endopelvic fascia; blue, the soft abdominal viscera; yellow, the abdominal wall.

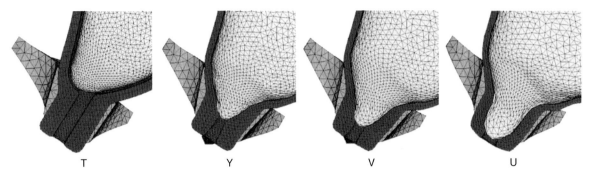

| T | Y | V | U |

Figure 8.3 TYVU progression of cervical funneling. The pattern of cervical deformation reflects the changing stress distribution within the cervical stroma.

objective way, common clinical questions like the structural features of cerclage, cervical loading of multiple gestation, and the physical connection between uterine contractions and cervical deformation.

INSIGHTS FROM ANIMAL STUDIES

Given the complexities and limitations of studying cervical biomechanics during human pregnancy, much insight has been gained by investigating nonhuman models. Several recent and intriguing studies are presented below.

A study of rat cervices using techniques of vascular mechanics addressed the following question: how can a remodeled cervix with nonaligned collagen be strong enough to remain closed? The study findings suggest that the answer lies in a dual mechanism: (i) the volume of the cervix, the collagen rearrangement and the growth of the cervix through an increase in glycosaminoglycans and water all increase compliance; but (ii) there is increasing wall stiffness that helps to keep the cervix closed and undilated until labor is initiated.[77] This study further suggests that the rearranged, unparallel collagen fibers seen in late gestation strengthen the cervical wall in a manner similar to that of reinforcing concrete with steel rods. When the rods are placed at various angles to each other, as opposed to rods placed parallel to each other, a concrete cylinder is strengthened.

TSP-2 affects the morphology of fibrils of type I collagen and causes skin and tendon laxity.[25,78] TSP-2 expression in the murine cervix is induced between day 10 and 14 of gestation. The TSP-2 null mice exhibited significantly increased extensibility (as measured by mechanical testing) on day 14 of pregnancy, which increased even further on day 18 suggesting that the lack of TSP-2 allowed a very rapid slippage of the collagen fibrils. TSP-2 null mouse cervices demonstrated an increased production of MMP. These cervices invariably broke at the time of mechanical testing. The findings strongly infer that TSP-2 induction in wild-type animals protected them from serious alterations in their cervical tissues. The changes in the TSP-2 null animals did not, however, result in preterm delivery of pups. The altered biomechanics of TSP-2 null mice cervical tissue is intriguing and strongly suggests that TSP-2 plays a role in maintaining cervical tensile strength. Taken together these findings suggest synthesis and degradation of existing matrix proteins may not be the sole factor in cervical remodeling.[5]

EP4, a prostaglandin (PG) E_2 receptor, mediates cervical ripening in the rat at term gestation.[79] Studies of the effects of this receptor in a rat model correlated biomechanical studies with determination of the morphology of collagen fibrils and their orientation in the cervix. Animals were pretreated with indomethacin on day 19 and day 20 of gestation to inhibit PG, and then PGE_2 receptor agonists were administered. When the cervices were observed by electron microscopy the average interfibrillary distance in animals treated with PGE_2 was significantly greater than the distance between fibrils in the control animals. Furthermore, no difference in fiber length was noted. The correlation of these findings with changes in biomechanical tensile strength points to a contribution of proteoglycan synthesis and degradation as mediators of collagen, and implies that collagenolysis plays relatively little part in ripening of the cervix.[79]

A second study of the biomechanical properties of the rat cervix also indicate that cervical ripening does not completely involve collagen degradation.[80] In this study, the tensile strength measurements in cervical tissue exposed to either PGE or MMP-1 revealed changes of increased extensibility and strength which could not be attributed to MMP-1 activity, as that decreased strength. These studies cast serious doubt on the role of collagen degradation in cervical remodeling. However, these studies should not be interpreted as indicating no role for MMP in cervical remodeling as these proteinases have numerous functions in tissues, such as cell surface and ECM protein activators.

INSIGHTS FROM HUMAN STUDIES

Measurement of cervical material properties in vivo is attracting increasing interest because the current strategy for diagnosing cervical insufficiency is problematic.[81] At present, the diagnosis of cervical insufficiency is made on clinical grounds. A patient is diagnosed with cervical insufficiency when a preterm delivery occurs and uterine contractions are not prominent. There are several difficulties with this diagnostic strategy. First, there is no way of knowing if a patient is at risk for cervical insufficiency in a first pregnancy because it is necessary to have a bad outcome in order to qualify for the diagnosis. Second, many patients present with multiple etiologies of spontaneous preterm birth at the same time, like premature rupture of membranes or preterm labor. It is difficult to distinguish a cervical etiology from other etiologies of spontaneous preterm birth. The core difficulty of diagnosing cervical insufficiency is this: the assumption of mechanical weakness underlies the existing paradigm, yet there is no way to measure structural function in these patients. Although cervical sonography can demonstrate progressive cervical shortening, intervention trials of cerclage for a short cervix have yielded conflicting results.[82–84]

Investigators are presently investigating three strategies for measuring cervical material properties in vivo: tonometry, fluorescence, and sonography. Tonometric methods measure cervical softness in a manner similar to clinical palpation. Cabrol et al[57] demonstrated a cervicotonometer which defined a cervical distensability index (CDI). In this device, two small tips were introduced into the cervical canal: the tips were slowly opened and the force needed to open the endocervical canal was measured. A force–displacement curve was generated and the slope of the curve was then defined as the CDI. Using this device, investigators were able to demonstrate a progressive increase in the CDI with increasing gestational age. They also showed that the CDI was higher in cases of preterm delivery compared to term delivery. In a more recent study, Mazza et al[85] proposed an aspiration device to measure softness of the cervical tissue. By creating a time-variable vacuum inside a tube, a small section of the cervical tissue at the site of the external os was aspirated into the device. The deformation of the tissue was recorded with a digital camera mounted on the far end of the device. A stiffness parameter was calculated from the data as the ratio of the applied relative negative pressure versus the vertical displacement of the superficial layer of the tissue. The aspiration experiments were conducted both in vivo and ex vivo (on the same organ, following hysterectomy), and demonstrated that the mechanical properties of the cervix do not change appreciably in vitro compared to in vivo. In an alternative strategy, Garfield et al[86] have constructed a noninvasive device that takes advantage of the changing fluorescence spectrum of cervical collagen with increasing cervical ripening. The device suggests that light-induced fluorescence is a measure of collagen cross-linking. Further, decreased light-induced fluorescence was measured following PG administration for term inductions in humans.[87]

Sonographic techniques which measure mechanical properties of soft tissue in vivo are attracting increasing interest, and may have applications in obstetrics. Ultrasound elastography refers to a new technique which aims to use sonographic information to determine mechanical properties of soft tissue.[88,89] Essentially, the transducer is used to compress the tissue, and the image-processing techniques are used to compare the precompression and postcompression images. Soft tissue deforms differently to firm tissue, and the sonographic images reflect this difference. In tissue with nonhomogeneous properties, 'elastograms' are derived, which are two-dimensional images that show tissue stiffness as a function of position. A clinical example is the diagnosis of breast disease. Elastograms of breast tissue show varying degrees of stiffness, and elastography may be useful in discriminating benign from cancerous masses.[90,91] Ultrasound elastography is making its way into many areas of medicine; human studies are ongoing in cardiology,[92] urology[93] and gastroenterology,[94] and pilot studies have begun in obstetrics.[95]

RECENT PROVOCATIVE STUDIES

The currently accepted model for cervical ripening, or the second phase of cervical remodeling, is that migration of inflammatory cells from the blood is the major regulatory event of cervical change.[49] These cells are considered to play a role in the secretion of cytokines and MMP that degrade cervical collagen. The most often cited studies to support this view are studies in C3H/HeN mice that describe increased macrophage numbers in the uterine cervix during gestation,[96] a study in nonpregnant women, women at term just prior to

Cesarean section and immediately postpartum,[97] and to one report that cervical fibroblasts do not secrete MMP.[98]

Nitric oxide (NO) acts in concert with progesterone to modulate cervical ripening and effects MMP production.[99,100] NO is produced when macrophages secrete inducible NO synthase (iNOS),[101] further supporting a role for leukocytes in cervical ripening.

In a study of three groups of women – nonpregnant, pregnant women at term, not in labor, and with clinical findings of an unripe cervix and women 15 min postpartum – investigators detected MMP-2 protein in cervical smooth muscle cells. MMP immunostaining and the number of positive cells increased in the stroma at term compared to the nonpregnant cervices. MMP-9 protein was only observed in leukocytes. This study evaluated the final phase of cervical remodeling, but the activity of the MMP-2 and MMP-9 was not able to be determined by this study protocol.[102] Thus, it is not apparent if the MMP degraded molecules prior to birth or in the postpartum period as the timing of activation is not known.

It is not clear, however, that immune cell action plays any role in cervical ripening, or in the dilatation of labor, as several studies previously cited in this chapter have reported that cervical cells are able to secrete MMP and that collagenase does not affect the biomechanical properties of the cervix.

A meticulous study challenges the traditional view of the role of immune cell migration as causative of cervical remodeling prior to parturition.[50] In this study, three strains of mice – C57Bl6/129 SvEv, C57Bl6 and NIH Swiss – as well as steroid 5α-reductase type 1 null mice (which do not undergo cervical ripening due to decreased local progesterone metabolism), were studied. On day 15 (prior to ripening), day 18 (during ripening), day 19, and day 19 2 h after birth (postpartum), the timing of migration and distribution of macrophages, monocytes, and neutrophils were studied. The activation of neutrophils was quantitated, and activity was measured by the presence of myeloperoxdidase and neutrophil chemoattractants. Tissue macrophages, myeloperoxidase activity and expression of proinflammatory molecules were not increased in the cervix until after birth. Neutrophil numbers did not change until after birth, and neutrohil depletion did not affect the timing of parturition. Thus, the role of these cells is most likely in postpartum remodeling of the cervix. The number of neutrophils was similar in cervical tissues from wild-type animals on days 15, 18 and postpartum day 19. One of the conclusions of this study is that proinflammatory gene expression timing and composition differed in fetal membranes compared to the cervix, and that the mechanisms of cervical ripening in normal labor are different from those of infection-induced labor. The investigators suggest that other determinants of collagen remodeling, such as the ability of proteoglycans, especially HA, to affect collagen fibrils can decrease tensile strength.

The increase in water content as gestation progresses is critical for cervical remodeling and function of many ECM proteins. First, it increases the biomechanically important cervical volume, and secondly it provides the necessary functioning of ECM proteins such as highly hydrophilic HA. Recently, the aquaporin (AQP) water channels were studied in CD-1 and 5α-reductase null mice, C57Bl6/129SvEv AQP-3 expression peaked at day 19 compared to nongravid and day 15 cervices. AQP-4 was low but trended upward at parturition, AQP-5 and AQP-8 increased on days 12–15 but fell to nongravid levels on day 19. Steroid 5α-reductase null mice had reduction in AQP-3, -4 and -8 on day 19, or post partum day 1 (PP1). These studies show that specific AQP water channels are involved in specific phases of cervical remodeling.[103]

While HA can release MMP and contribute to leukocyte migration, it promotes tissue hydration. It has been shown that PGE_2 induced the expression of an HA-binding protein, tumor necrosis factor-stimulated gene-6, in cervical smooth muscle cells in vitro implicating HA in cervical ripening. However, this increased expression was not as great as that seen with tumor necrosis factor (TNF)α.[104]

Two intriguing studies suggest a role for mechanotransduction of ECM components in uterine cells. HA synthesis, and HAS1, -2, -3, are enhanced by cyclic mechanical stretch in an in vitro system suggesting that, in labor, the final phase of cervical remodeling, the mechanical stretch of the presenting part on the cervix increased secretion of HA.[105] Mechanical stretch, $PGF_{2\alpha}$ and cytokines have been observed to augment MMP-1 secretion from cultured human cervical cells.[30] This study clearly demonstrates that human cervical fibroblasts can produce pro-MMP-1.

TRANSCRIPT PROFILING STUDIES

A study of tissue obtained from the LUS reported 56 differentially expressed genes on a 6912 gene platform cDNA array. Selected gene expression was confirmed by polymerase chain reaction (PCR). Among those of interest to matrix biology, the genes of transforming growth factor (TGF) β_2, TSP-2 and TIMP-2 were found to have increased expression.[106] Another genome-wide microarray study of 9182 genes revealed that cyclooxygenase (COX) 2 was highly expressed in the endocervical epithelial cells prior to labor. However, the stromal expression of COX-2 was either absent or weak at that time point. In tissue obtained after onset of labor, COX-2 was localized in the endocervical cells, but some expression was noted in stromal fibroblasts and smooth muscle cells, occasional tissue macrophages and the endothelial cells of small arterioles. COX-2 was not seen infiltrating leukocytes or vascular smooth muscle cells. COX-2 appeared to be constitutively present as immunoreactivity was present in tissues at 13 and 28 weeks of gestation, but was less intense which suggests that the level of COX-2 expression is regulated throughout pregnancy. The same array study revealed the differential expression of the S100A9 (calgranulin A) gene in cervical tissue. Immunolocalization showed that this gene is expressed in neutrophils and to a lesser degree in tissue macrophages. These immunoreactive cells increased in the cervical tissues in labor. S100A9 was found in the vascular endothelium near marginating neutrophils, suggesting secretion into vessels involved in leukocyte migrations in laboring women.[70]

Utilizing a human cancer cDNA array, expression of 588 genes (Atlas Human Cancer Array is cited by company website as having a platform of 588 genes) was evaluated during cervical effacement, another group pooled specimens from ten women immediately after delivery and women prior to Cesarean section. Several genes were confirmed by real time (RT)-PCR. Altered genes in postpartum specimens included interleukin (IL) 8 precursor, vascular endothelial growth factor (VEGF), and monocyte chemoattractant protein (MCP) 1. The transcripts found in ripe cervix were genes involved in mechanisms of mitosis, cell cycle regulation and cell metabolism, cell–cell interaction and apoptosis-related genes.[107]

FETAL MEMBRANES

Spontaneous rupture of the fetal membranes occurring before the onset of labor is defined as 'premature rupture of membranes' (PROM). Prior to 37 weeks of gestation spontaneous membrane rupture is referred to as preterm PROM (PPROM). PPROM occurs in 3% of pregnancies and is responsible for approximately one third of all preterm births. Due to its association with perinatal infection, oligohydramnios, resultant compression of the umbilical cord and the ultimate progression to preterm birth, PPROM is a significant cause of perinatal morbidity and mortality.[108,109] Additionally, many conditions occur with increased frequency in the context of PPROM, including amnionitis, placental abruption, fetal inflammatory response syndrome, and other complications specific to the age of the delivered fetus (necrotizing enterocolitis, intraventricular hemorrhage, cerebral palsy, and respiratory distress).[108]

NORMAL PROCESSES OF MEMBRANE RUPTURE AT TERM

Before there can be full understanding of the pathophysiology of PPROM, the normal process of membrane rupture must be understood. The normal spontaneous rupture of membranes following the initiation of labor occurs in about 90% of pregnancies at term. Rupture most likely occurs due to a combination of altered membrane integrity and increased pressure placed on the membranes by a contracting uterus. Knowledge concerning the exact mechanism of membrane rupture is growing, and it appears that the process is indeed interplay of both physical and biochemical stresses on the membrane. Early in the study of membrane rupture it was thought to be due entirely to the increased stress of uterine contractions which caused the membrane to stretch and rupture. It is now clear that there are numerous other factors, including the effect of apoptosis, matrix remodeling and consequent alterations in the presence of inflammation, and inherent structural predispositions to rupture.

Recent work has shown that the principle site for membrane rupture is described as being a 'zone of altered morphology' (ZAM).[110] This is a region of fetal membrane that overlies the cervix. It is significant for its response to (or generation of) inflammation and ECM remodeling, and is the site of significant biochemical and histological changes. It is currently understood that there is an increase in activity of various key players in membrane integrity at this zone that contribute to its propensity to rupture.[111] Although inflammation is the most understood, and most commonly accepted, contributor to membrane rupture at the ZAM, other processes, including apoptosis[112] and increased MMP expression,[113] have been shown to be crucial elements as well, and most likely represent an extension of this common inflammatory response. It has even been proposed that the ZAM is an initiator of labor and parturition, but this important relationship is disputed.[114] The role that the ZAM has on rupture (separate from the parturition mechanism), however, is currently accepted as being a crucial development for the spontaneous rupture of fetal membranes.

There is growing knowledge related to the mechanics and distinct events that lead to the rupture of the fetal membranes. Previously it has been established that two distinct layers of the fetal membranes (the amnion and choriodecidual layers) rupture separately. Recent work by Arikat et al[115] has documented the order in which the layers of fetal membranes rupture by the use of video documentation of membrane samples placed under physical stress. This study has shown that the amniotic layer and the choriodecidual layer first separate prior to the rupture of the membranes. This likely occurs due to a combination of sheer stress and altered matrix integrity between the two layers.[115] Once this separation occurs, the weaker choriodecidual layer ruptures leaving the inner amniotic layer intact. Following the formation of this defect in the outer chroriodecidua, the amniotic membrane is able to herniate through the defect (observed in vitro as a 'bubble' of membrane), followed by its eventual rupture when increased pressure is applied.[115] This research showed that not only does the outer choriodecidua rupture first, but that separation of the choriodecidua from the amnion is a crucial initial step in the weakening of the membranes.

In addition to the work investigating regional differences of the fetal membranes, other research has demonstrated that important biological messengers have influence over the integrity and strength of the membrane tissue.[110,116] This research was conducted with normal membrane fragments cultured with TNFα and IL-1β, and then analyzed using industrial rupture strength testing equipment. The study by Kumar et al[116] demonstrated a dose-dependant decrease in strength and work required to produce membrane rupture with both TNF-α and Il-1β. In addition to this demonstration of strength reduction, membrane samples that were cultured with either of these two proinflammatory cytokines showed an increased expression of MMP-9, a decreased expression of TIMP-3, and an increase in poly-(ADP-ribose)-polymerase (PARP) 1 cleavage. Each of these proteins and actions suggest an increase in collagen remodeling and apoptosis.[116]

LOX, the enzyme responsible for cross-linking collagen and elastin, may also play a significant role in normal membrane maintenance, integrity, and eventual rupture. A study of LOX in normal placental and membrane tissues revealed that there are at least three different subtypes of the LOX enzyme (LOX, LOXL, and LOXL-2).[117] Although each enzyme shows very similar expression patterns early in gestation, the expression pattern diverges as gestation advances. These differences in enzyme expression may then allow those tissues to change in character in order to facilitate the maintenance of pregnancy, or the initiation of parturition. Despite showing similar expression patterns early in gestation, LOX shows the greatest level of expression in the amnion and qualitatively less expression in the placenta at term, and LOXL-1 is seen primarily in the placenta and has lower levels of expression in the amnion at term. Uniquely, LOXL-2 is predominantly expressed in the chorion, the layer of membrane which has been shown to rupture first.[111,117] Whether alterations in the expression or activity of these enzymes involves post-translational modification of the ECM,

influencing the risk of PROM or PPROM, has yet to be determined.

PREMATURE RUPTURE OF THE MEMBRANES: DEFINITIONS AND DIAGNOSIS

Definitions

Due to the differences in recommended management of PPROM based on the gestational age at occurrence, there must be clear guidelines as to when conservative measures are appropriate or when an expeditious delivery is warranted. Patients, for this purpose, can be assigned to functional categories which will aid in determining the most appropriate treatment. The following definitions proposed by Mercer[108] are based on clinically significant outcomes, and thus offer relevant management directions based on the gestational age at the time of rupture (Table 8.2).

PPROM that occurs prior to 23 weeks of gestation poses difficult dilemmas for the management of the patient. Ultimately, the choice to deliver the fetus immediately or pursue conservative management rests with the patient and the condition of the fetus. Thus, it is imperative to monitor the fetus for infection and pulmonary hypoplasia secondary to oligohydramnios, as well as other physical abnormalities which may be related to the rupture of membranes in order for fully informed consent to be obtained. Additionally, because of its association with infection and inflammation, the risks of periventricular leukomalasia (and subsequent cerebral palsy) are very high and must be considered in the management strategy. Prolongation of latency, however, may be able to lead to a viable birth with a relatively low incidence of fetal morbidities and mortality, and may be an acceptable choice for the patient. Thus, all of the risks must be carefully weighed against the potential benefits connected to the management strategy.

Table 8.2 Preterm premature rupture of membranes (PPROM) definitions (Mercer, Obstet Gynecol 2003; 101: 178–93)

	No. of weeks gestation
Pre-viability PROM	<23
PPROM remote from term	23–31
PROM near term	>32

The second category is that of PPROM remote from term. This is defined as gestational age of 23–31 weeks.[118] Once the fetus has attained the 23rd week of gestation the benefits of conservative management increase secondary to the maturity of the fetus. With patients in this category, serial assessments of fetal condition should be performed, as well as the continuance of other preventative measures. Such measures would include the avoidance of digital examinations, and the institution of bed rest and pelvic rest. Other specific management strategies are discussed later.

Finally, there is PPROM near term, which is defined by the rupture of membranes after 32 weeks and before term (37 weeks). Within this category the aim is to determine the maturity of the fetus in order to deliver as soon as possible. At 32 weeks of gestation assessment should be made of fetal lung maturity because the risk of the respiratory distress is the most significant morbidity at this developmental age, other than that of infection. It is infection that prompts the immediate delivery of all fetuses that have demonstratable lung maturity before 34 weeks and the delivery of all pregnancies greater than 34 weeks.

Diagnostic evaluation

Often the diagnosis of PPROM is evident at presentation but many times, due to ambiguities in the patient history, the diagnosis can only result from clinical and laboratory examination. The initial step in obtaining a diagnosis of PROM is a complete patient history followed by the observation of pooling amniotic fluid in the vagina using a sterile speculum. As part of normal protocol the fluid should also be obtained and sent for maturity studies and culture (group B streptococci, chlamydia, and gonorrhea). Definitive diagnosis of PROM can be made when amniotic fluid, meconium, fetal vernix or dye (after injection into the amniotic cavity) is seen flowing from the cervical os. The fluid collected at the time of examination may also be dried on a glass slide for the observation of 'ferning' – a crystal formation that develops due to the physical interplay of the salt and protein content of the amniotic fluid – but more often the fluid is applied to Nitrazine paper to determine pH. When the pH of the fluid obtained is alkaline (pH > 6.0) the Nitrazine paper develops a blue color. Because amniotic fluid has an alkaline pH, a positive Nitrazine blue test infers rupture of membranes. Although these tests are easy to perform, they are less reliable indicators of membrane rupture due to interference of any number of chemicals or products to the sample of fluid obtained (including blood, semen, or vaginitis). However, a study conducted on the diagnosis of PROM using the aforementioned techniques showed that, above all other laboratory tests, detection of alpha-fetal protein (AFP) can be used to reliably diagnose rupture, due to its high sensitivity and specificity, when other methods proved unreliable.[119] Importantly, while the diagnosis of PROM is entertained, digital examination of the cervix should not be performed. Digital examinations increase the risk of infection and consistently decrease pregnancy latency following rupture.[120]

Histology

The fetal membranes consist of two distinct layers; the amnion and the chorion. The amnion provides the majority of the tensile strength to the membranes due to its production and maintenance of a rich ECM. The amnion consist of five layers; amniotic epithelial cells, basement membrane, and compact, fibroblastic and intermediate layers. The first layer of epithelial cells is responsible for the production of collagen types III and IV, as well as other components of the second, basement membrane layer.[121,122] The compact layer consists of mesenchymal cells that produce types I, III, V and VI collagen, which serves (in connection with the products of the first two layers) to provide the large tensile strength of the membrane.[123,124] The fourth, fibroblastic, layer provides the greatest amount of bulk to the amnion, and consists of both mesenchymal cells and macrophages. This layer is unique because if its production of MMPs and TIMPs.[121] The final intermediate layer has a histological spongy appearance due to its heavy meshwork of glycoprotein, type III collagen, and proteoglycans. This layer allows movement to occur between the amnion and chorion layers, secondary to sheer mechanical stress or to the effects of digestion by MMPs.[115,121]

Through the histological study of the fetal membranes, an ZAM was described that directly overlies the internal cervical os.[125,126] This zone has been defined as having both biochemical and histological distinctions, namely increased MMP[113] and apoptotic activity[112] as parturition approaches. Recent work has demonstrated that the expression patterns of important proteins – MMPs, TIMP-3 and PARP – differ as gestation advances in this zone, and that these changes are in fact associated with decreased membrane strength when compared to distant membrane samples.[110,111] Interestingly, this observation of weakness in the fetal membranes overlying the cervix is not unique to membranes following rupture. Of membranes sampled, exposed to different modes of delivery (including elective Cesarean section), there was demonstrated a weak zone of membrane overlying the cervix in both unruptured and ruptured cases.

This area of membrane – ZAM – is unique when compared to other membrane regions. These differences are not only based on exposure to stress, but also on demonstrated cellular differences which develop either independently or in response to those pressures. For example, work by McParland et al[127] showed there to be a differentiation of myofibroblasts during the labor process in the membrane sections that immediately overly the cervix. This differentiation caused a significantly increased expression pattern of α smooth muscle actin (α-sma) in reticular layers near the rupture sites compared to midline tissues. There was also a trend of increased α-sma expression, prior to clinically apparent labor, in the membrane of the lower uterine pole compared to midline tissues, suggesting that this process may precede labor. The authors make note that the sma, studied here from the reticular layer, is analogous to the myofibroblast phenotype that is seen in the wound response. Thus, functions such as turnover of ECM and contraction can be attributed to these cells in the fetal membrane.

PATHOLOGY OF THE PREMATURE RUPTURE OF FETAL MEMBRANES

The maintenance of fetal membranes is a physiologic process involving equilibrium of ECM synthesis and degradation. While there is a constant process of remodeling of the matrix throughout gestation, premature rupture of membranes can be thought of as a simple disequilibrium which leads to critical weakening of the tissue and resultant rupture. The causes of the disequilibrium are many, and are in the forefront of current matrix and fetal membrane research. It is now clear from the body of literature available that not just one process dominates in the development of PROM, but instead there appears to be multiple paths which lead to the weakening of the membranes through disruption of the normal physiologic balance. Of those documented paths there is a consistent genetic determination of risk, and an unquestionable association with infection and inflammation. But the pattern of PPROM also shows an interesting predilection to those who smoke and are of a poor socioeconomic status. It is also interesting to note that the risk of recurrent PPROM is nearly 20 times higher than that of an individual's first PPROM.[128] This, in addition to offering clues to the pathology of rupture, suggests that investigation into the etiology of PPROM may yield information which would allow prevention of recurrence. Overall, the proposed mechanisms of premature rupture of the fetal membranes is that of infection, inflammation, stretch/trauma/abruption, disregulated MMP, and inherited (or acquired) collagen pathology.

Subclinical intrauterine infection has long been implicated in the pathogenesis and subsequent maternal and neonatal morbidity in PPROM.[129–132] Infection not only exposes the membranes to pathogens that are responsible for the production and secretion of proteases (which disrupt the membrane structure), but is also involved in the initiation of membrane modulation by the inflammatory response. The organisms involved are generally vaginal in origin and appear to ascend first into the choriodecidual space.[132] Once clinical (or subclinical) chorioamnionitis has occurred it is believed that the pathogens are able to cross the intact chorioamniotic membrane into the amniotic fluid, resulting in amnionitis and, more rarely, lead to direct infection of the fetus.[130,133]

The organisms that are epidemiologically consistently associated with PPROM are group B streptococci, Chlamydia trachomatis, Neisseria gonorrheae, and Gardnerella vaginalis.[134,135] Another organism has been demonstrated to have an impact on the development of rupture. In a study of 207 women between 23 and 34 weeks of gestation, where Cesarean delivery was undertaken, three groups were established in order to compare the association of Ureaplasma urealyticum in the pathogenesis of preterm labor and PPROM. Amniotic fluid, amniotic membrane and placenta samples were taken in a sterile fashion at the time of Cesarean delivery, ensuring that the samples were representative of the actual uterine environment without vaginal contamination. The study reported that 43.9% (58/132) of the patients undergoing Cesarean delivery following preterm labor and PPROM had tissue or amniotic fluid samples positive for U urealyticum infection. This is compared to 2.7% (2/75) of the control group who had a positive identification of U urealyticum at Cesarean delivery.[136] The study was interesting in that it showed that there was not a significant difference between the prevalence of U urealyticum in the patients with preterm labor and those with PPROM. This suggests that the microbes were present prior to rupture, and play a role in the initiation of preterm labor and PPROM and do not simply result from it. Other work has shown that invasion of the amnion by an infective agent may precede PPROM well before the clinical manifestation of infection.[127] Thus, current evidence supports the conclusion that infection of the amnionic cavity is not dependant upon, nor does it by necessity follow, the rupture of the fetal membranes. This offers clinicians the potential to prevent PPROM through the use of antimicrobial therapy.

To further support the association of infection to membrane rupture, it has been shown that treatment of infected women with antibiotics decreased the rate of PPROM.[135] It has also been shown that in women with PROM without labor, the initiation of antimicrobial treatment reduced maternal and neonatal morbidity and mortality.[137] Thus, antimicrobial therapy is a relevant management of PPROM.

An additional insight can be gained from a study of U urealyticum showing an association of infection with this microbe to the development of spontaneous abortion.[138] This association suggests that the role of infection may be to initiate a powerful inflammatory cascade, which ultimately results in the untimely initiation of parturition as well as the rupture of the fetal membranes. It has been demonstrated previously that cytokines play significant roles in the normal development of ovulation, implantation and parturition,[139,140] which makes it is reasonable to deduce that an exaggeration of cytokine expression may result in the pathology of such processes. Infection, and other conditions, may then serve as catalysts of a detrimental inflammatory environment, leading to the degradation and weakening of the fetal membranes. Finding the exact mechanisms through which inflammation has its effect on membrane integrity is an important step to fully understanding PPROM.

Normally during labor and parturition there is an increase in the inflammatory cytokines TNF-α and IL-1β. It has also been shown that placental tissue following PROM is associated with increased expression of proinflammatory cytokines compared to tissue obtained after normal delivery. In one such study IL-2, IL-12 and interferon-γ were measured, and were shown to be expressed in both the placenta of patients with preterm delivery and PPROM at a higher level than in controls.[141] Increases in cytokine levels have previously been shown to play a role in the weakening of the fetal membranes by inducing apoptosis, and increasing MMP-1 and MMP-3 expression levels.[142] Work done by Kumar et al[116] described the experimental weakening of healthy fetal membranes obtained from elective Cesarean section after in vitro exposure to high concentrations of TNFα and IL-1B. In this study, the weakening of the membranes, when exposed to TNF-α and IL-1β, were demonstrated by measuring the work required to obtain membrane rupture using modified industrial rupture testing equipment. The results of the study showed that the higher the cytokine concentration the membranes were exposed to in culture then the smaller the degree of work required to obtain rupture of the membranes. Additionally, this study demonstrated the expression patterns of MMP-9, TIMP-3 and PARP-1 when exposed to TNF-α in culture. TNF-α increased the expression of MMP-9 and PARP-1 (a marker of apoptosis) in a dose-dependant manner, and

simultaneously decreased the expression of TIMP-3 in a similar fashion. This study not only demonstrates the role inflammation in the development of PPROM but also implicates the influence of the proinflammatory cytokines on the control of expression of important biological mediators of membrane metabolism.

PARP, mentioned earlier for its induced expression in human placenta tissue following cytokine exposure, is an apoptotic nuclear enzyme. It is cleaved during the course of activation and is used as a marker of programmed cell death. Study of this enzyme has shown that apoptosis normally occurs at a greater rate in the section of fetal membrane overlying the internal cervical os than other membrane sites. Additionally, this enzyme's relative concentration has been shown to have an inverse linear relationship with membrane strength,[143] and concentrations are seen in higher amounts in the ZAM. Because of these observations, apoptosis is believed to be a part of the normal process of membrane rupture and, because if its role in membrane integrity, may contribute to the development and risk of premature rupture. Recent work evaluating the biochemical distinctions between preterm labor and PPROM found there to be multiple differences in regard to the pro-apoptotic pathways.[144,145] In one such study looking at pro-apoptotic pathways in PPROM, it was shown that there is a significant increase in the -670 AG genotype of Fas in those with PPROM compared with controls,[144] suggesting that a polymorphism in this molecule in the apoptotic cascade is associated with the development of membrane pathology. In another study, the membranes involved in PPROM, compared to those of preterm labor, showed an increase in mRNA (shown by quantitative PCR) of the p53 and bax genes, and an increase of IL-18 in amniotic fluid (each of which has pro-apoptotic effects). There was also seen an increase in Bcl-2 expression (an anti-apoptotic gene) in the preterm labor group when compared to PPROM.[145] It is interesting that, although inflammation is an inducer of apoptosis,[146] and that TNFα levels are increased in both preterm labor and PPROM, increased apoptosis is only seen in the one group. This suggests that there is a biochemical or genetic predisposition to premature rupture of fetal membranes, in regards to programmed cell death, which is distinct from other causes of preterm birth.

Apoptosis is clearly not the only result of increased cytokine exposure of the membranes; a much more extensively studied phenomenon is the upregulation of specific proteases. As mentioned previously, MMP (when left unchecked) function to cleave the ECM of the fetal membrane and leave the structure physically weaker than healthy tissue.[116]

The MMP families of proteins, along with the TIMP proteins, serve to develop equilibrium in the fetal membranes. During the development and growth of the fetus there is an interplay of these two classes of proteins, which allows for remodeling, growth, and the eventual natural rupture of the membranes. After a continual increase in the synthetic processes of the ECM, production and growth of the ECM peaks at around 20 weeks of gestation;[123,147] after such time there is an increase in the processes of membrane degradation, seen as a change in quantity and strength of the ECM. The degradation of the ECM occurs specifically to an increased expression and activity of several MMPs. For example, MMP-1 and MMP-8 are key to the cleavage of fibrillar collagens,[121] and are termed the interstitial collagenases. The gelatinases consist of MMP-2 and MMP-9, expression of which leads to the eventual degradation of type IV collagen, fibronectin, and proteoglycans.[147] The primary source of MMP and tissue inhibitors of metalloproteinases is the dominant fibroblastic layer of the amnion,[121] which suggest a regulatory function of this tissue layer. The control mechanisms of MMP expression are currently a topic of research, which may give us insight into the ultimate control of fetal membrane integrity and function.

One such mechanism is that of TNF-α and IL-1B influence on membrane strength. It was discussed earlier that increasing concentrations of these two cytokines in culture with healthy fetal membranes (obtained from Cesarean section) increase the expression of MMP-9 and decrease the expression of TIMP in a dose-dependant fashion,[116] showing the responsiveness of MMP expression to inflammation. Another mechanism is that of thrombin-induced expression of MMP-1 and MMP-3, which offers an explanation as to how placental abruption leads to the premature rupture of fetal membranes.[148]

Overall, the changes in MMP/TIMP concentration ratios – an increase in MMP with a parallel suppression of TIMP – represent an imbalance in an important physiologic process, and makes rupture of the fetal membranes more likely to occur.[149] This imbalance has not only been shown to develop from the presence of cytokines, but has also been shown to be associated with the detection of decreased expression of TIMP-3 as gestation advances.[150] This finding suggests that programmed expression patterns favor weakening of the membranes near term, which then allows rupture to occur and may precipitate premature rupture. Another study looking to assess the utility of genome-wide survey analysis in the context of PROM used a microarray experiment to demonstrate a deficiency of proteinase inhibitor 3 in individuals with PROM compared to those with preterm deliveries and intact membranes.[151]

Due to its association with PPROM, researchers have been also been interested in using MMP as a marker for subsequent PPROM. In one such study there was an association found with MMP-8 and PPROM, but not one that yielded any clinical usefulness. The association was with MMP-8 concentrations above the 90th percentile and subsequent PPROM.[152] This showed a clear role of MMP-8 in PROM but did not give any additional information. Although these and other interesting associations are being made to PPROM, there still remain many unanswered questions regarding causation. There also has yet to be determined a genetic screen to predict future PROM despite the growing number of such associations.

Fetal membrane integrity is dependant upon structurally sound collagen (and other matrix components) with the appropriate structure and helical arrangements (see discussion on ECM). When conditions are present which weaken the collagen matrix, PPROM is an event that occurs with greater frequency. In addition to increased degradation by proteases, the collagen matrix may be reduced due to disruptions in collagen metabolism, which prevents full expression[153] and other structural abnormalities in morphology. For example, it has been shown that women with recurrent PPROM are more likely to have a connective tissue abnormality of dermal tissue, as seen by optic microscopy, and electron microscopy, compared to women with uncomplicated pregnancies, and compared to nonpregnant women. This abnormality is described as follows.

Collagen bundles appeared thin, separated from each other, and little interconnected. The distribution of elastic fibers was anarchic with clumps of thicker, irregularly shaped fibers interspersed with other foci containing only thin and delicate elastic fibers. Deposits of acidic proteoglycans were occasionally found in the reticular dermis.[154] These changes were described by the authors as being an Ehlers-Danlos-like dermal abnormality. The dysfunction that they describe is one interesting example of how inherited collagen abnormalities, even though not otherwise evident, may yet play a role in the premature rupture of membranes.

A recent report revealed that a polymorphism in the *SERPINH1* gene, which encodes heat shock protein 47, a chaperone that directly influences collagen production, is associated with risk of PPROM in African Americans.[155] The risk allele is located in the *SERPINH1* promoter and reduces promoter activity, which would lead to less HSP47 and consequently less amnion collagen and thus weakened fetal membranes.

Another interesting look at collagen integrity and balance is with the influence of ascorbic acid and its variable availability during gestation. The concentration of vitamin C naturally declines in women during pregnancy, which probably occurs due to a hemodilutional effect and active transport of the vitamin to the fetus.[156] This decline is normal and does not appear to have any adverse affects on the pregnancy. Ascorbic acid consumption by the body is also increased in response to intrauterine or vaginal infections (both of which are independent risk factors for PPROM), which contributes to a potentially significant nutritional deficit. This consumption of ascorbic acid in response to the oxidative respiratory burst by leukocytes may lead to a significant reduction in available vitamin for maintenance of the collagen matrix in the fetal membranes. Casanueva et al[157] found that when ascorbic acid was supplemented into the diet of pregnant women there was a significant decrease in PPROM compared to controls. This finding further substantiates the role that normal collagen synthesis and maintenance plays in membrane integrity.[157]

LOX, which cross-links collagen and elastin bundles, could play a significant role in its integrity and maintenance. It has been shown that the maternal blood level of copper (the co-factor for LOX) is lower when PROM occurred compared with controls.[158] Additionally, cadmium exposure from cigarette smoke, which induces metalothionein expression, would reduce copper availability, as potentially reducing LOX activity and as a result collagen coss-linking. These are yet other mechanisms that effect the structure of the collagen matrix and could contribute to risk of PPROM.

One effect infection has on the maintenance of the fetal membrane is to expose it to a large amount of reactive oxygen species (ROS) secondary to the recruitment, and respiratory bursts, of leukocytes. In such instances, the anti-oxidant ascorbic acid is depleted, which leads to an effective nutritional deficit. Interestingly, the administration of vitamin C to pregnant women has been shown to decrease the rate of PPROM significantly. This is likely due to the oxidative stress caused by an ascending infection[130] and the resulting damage to the collaginous matrix. Evidence suggests a beneficial role of vitamins C and E to prevent the rupture of membranes.[159] Other treatments include the administration of n-acetylcysteine, which further serves to prevent excessive oxidative stress.

Research has recently been performed to assess the protective role of vitamin C against ROS-induced apoptosis.[160] This work showed that Hydrogen peroxide (serving as the ROS) induced apoptosis in amnionderived WISH cells. This occurred, however, even after incubating the cells with vitamin C. Presumably, the protective effect of vitamin C is not in the prevention of apoptosis but rather by facilitating ECM regeneration after physiologic turnover. And so the administration of ascorbic acid for the prevention of PROM may only

have application in those populations where nutritional deficiencies are common.

Imbalance of the MMP concentrations is not only seen in the context of inflammation, but there is also a genetic predisposition which increases the concentration of this significant protease. Both the expression of MMP-1 and MMP-9 have been linked to polymorphisms that not only lead to increased expression of the enzymes but also to an association with PPROM.[161,162] The most significant single genetic factor involved in the development of PPROM appears to be a polymorphism of the TNF-α cytokine.

The polymorphism predominantly described is the TNF-2 (-308A) polymorphism, which has been shown to cause a higher production of TNF-α than in individuals with the major allele.[163] It is assumed that this increased production of cytokine leads to an exadurated response to infection or stress partly due to the observations that those with this allele experience greater complications when infected with human papilloma virus, cerebral malaria, mucocutaneous leishmaniasis, and sepsis.[164–167] Studies have shown that the -308A allele was found in a significantly higher proportion of women who underwent preterm birth[168] and PPROM[169] than in controls.

Another inducer of MMP production is the systemic hormone relaxin. Relaxin is produced by the corpus luteum of pregnancy, which functions to remodel and allow the reproductive tissues to accommodate the pregnancy, and to allow for the delivery of the fetus.[170] In addition to the corpus luteum, relaxin production occurs in the decidua and placenta, where it has been implicated in the pathophysiology and development of PPROM. This mechanism has been proposed by Bryant-Greenwood et al[170] to be similar to the development and rupture of the follicle where both systems (ovulation and parturition) are controlled with similar endocrine and paracrine mechanisms, are nonreversible, and take place within a closed environment. Because of these similarities, work was performed to assess the role of relaxin in the development of the rupture of fetal membranes by in vitro incubation of the membranes with relaxin. This study showed a dose-dependant increase in expression of MMP-1, MMP-3, and MMP-9[171,172] within the membrane tissue when exposed to relaxin. Others have shown that relaxin expression was not increased in term membranes or in membranes exposed to chorioamnionitis, showing that its expression is relatively specific to the clinical presentation of PPROM.[173]

The most intuitive causes of PROM are those caused by trauma, or as complications of a procedure. The risks of amniocentesis, fetoscopy, chorionic villus sampling (CVS), and a variety of other intra-amniotic procedures include a clinical rupture of the fetal membranes. Most often the rupture caused by the procedure is resolved through normal regeneration of the tissue layers and supporting collagen matrix. However, it the defect is in association with an underlying predisposition for rupture the defect may be unable to be resolved. One of the mechanisms associated with traumatic rupture of membranes, other than the production of a primary defect, is exemplified by thrombin's effects following placental abruption.

Thrombin, in addition to its role in the coagulation cascade, is an activator of MMP-3.[174] Following decidual hemorrhage, thrombin begins to play this role by binding to protease-activated membrane receptors (PAR) to initiate the synthesis and secretion of the MMP. This occurs at the membrane level but also through the recruitment of neutrophils to the area by the expression of IL-8, a potent neutrophil chemoattractant.[148] The consequent migration into the decidual layer allows the protease-rich neutrophils to serve as an important factor in the membranes loss of integrity. Thus, trauma can not only lead to localized defects in the membrane but it also contributes to the interplay of the homeostatic proteins responsible for maintenance of the fetal membranes. Interestingly, in a study of thrombin's effects on the integrity of the fetal membranes, addition of progestin's had a protective effect. When exposure to relaxin and MMP was then analyzed, it was shown that the protective function of the progestin was overcome, and ultimately membrane integrity was compromised.

SUMMARY

Uterine cervix remodeling occurs in three phases: cervical softening of early gestation, cervical ripening in late gestation, and in a final phase occurring in labor and delivery. Recent studies indicate that MMP-1 is produced by human cervical cells. The timing and activation of leukocytes that migrate into the cervix during gestation in a murine model suggests a role for MMP in postpartum remodeling, but not remodeling prior to parturition or even during labor. Further progress in the complete understanding of cervical remodeling will only occur by careful correlative studies by physicians-scientists, biomechanical engineers and matrix biologists. The roles of proteoglycans, especially HA and decorin (a small dermatan sulfate), in prepartum cervical remodeling should be further elucidated.

The fetal membranes during gestation undergo extensive remodeling and growth in order to accommodate the growing fetus, while maintaining the tensile strength required to contain the fetus and amniotic fluid throughout. Then, as gestation progresses to term, the membranes undergo physiologic and histological changes in a location-specific manner which allows for their timely and spontaneous rupture. These processes occur in response to a variety of complex signals and pathways, including those of hormonal and developmental origins. In addition to these fundamental actions and responses, the membranes appear to function as a protective barrier to the fetus from ascending infection. Much of what we know about the normal processes of parturition and rupture of membranes, however, comes from the study of its pathology. Thus, a more detailed discussion of the mechanisms of membrane rupture will be entertained in the context of PPROM.

There are many predisposing conditions to the development of PPROM – cytokine gene variants, increased proteolytic activity, decreased concentration or availability of nutritional factors, inherited collagen pathology – when introduced to the environment of infection, inflammation, or stress, leading to the rupture of the fetal membranes. A case in point is that of TNF-α and its upregulation. TNF-α is synthesized in a pro-form that is not biologically active. This pro-form requires cleavage by a TNF-α converting enzyme in order to be activated. Having this level of control on the activation of TNFα allows for the possibility of environmental cues to help regulate the activity of the cytokine (i.e. gene–environment interactions). Thus, the potential for increased production of key proteins resulting from genetic polymorphisms may not be sufficient to create an exaggerated response; it may require the additional cues of infection or inflammation.[163,175]

REFERENCES

1. Alberts B, Johnson A, Lewis J et al. In: Anon, ed. Molecular Biology of the Cell. New York: Garland Science, Taylor & Francis Group, 2002; 1065–127.
2. Kleissl HP, van der Rest M, Naftolin F, Glorieux FH, de Leon A. Collagen changes in the human uterine cervix at parturition. Am J Obstet Gynecol 1978; 130(7): 748–53.
3. Kao KY, Leslie JG. Polymorphism in human uterine collagen. Connect Tissue Res 1977; 5(2): 127–9.
4. Leppert PC, Yu SY. Three-dimensional structures of uterine elastic fibers: scanning electron microscopic studies. Connect Tissue Res 1991; 27(1): 15–31.
5. Kokenyesi R, Armstrong LC, Agah A, Artal R, Bornstein P. Thrombospondin 2 deficiency in pregnant mice results in premature softening of the uterine cervix. Biol Reprod 2004; 70(2): 385–90.
6. Langevin HM, Cornbrooks CJ, Taatjes DJ. Fibroblasts form a body-wide cellular network. Histochem Cell Biol 2004; 122(1): 7–15.
7. Leppert PC. The biochemistry and physiology of the uterine cervix during gestation and parturition. Prenat Neonatal Med 1998; 3: 103–6.

8. Ricard-Blum S, Ruggiero F. The collagen superfamily: from the extracellular matrix to the cell membrane. Pathol Biol 2005; 53(7): 430–42.

9. Uldbjerg N, Forman A, Peterson LK et al. Biomechanical and biochemical changes of the uterus and cervix during pregnancy. In: Anon, ed. Medicine of the Fetus and Mother. Philadelphia: JB Lippincott Co, 1992; 849–69.

10. Yu SY, Leppert PC, Leppert PC, Woessner F. The collagenous tissue of the cervix during pregnancy. In: Anon, ed. The Extracellular Matrix of the Uterus, Cervix and Fetal Membranes. Ithaca: Perinatology Press, 1991; 68–76.

11. Petersen LK, Uldbjerg N. Cervical collagen in non-pregnant women with previous cervical incompetence. Eur J Obstet Gynecol Reprod Biol 1996; 67(1): 41–5.

12. Kokenyesi R, Tan L, Robbins JR, Goldring MB. Proteoglycan production by immortalized human chondrocyte cell lines cultured under conditions that promote expression of the differentiated phenotype. Arch Biochem Biophys 2000; 383(1): 79–90.

13. Camenisch TD, McDonald JA. Hyaluronan: is bigger better? Am J Respir Cell Mol Biol 2000; 23(4): 431–3.

14 Iozzo RV. The family of the small leucine-rich proteoglycans: key regulators of matrix assembly and cellular growth. Crit Revi Biochem Mol Biol 1997; 32(2): 141–74.

15. Kokenyesi R, Woessner Jr JF. Effects of hormonal perturbations on the small dermatan sulfate proteoglycan and mechanical properties of the uterine cervix of late pregnant rats. Connect Tissue Res 1991; (3): 199–205.

16. Kokenyesi R, Woessner Jr JF. Relationship between dilatation of the rat uterine cervix and a small dermatan sulfate proteoglycan. Biol Reprod 1990; 42(1): 87–97.

17. Leppert PC, Kokenyesi R, Klemenich CA, Fisher J. Further evidence of a decorin-collagen interaction in the disruption of cervical collagen fibers during rat gestation. Am J Obstet Gynecol 2000; 182(4): 805–11; discussion 811–2.

18. Golichowski AM, King SR, Mascaro K. Pregnancy-related changes in rat cervical glycosaminoglycans. Biochem J 1980; 192(1): 1–8.

19. Straach KJ, Shelton JM, Richardson JA, Hascall VC, Mahendroo MS. Regulation of hyaluronan expression during cervical ripening. Glycobiology 2005; 15(1): 55–65.

20. Sandberg LB, Soskel NT, Leslie JG. Elastin structure, biosynthesis, and relation to disease states. N Engl J Med 1981; 304(10): 566–79.

21. Czirok A, Zach J, Kozel BA et al. Elastic fiber macro-assembly is a hierarchical, cell motion-mediated process. J Cell Physiol 2006; 207(1): 97–106.

22. Leppert PC, Cerreta J, Mandl I. The anatomical orientation of elastic fibers in the human uterine cervix. Am J Obstet Gynecol 1986; 155: 219–24.

23. Leppert PC, Yu SY, Keller S, Cerreta J, Mandl I. Decreased elastic fibers and desmosine content in incompetent cervix. Am J Obstet Gynecol 1987; 157(5): 1134–9.

24. Thomassin L, Werneck CC, Broekelman TJ et al. The proregions of lysyl oxidase-like 1 are required for deposition into elastic fibers. J Biol Chem 2005; 280: 42848–55.

25. Bornstein P. Thrombospondins as matricellular modulators of cell function. J Clin Invest 2001; 107(8): 929–34.

26. Alford AI, Hankenson KD. Matricellular proteins: Extracellular modulators of bone development, remodeling, and regeneration. Bone 2006 (in press).

27. Nagase H, Visse R, Murphy G. Structure and function of matrix metalloproteinases and TIMPs. Cardiovasc Res 2006; 69(3): 562–73.

28. Sluijter JP, de Kleijn DP, Pasterkamp G. Vascular remodeling and protease inhibition – bench to bedside. Cardiovasc Res 2006; 69(3): 595–603.

29. Reuben PM, Cheung HS. Regulation of matrix metalloproteinase (MMP) gene expression by protein kinases. Front Biosci 2006; 11: 1199–215.

30. Yoshida M, Sagawa N, Itoh H et al. Prostaglandin F(2alpha), cytokines and cyclic mechanical stretch augment matrix metalloproteinase-1 secretion from cultured human uterine cervical fibroblast cells. Mol Hum Reprod 2002; 8(7): 681–7.

31. Watari M, Watari H, Fujimoto T et al. Lipopolysaccharide induces interleukin-8 production by human cervical smooth muscle cells. J Soc Gynecol Invest 2003; 10(2): 110–17.

32. Guo H, Zucker S, Gordon MK, Toole BP, Biswas C. Stimulation of matrix metalloproteinase production by recombinant extracellular matrix metalloproteinase inducer from transfected Chinese hamster ovary cells. J Biol Chem 1997; 272(1): 24–7.

33. Vincenti MP, Brinckerhoff CE. Transcriptional regulation of collagenase (MMP-1, MMP-13) genes in arthritis: integration of complex signaling pathways for the recruitment of gene-specific transcription factors. Arthritis Res 2002; 4(3): 157–64.

34. Suzuki K, Enghild JJ, Morodomi T, Salvesen G, Nagase H. Mechanisms of activation of tissue procollagenase by matrix metalloproteinase 3 (stromelysin). Biochemistry 1990; 29(44): 10 261–70.

35. Chung L, Dinakarpandian D, Yoshida N et al. Collagenase unwinds triple-helical collagen prior to peptide bond hydrolysis. EMBO J 2004; 23(15): 3020–30.

36. Pham DN, Chu HW, Martin RJ, Kraft M. Increased matrix metalloproteinase-9 with elastolysis in nocturnal asthma. Ann Allergy Asthma Immunol 2003; 90(1): 72–8.

37. Jeyabalan A, Kerchner LJ, Fisher MC et al. Matrix metalloproteinase-2 activity, protein, mRNA and tissue inhibitors in small arteries from pregnant and relaxin-treated nonpregnant rats. J Appl Physiol Respir Environ Exercise Physiol 2006; 100: 1955–63.

38. Curry Jr TE, Osteen KG. The matrix metalloproteinase system: changes, regulation, and impact throughout the ovarian and uterine reproductive cycle. Endocr Rev 2003; 24(4): 428–65.

39. Danforth DN. The distribution and functional activity of the cervical musculature. Am J Obstet Gynecol 1954; 68(5): 1261–71.

40. Leppert PC, Cerreta JM, Mandl I. Orientation of elastic fibers in the human cervix. Am J Obstet Gynecol 1986; 155(1): 219–24.

41. von Maillot K, Stuhlsatz HW, Mohanaradhakrishnan V, Greiling H. Changes in the glycosaminoglycans distribution pattern in the human uterine cervix during pregnancy and labor. Am J Obstet Gynecol 1979; 135(4): 503–6.

42. Leppert PC, Yu SY. Apoptosis in the cervix of pregnant rats in association with cervical softening. Gynecol Obstet Invest 1994; 37(3): 150–4.

43. Leppert PC. Proliferation and apoptosis of fibroblasts and smooth muscle cells in rat uterine cervix throughout gestation and the effect of the antiprogesterone onapristone. Am J Obstet Gynecol 1998; 178(4): 713–21.

44. Allaire AD, D'Andrea N, Truong P, McMahon MJ, Lessey BA. Cervical stroma apoptosis in pregnancy. Obstet Gynecol 2001; 97(3): 399–403.

45. Zhao S, Fields PA, Sherwood OD. Evidence that relaxin inhibits apoptosis in the cervix and the vagina during the second half of pregnancy in the rat. Endocrinology 2001; 142(6): 2221–9.

46. Danforth DN, Veis A, Breen M et al. The effect of pregnancy and labor on the human cervix: changes in collagen, glycoproteins, and glycosaminoglycans. Am J Obstet Gynecol 1974; 120(5): 641–51.

47. Danforth DN. The fibrous nature of the human cervix and its relation to the isthmic segment in gravid and nongravid uteri. Am J Obstet Gynecol 1947; 53: 541–57.

48. Yu SY, Tozzi CA, Babiarz J, Leppert PC. Collagen changes in rat cervix in pregnancy – polarized light microscopic and electron microscopic studies. Proc Soc Exp Biol Med 1995; 209(4): 360–8.

49. Yellon SM, Mackler AM, Kirby MA. The role of leukocyte traffic and activation in parturition. J Soc Gynecol Invest 2003; 10(6): 323–38.

50. Timmons BC, Mahendroo MS. Timing of neutrophil activation and expression of proinflammatory markers do not support a role for neutrophils in cervical ripening in the mouse. Biol Reprod 2006; 74(2): 236–45.

51. Ramos JG, Varayoud J, Bosquiazzo VL, Luque EH, Munoz-de-Toro M. Cellular turnover in the rat uterine cervix and its relationship to estrogen and progesterone receptor dynamics. Biol Reprod 2002; 67(3): 735–42.

52. Takamoto N, Leppert PC, Yu SY. Cell death and proliferation and its relation to collagen degradation in uterine involution of rat. Connect Tissue Res 1998; 37(3–4): 163–75.

53. Kerr JF, Wyllie AH, Currie AR. Apoptosis: a basic biological phenomenon with wide-ranging implications in tissue kinetics. Br J Cancer 1972; 26(4): 239–57.

54. Esko JD, Lindahl V. Molecular diversity of heparin sulfate. J Clin Invest 2001; 108: 169–73.

55. Vuoristo MM, Pihlajamaa T, Vandenberg P et al. Complete structure of the human COL11A2 gene: the exon sizes and other features indicate the gene has not evolved with genes for other fibriller collagens. Ann NY Acad Sci 1996; 785: 343–4.

56. Myles MF. In: Anon, ed. Textbook for Midwives. Edinburgh: Churchill Linvingstone, 1975; 67.

57. Cabrol D, Jannet D, Le Houezec R et al. Mechanical properties of the pregnant human uterine cervix use of an instrument to measure the index of cervical distensibility. Gynecol Obstet Invest 1990; 29(1): 32–6.

58. Leppert PC. Anatomy and physiology of cervical ripening. Clin Obstet Gynecol 1995; 38(2): 267–79.

59. Winkler M. Role of cytokines and other inflammatory mediators. Br J Obstet Gynaecol 2003; 110 (Suppl 20): 118–23.

60. Stjernholm-Vladic Y, Stygar D, Mansson C et al. Factors involved in the inflammatory events of cervical ripening in humans. Reprod Biol Endocrinol 2004; 2(1): 74.

61. Calkins LA. On predicting the length of labor. Am J Obstet Gynecol 1941; 42(802).

62. Cocks DP. Significance of initial condition of cervix uteri to subsequent course of labour. BMJ 1955; 4909: 327–8.

63. Dutton WA. The assessment of the cervix at surgical induction. Canadian Med Assoc J 1958; 79(6): 463–7.

64. Friedman EA. Primigravid labor; a graphicostatistical analysis. Obstet Gynecol 1955; 6(6): 567–89.

65. Leppert PC. Cervical softening, effacement and dilation: a complex biochemical cascade. J Matem Fetal Med 1992; 1: 213–23.

66. O'Brien WF. Cervical ripening and labor induction: progress and challenges. Clin Obstet Gynecol 1995; 38(2): 221–3.

67. Romero R, Espinoza J, Erez O, Hassan S. The role of cervical cerclage in obstetric practice: can the patient who could benefit from this procedure be identified? Am J Obstet Gynecol 2006; 194(1): 1–9.

68. Iams JD, Goldenberg RL, Meis PJ et al. The length of the cervix and the risk of spontaneous premature delivery. National Institute of Child Health and Human Development Maternal Fetal Medicine Unit Network. New Engl J Med 1996; 334(9): 567–72.

69. Hassan SS, Romero R, Maymon E et al. Does cervical cerclage prevent preterm delivery in patients with a short cervix? Am J Obstet Gynecol 2001; 184(7): 1325–9; discussion 1329–31.

70. Havelock JC, Keller P, Muleba N et al. Human myometrial gene expression before and during parturition. Biol Reprod 2005; 72(3): 707–19.

71. Aspden RM. The theory of fibre-reinforced composite materials applied to changes in the mechanical properties of the cervix during pregnancy. J Theor Biol 1988; 130(2): 213–21.

72. Aspden RM. Collagen organisation in the cervix and its relation to mechanical function. Coll Rela Res 1988; 8(2): 103–12.

73. Fabvey S, Socrate S, House M. Biomechanical modeling of cervical tissue: a quantitiative investigation of cervical funneling. In: International Mechanical Engineering Congress and Exposition. Washington DC: 2003.

74. Petersen LK, Oxlund H, Uldbjerg N, Forman A. In vitro analysis of muscular contractile ability and passive biomechanical properties of uterine cervical samples from nonpregnant women. Obstet Gynecol 1991; 77(5): 772–6.

75. House M, Paskaleva A, Favey S, Myers K, Socrate S. The biomechanics of cervical funneling: the effect of stroma properties, anatomic geometry and pelvic forces on funnel formation. Am J Obstet Gynecol 2004; 191(6): 36.

76. House M, O'Callaghan M, Bahrami S et al. Magnetic resonance imaging of the cervix during pregnancy: effect of gestational age and prior vaginal birth. Am J Obstet Gynecol 2005; 193(4): 1554–60.

77. Drzewiecki G, Tozzi C, Yu SY, Leppert PC. A dual mechanism of biomechanical change in rat cervix in gestation and postpartum: applied vascular mechanics. Cardiovasc Eng 2005; 5: 187–93.

78. Kyriakides TR, Zhu YH, Smith LT et al. Mice that lack thrombospondin 2 display connective tissue abnormalities that are associated with disordered collagen fibrillogenesis, an increased vascular density, and a bleeding diathesis. J Cell Biol 1998; 140(2): 419–30.

79. Feltovich H, Ji H, Janowski JW et al. Effects of selective and nonselective PGE2 receptor agonists on cervical tensile strength and collagen organization and microstructure in the pregnant rat at term. Am J Obstet Gynecol 2005; 192(3): 753–60.

80. Buhimschi IA, Dussably L, Buhimschi CS, Ahmed A, Weiner CP. Physical and biomechanical characteristics of rat cervical ripening are not consistent with increased collagenase activity. Am J Obstet Gynecol 2004; 191(5): 1695–704.

81. Alfirevic Z. Cerclage: we all know how to do it but can't agree when to do it. Obstet Gynecol 2006; 107(2 Pt 1): 219–20.

82. Rust OA, Atlas RO, Jones KJ, Benham BN, Balducci J. A randomized trial of cerclage versus no cerclage among patients with ultrasonographically detected second-trimester preterm dilation of the internal os. Am J Obstet Gynecol 2000; 183(4): 830–5.

83. To MS, Alfirevic Z, Heath VC et al. Cervical cerclage for prevention of preterm delivery in women with short cervix: randomised controlled trial. Lancet 2004; 363(9424): 1849–53.

84. Althuisius SM, Dekker GA, Hummel P, Bekedam DJ, van Geijn HP. Final results of the Cervical Incompetence Prevention Randomized Cerclage Trial (CIPRACT): therapeutic cerclage with bed rest versus bed rest alone. Am J Obstet Gynecol 2001; 185(5): 1106–12.

85. Mazza E, Nava A, Bauer M et al. Mechanical properties of the human uterine cervix: an in vivo study. Med Image Anal 2006; 10(2): 125–36.

86. Garfield RE, Maul H, Maner W et al. Uterine electromyography and light-induced fluorescence in the management of term and preterm labor. J Soc Gynecol Investi 2002; 9(5): 265–75.

87. Fittkow CT, Maul H, Olson G et al. Light-induced fluorescence of the human cervix decreases after prostaglandin application for induction of labor at term. Eur J Obstet Gynecol Reprod Biol 2005; 123(1): 62–6.

88. Ophir J, Garra B, Kallel F et al. Elastographic imaging. Ultrasound Med Biol 2000; 26 (Suppl 1): S23–9.

89. Greenleaf JF, Fatemi M, Insana M. Selected methods for imaging elastic properties of biological tissues. Annu Rev Biomed Eng 2003; 5: 57–78.

90. Hiltawsky KM, Kruger M, Starke C et al. Freehand ultrasound elastography of breast lesions: clinical results. Ultrasound Med Biol 2001; 27(11): 1461–9.

91. Krouskop TA, Younes PS, Srinivasan S, Wheeler T, Ophir J. Differences in the compressive stress–strain response of infiltrating ductal carcinomas with and without lobular features – implications for mammography and elastography. Ultrason Imaging 2003; 25(3): 162–70.

92. de Korte CL, van der Steen AF. Intravascular ultrasound elastography: an overview. Ultrasonics 2002; 40(1–8): 859–65.

93. Souchon R, Rouviere O, Gelet A et al. Visualisation of HIFU lesions using elastography of the human prostate in vivo: preliminary results. Ultrasound Med Biol 2003; 29(7): 1007–15.

94. Takeda T, Kassab G, Liu J et al. A novel ultrasound technique to study the biomechanics of the human esophagus in vivo. Am J Physiol Gastrointest Liver Physiol 2002; 282(5): G785–93.

95. McFarlin B, O'Brien WD, Oelze ML, Zachary JF, White-Traut R. Quantitative ultrasound predicts cervical riepining in the rat. Am J Obstet Gynecol 2005; 196(6): s153–534.

96. Mackler AM, Iezza G, Akin MR, McMillan P, Yellon SM. Macrophage trafficking in the uterus and cervix precedes parturition in the mouse. Biol Reprod 1999; 61(4): 879–83.

97. Bokstrom H, Brannstrom M, Alexandersson M, Norstrom A. Leukocyte subpopulations in the human uterine cervical stroma at early and term pregnancy. Hum Reprod 1997; 12(3): 586–90.

98. Osmers R, Rath W, Adelmann-Grill BC et al. Origin of cervical collagenase during parturition. Am J Obstet Gynecol 1992; 166(5): 1455–60.

99. Chwalisz K, Garfeild RE. New molecular challenges in the induction of cervical ripening. Hum Reprod 1998; 13: 245–52.

100. Chwalisz K, Garfield RE. Role of nitric oxide in the uterus and cervix: implications for the management of labor. J Perinat Med 1998; 26(6): 448–57.

101. Buhimschi I, Ali M, Jain V, Chwalisz K, Garfield RE. Differential regulation of nitric oxide in the rat uterus and cervix during pregnancy and labour. Hum Reprod 1996; 11(8): 1755–66.

102. Stygar D, Wang H, Vladic et al. Increased level of matrix metalloproteinases 2 and 9 in the ripening process of the human cervix. Biol Reprod 2002; 67(3): 889–94.

103. Anderson J, Brown N, Mahendroo MS, Reese J. Utilization of different aquaporin water channels in the mouse cervix during pregnancy and parturition and in models of preterm and delayed cervical ripening. Endocrinology 2006; 147(1): 130–40.

104. Fujimoto T, Savani RC, Watari M, Day AJ, Strauss 3rd JF. Induction of the hyaluronic acid-binding protein, tumor necrosis factor-stimulated gene-6, in cervical smooth muscle cells by tumor necrosis factor-alpha and prostaglandin E(2). Am J Pathol 2002; 160(4): 1495–502.

105. Takemura M, Itoh H, Sagawa N et al. Cyclic mechanical stretch augments hyaluronan production in cultured human uterine cervical fibroblast cells. Mol Hum Reprod 2005; 11(9): 659–65.

106. Esplin MS, Fausett MB, Peltier MR et al. The use of cDNA microarray to identify differentially expressed labor-associated genes within the human myometrium during labor. Am J Obstet Gynecol 2005; 193(2): 404–13.

107. Huber A, Hudelist G, Czerwenka K et al. Gene expression profiling of cervical tissue during physiological cervical effacement. Obstet Gynecol 2005; 105(1): 91–8.

108. Mercer BM. Preterm premature rupture of the membranes. Obstet Gynecol 2003; 101(1): 178–93.

109. Polzin WJ, Brady K. The etiology of premature rupture of the membranes. Clin Obstet Gynecol 1998; 41(4): 810–16.

110. El Khwad M, Stetzer B, Moore RM et al. Term human fetal membranes have a weak zone overlying the lower uterine pole and cervix before onset of labor. Biol Reprod 2005; 72(3): 720–6.

111. Moore RM, Mansour JM, Redline RW, Mercer BM, Moore JJ. The physiology of fetal membrane rupture: insight gained from the determination of physical properties. Placenta 2006 (in press).

112. McLaren J, Taylor DJ, Bell SC. Increased incidence of apoptosis in non-labour-affected cytotrophoblast cells in term fetal membranes overlying the cervix. Hum Reprod 1999; 14(11): 2895–900.

113. McLaren J, Taylor DJ, Bell SC. Increased concentration of promatrix metalloproteinase 9 in term fetal membranes overlying the cervix before labor: implications for membrane remodeling and rupture. Am J Obstet Gynecol 2000; 182(2): 409–16.

114. Osman I, Young A, Jordan F, Greer IA, Norman JE. Leukocyte density and proinflammatory mediator expression in regional human fetal membranes and decidua before and during labor at term. J Soc Gynecol Invest 2006; 13(2): 97–103.

115. Arikat S, Novince RW, Mercer BM et al. Separation of amnion from choriodecidua is an integral event to the rupture of normal term fetal membranes and constitutes a significant component of the work required. Am J Obstet Gynecol 2006; 194(1): 211–17.

116. Kumar D, Fung W, Moore RM, Pandey V, Fox J, Stetzer B, et al. Proinflammatory cytokines found in amniotic fluid induce collagen remodeling, apoptosis, and biophysical weakening of cultured human fetal membranes. Biol Reprod 2006; 74(1): 29–34.

117. Hein S, Yamamoto SY, Okazaki K et al. Lysyl oxidases: expression in the fetal membranes and placenta. Placenta 2001; 22(1): 49–57.

118. Alexander JM, Cox SM. Clinical course of premature rupture of the membranes. Semin Perinatol 1996; 20(5): 369–74.

119. Ni CY, Jia WX, Yi WM, Feng LH, Yu LZ. Practicability of using vaginal fluid markers in detecting premature rupture of membranes. Ann Clin Biochem 2003; 40(Pt 5): 542–5.

120. Alexander JM, Mercer BM, Miodovnik M et al. The impact of digital cervical examination on expectantly managed preterm rupture of membranes. Am J Obstet Gynecol 2000; 183(4): 1003–7.

121. Parry S, Strauss 3rd JF Premature rupture of the fetal membranes. New Engl J Med 1998; 338(10): 663–70.

122. Schmidt W. The amniotic fluid compartment: the fetal habitat. Adv Anat Embryol Cell Biol 1992; 127: 1–100.

123. Casey ML, MacDonald PC. Interstitial collagen synthesis and processing in human amnion: a property of the mesenchymal cells. Biol Reprod 1996; 55(6): 1253–60.

124. Aagaard-Tillery KM, Nuthalapaty FS, Ramsey PS, Ramin KD. Preterm premature rupture of membranes: perspectives surrounding controversies in management. Am J Perinatol 2005; 22(6): 287–97.

125. Malak TM, Bell SC. Differential expression of the integrin subunits in human fetal membranes. J Reprod Fertil 1994; 102(2): 269–76.

126. McLaren J, Malak TM, Bell SC. Structural characteristics of term human fetal membranes prior to labour: identification of an area of altered morphology overlying the cervix. Hum Reprod 1999; 14(1): 237–41.

127. McParland PC, Taylor DJ, Bell SC. Myofibroblast differentiation in the connective tissues of the amnion and chorion of term human fetal membranes – implications for fetal membrane rupture and labour. Placenta 2000; 21(1): 44–53.

128. Lee T, Carpenter MW, Heber WW, Silver HM. Preterm premature rupture of membranes: risks of recurrent complications in the next pregnancy among a population-based sample of gravid women. Am J Obstet Gynecol 2003; 188(1): 209–13.

129. Regan JA, Chao S, James LS. Premature rupture of membranes, preterm delivery, and group B streptococcal colonization of mothers. Am J Obstet Gynecol 1981; 141(2): 184–6.

130. Romero R, Mazor M. Infection and preterm labor. Clin Obstet Gynecol 1988; 31(3): 553–84.

131. Ekwo EE, Gosselink CA, Woolson R, Moawad A. Risks for premature rupture of amniotic membranes. Int J Epidemiol 1993; 22(3): 495–503.

132. Goldenberg RL, Hauth JC, Andrews WW. Intrauterine infection and preterm delivery. New Engl J Med 2000; 342(20): 1500–7.

133. Gomez R, Romero R, Ghezzi F et al. The fetal inflammatory response syndrome. Am J Obstet Gynecol 1998; 179(1): 194–202.

134. Alger LS, Lovchik JC, Hebel JR, Blackmon LR, Crenshaw MC. The association of Chlamydia trachomatis, Neisseria gonorrhoeae, and group B streptococci with preterm rupture of the membranes and pregnancy outcome. Am J Obstet Gynecol 1988; 159(2): 397–404.

135. McGregor JA, French JI, Parker R et al. Prevention of premature birth by screening and treatment for common genital tract infections: results of a prospective controlled evaluation. Am J Obstet Gynecol 1995; 173(1): 157–67.

136. Witt A, Berger A, Gruber CJ et al. Increased intrauterine frequency of Ureaplasma urealyticum in women with preterm labor and preterm premature rupture of the membranes and subsequent cesarean delivery. Am J Obstet Gynecol 2005; 193(5): 1663–9.

137. Mercer BM, Arheart KL. Antimicrobial therapy in expectant management of preterm premature rupture of the membranes. Lancet 1995; 346(8985): 1271–9.

138. Joste NE, Kundsin RB, Genest DR. Histology and ureaplasma urealyticum culture in 63 cases of first trimester abortion. Am J Clin Pathol 1994; 102(6): 729–32.

139. Bowen JM, Chamley L, Keelan JA, Mitchell MD. Cytokines of the placenta and extra-placental membranes: roles and regulation during human pregnancy and parturition. Placenta 2002; 23(4): 257–73.

140. Bowen JM, Chamley L, Mitchell MD, Keelan JA. Cytokines of the placenta and extra-placental membranes: biosynthesis, secretion and roles in establishment of pregnancy in women. Placenta 2002; 23(4): 239–56.

141. El-Shazly S, Makhseed M, Azizieh F, Raghupathy R. Increased expression of pro-inflammatory cytokines in placentas of women undergoing spontaneous preterm delivery or premature rupture of membranes. Am J Reprod Immunol 2004; 52(1): 45–52.

142. So T, Ito A, Sato T, Mori Y, Hirakawa S. Tumor necrosis factor-alpha stimulates the biosynthesis of matrix metalloproteinases and plasminogen activator in cultured human chorionic cells. Biol Reprod 1992; 46(5): 772–8.

143. McParland PC, Taylor DJ, Bell SC. Mapping of zones of altered morphology and chorionic connective tissue cellular phenotype in human fetal membranes (amniochorion and decidua) overlying the lower uterine pole and cervix before labor at term. Am J Obstet Gynecol 2003; 189(5): 1481–88.

144. Fuks A, Parton LA, Polavarapu S et al. Polymorphism of Fas and Fas ligand in preterm premature rupture of membranes in singleton pregnancies. Am J Obstet Gynecol 2005; 193(3 Pt 2): 1132–36.

145. Fortunato SJ, Menon R. Distinct molecular events suggest different pathways for preterm labor and premature rupture of membranes. Am J Obstet Gynecol 2001; 184(7): 1399–405; discussion 1405–6.

146. Menon R, Lombardi SJ, Fortunato SJ. TNF-alpha promotes caspase activation and apoptosis in human fetal membranes. J Assist Reprod Genet 2002; 19(4): 201–4.

147. Arias F, Gonzalez-Ruiz AR, Jacobson RL. Recent advances in the pathophysiology and management of preterm premature rupture of the fetal membranes. Curr Opin Obstet Gynecol 1999; 11(2): 141–7.

148. Lockwood CJ, Toti P, Arcuri F et al. Mechanisms of abruption-induced premature rupture of the fetal membranes: thrombin-enhanced interleukin-8 expression in term decidua. Am J Pathol 2005; 167(5): 1443–9.

149. Edwards DR, Beaudry PP, Laing TD et al. The roles of tissue inhibitors of metalloproteinases in tissue remodelling and cell growth. Int J Obes Relat Metab Disord 1996; 20 (Suppl 3): S9–15.

150. Marvin KW, Keelan JA, Eykholt RL, Sato TA, Mitchell MD. Use of cDNA arrays to generate differential expression profiles for inflammatory genes in human gestational membranes delivered at term and preterm. Mol Hum Reprod 2002; 8(4): 399–408.

151. Tromp G, Kuivaniemi H, Romero R et al. Genome-wide expression profiling of fetal membranes reveals a deficient expression of proteinase inhibitor 3 in premature rupture of membranes. Am J Obstet Gynecol 2004; 191(4): 1331–8.

152. Biggio Jr JR, Ramsey PS, Cliver SP et al. Midtrimester amniotic fluid matrix metalloproteinase-8 (MMP-8) levels above the 90th percentile are a marker for subsequent preterm premature rupture of membranes. Am J Obstet Gynecol 2005; 192(1): 109–13.

153. Hampson V, Liu D, Billett E, Kirk S. Amniotic membrane collagen content and type distribution in women with preterm premature rupture of the membranes in pregnancy. Br J Obstet Gynaecol 1997; 104(9): 1087–91.

154. Hermanns-Le T, Pierard G, Quatresooz P. Ehlers-Danlos-like dermal abnormalities in women with recurrent preterm premature rupture of fetal membranes. Am J Dermatopathol 2005; 27(5): 407–10.

155. Wang H, Parry S, Macones G, et al. A functional SNP in the promoter of the SERPINH1 gene increases risk of preterm premature rupture of membranes in African Americans. Proc Natl Acad Sci USA 2006; 103(36): 13463–7.

156. Monsen ER. Dietary reference intakes for the antioxidant nutrients: vitamin C, vitamin E, selenium, and carotenoids. J Am Diet Assoc 2000; 100(6): 637–40.

157. Casanueva E, Ripoll C, Tolentino M et al. Vitamin C supplementation to prevent premature rupture of the chorioamniotic membranes: a randomized trial. Am J Clin Nutr 2005; 81(4): 859–63.

158. Artal R, Burgeson R, Fernandez FJ, Hobel CJ. Fetal and maternal copper levels in patients at term and without premature rupture of membranes. Obstet Gynecol 1979; 53(5): 608–10.

159. Romero R, Chaiworapongsa T, Espinoza J. Micronutrients and intrauterine infection, preterm birth and the fetal inflammatory response syndrome. J Nutr 2003; 133(5 Suppl 2): 1668S–1673S.

160. Kumar D, Lundgren DW, Moore RM, Silver RJ, Moore JJ. Hydrogen peroxide induced apoptosis in amnion-derived WISH cells is not inhibited by vitamin C. Placenta 2004; 25(4): 266–72.

161. Fujimoto T, Parry S, Urbanek M et al. A single nucleotide polymorphism in the matrix metalloproteinase-1 (MMP-1) promoter influences amnion cell MMP-1 expression and risk for preterm premature rupture of the fetal membranes. J Biol Chem 2002; 277(8): 6296–302.

162. Ferrand PE, Parry S, Sammel M et al. A polymorphism in the matrix metalloproteinase-9 promoter is associated with increased risk of preterm premature rupture of membranes in African Americans. Mol Hum Reprod 2002; 8(5): 494–501.

163. Crider KS, Whitehead N, Buus RM. Genetic variation associated with preterm birth: a HuGE review. Genet Med 2005; 7(9): 593–604.

164. Hedberg CL, Adcock K, Martin J et al. Tumor necrosis factor alpha – 308 polymorphism associated with increased sepsis mortality in ventilated very low birth weight infants. Pediatr Infect Dis J 2004; 23(5): 424–8.

165. McGuire W, Hill AV, Allsopp CE, Greenwood BM, Kwiatkowski D. Variation in the TNF-alpha promoter region associated with susceptibility to cerebral malaria. Nature 1994; 371(6497): 508–10.

166. Cabrera M, Shaw MA, Sharples C et al. Polymorphism in tumor necrosis factor genes associated with mucocutaneous leishmaniasis. J Exp Med 1995; 182(5): 1259–64.

167. Kirkpatrick A, Bidwell J, van den Brule AJ et al. TNF alpha polymorphism frequencies in HPV-associated cervical dysplasia. Gynecol Oncol 2004; 92(2): 675–9.

168. Moore S, Ide M, Randhawa M et al. An investigation into the association among preterm birth, cytokine gene polymorphisms and periodontal disease. Br J Obstet Gynaecol 2004; 111(2): 125–32.

169. Roberts AK, Monzon-Bordonaba F, Van Deerlin PG et al. Association of polymorphism within the promoter of the tumor necrosis factor alpha gene with increased risk of preterm premature rupture of the fetal membranes. Am J Obstet Gynecol 1999; 180(5): 1297–302.

170. Bryant-Greenwood GD, Millar LK. Human fetal membranes: their preterm premature rupture. Biol Reprod 2000; 63(6): 1575–9.

171. Qin X, Chua PK, Ohira RH, Bryant-Greenwood GD. An autocrine/paracrine role of human decidual relaxin. II. Stromelysin-1 (MMP-3) and tissue inhibitor of matrix metalloproteinase-1 (TIMP-1). Biol Reprod 1997; 56(4): 812–20.

172. Qin X, Garibay-Tupas J, Chua PK, Cachola L, Bryant-Greenwood GD. An autocrine/paracrine role of human decidual relaxin. I. Interstitial collagenase (matrix metalloproteinase-1) and tissue plasminogen activator. Biol Reprod 1997; 56(4): 800–11.

173. Millar LK, Boesche MH, Yamamoto SY et al. A relaxin-mediated pathway to preterm premature rupture of the fetal membranes that is independent of infection. Am J Obstet Gynecol 1998; 179(1): 126–34.

174. Mackenzie AP, Schatz F, Krikun G et al. Mechanisms of abruption-induced premature rupture of the fetal membranes: thrombin enhanced decidual matrix metalloproteinase-3 (stromelysin-1) expression. Am J Obstet Gynecol 2004; 191(6): 1996–2001.

175. Macones GA, Parry S, Elkousy M et al. A polymorphism in the promoter region of TNF and bacterial vaginosis: preliminary evidence of gene-environment interaction in the etiology of spontaneous preterm birth. Am J Obstet Gynecol 2004; 190(6): 1504–8; discussion 3A.

9

Nitric oxide

Jane E Norman and Inass Osman

INTRODUCTION

Although the existence of the molecule nitric oxide (NO) – a single nitrogen molecule bound to a single oxygen molecule, which together forms a free radical gas – has been known for years, it was only with the publication of a series of papers in the 1980s that the biological importance of this mediator was appreciated. In 1980, Furchgott[1] showed that blood vessel endothelium actively released a factor which maintained vessels in a moderately dilated state. This factor was highly unstable, and its chemical properties were initially undefined. In view of its biological properties it was named endothelium-derived relaxing factor (EDRF). In the few years following, both Furchgott[2] and Ignarro[3] independently showed that EDRF was similar in its properties to NO. Thereafter, in 1987, Palmer et al[4] showed that EDRF released from endothelial cells by stimulation with bradykinin was found to have identical effects to NO on contraction of rat aorta that had been denuded of endothelium. Furthermore, the sensitivity of rat aorta to EDRF and to NO declined at similar rates, the half-life of both agents was identical, both were inhibited in a similar manner and amount by hemoglobin, and the activity of both was prolonged by superoxide dismutase. Lastly, L-arginine was the precursor to both NO and EDRF production. Thus, EDRF and NO are biologically and chemically identical. Ignarro et al[5] published similar results that same year, and Ignarro ultimately received the Nobel prize for medicine for his work on NO together with Furchgott and Murad.

NO is formed from L-arginine by one of three NO synthases (NOS) which convert L-arginine to NO and L-citrulline. L-citrulline can then be recycled back to L-arginine.[6,7] In blood vessel endothelium, NOS is activated by each of acetylcholine, bradykinin and shear stress. NO then diffuses into the smooth muscle cell underlying the blood vessel endothelium to activate soluble guanylate cyclase, generating cyclic guanosine monophosphate (GMP). Cyclic GMP activates protein kinases, which dephosphorylate myosin light chains and cause smooth muscle relaxation.

The three (known) forms of NOS are termed endothelial (e) NOS, neuronal (n) NOS (sometimes called brain (b) NOS) and inducible (i) NOS. As one might expect from its name, eNOS is the specific NOS present in the endothelium. Like nNOS, it is considered to be a constitutive enzyme that requires calcium as a cofactor, and generates small amounts of NO continuously.

The physiological effects of NO can be replicated pharmacologically by use of the class of drugs called NO donors. These are a heterogenous class of drugs which include the nitrosothiols, such as sodium nitroprusside (SNP) which releases NO spontaneously, and the organic nitrates, such as glyceryl trinitrate and isosorbide mono- or dinitrate, which require two distinct bioactivation pathways (one enzymatic and one nonenzymatic) for their conversion to NO.

iNOS, in contrast to eNOS and brain (b) NOS, is calcium independent.[5] Again, as its name suggests, it is not released constitutively, but is induced by inflammatory mediators such as lipopolysaccharide and cytokines. When iNOS is induced, it releases much larger amounts of NO than the constitutive isoforms. Physiologically, iNOS plays a major role in host defence. However, iNOS is also an important pathophysiological mediator. For example in septic shock associated with inflammation, iNOS is induced in both endothelial cells and in vascular smooth muscle cells. It also releases large quantities of NO, which activate guanylate cyclase in vascular smooth muscle, causing profound vasodilation leading to hypotension and shock. The induction of iNOS can be inhibited by glucocorticoids, and this is in part the mechanism by which glucocorticoids exert their anti-inflammatory action.

NO and the NO synthases have been proposed to have a variety of roles in the female reproductive system.[7–9] In this chapter, we focus on the role of NO in the inhibition and initiation of preterm labor.

NITRIC OXIDE (NO) IN THE INHIBITION OF PRETERM LABOR

Preliminary study showing use of NO donors as tocolytic agents

Interest in the role of NO as a potential tocolytic was sparked by the work of Lees and colleagues. They published a seminal paper in The Lancet in 1994 suggesting that NO might be an effective tocolytic agent with minimal side effects.[10] They recruited 13 women in preterm labor between 23 and 33 weeks of gestation. These 13 women had a total of 20 episodes of preterm labor in total. Women were defined to be in preterm labor if they had two or more painful uterine contractions in 10 min over a period of 1 h. Treatment was in the form of glyceryl trinitrate (GTN) patches applied to the laboring abdomen. Each of the GTN patches released 10 mg of GTN over the course of 24 h. If contractions did not stop after application of the first patch, a second patch was applied, up to a maximum of two patches in 24 h. Treatment was continued until contractions stopped.

Impressively, all 20 episodes of preterm labor responded to treatment, with an average prolongation of pregnancy of 34 days. Only one patient delivered during the index episode of preterm labor, but she was known to have cervical incompetence and had had a cervical suture removed immediately prior to GTN administration. Although her contractions ceased she still delivered – an event ascribed to cervical incompetence rather than inappropriate uterine activity. There were no adverse fetal effects identified amongst the eight babies who had delivered at the time of publication. Importantly, for a drug that is conventionally given to treat cardiac failure due to excessive preload and which is known to reduce blood pressure, only one woman became hypotensive. She quickly responded to removal of the patches and there were no other significant hemodynamic effects. One third of the women reported headache (again a known side effect of NO donors) but there were no other adverse effects. Although this was an uncontrolled trial, in a clinical condition notoriously difficult to diagnose confidently unless preterm delivery does occur, these data are strongly suggestive that NO donors might prove to be useful tocolytic agents in clinical practice.

Inhibitory effects of NO donors on myometrial contractility in vitro

Further support for the rationale that NO donors might be useful tocolytic agents has emerged from animal studies. In 1993, Yallampalli et al[11] showed that the NO donor sodium nitroprusside, in a concentration of 5 mM, completely abolished the spontaneous contractions of myometrium taken from pregnant rats in vitro. These data suggested that NO donors might be useful pharmacologically as tocolytic agents. They also showed that this pharmacological action of NO donors might mirror physiological events inhibiting uterine contractions in vivo. For example, when L-arginine was added to myometrium removed from pregnant rats, spontaneous contractile activity again declined. These inhibitory effects of L-arginine were abolished by concomitant addition of the NOS inhibitor L-nitro L-arginine methyl ester (L-NAME). Together these data suggest that rat myometrium is able to convert L-arginine to a uterine relaxant, and thus the pregnant rat uterus must contain enzymes with this capability. Since a specific inhibitor of NO synthesis inhibits the enzyme synthesis, it implies that the endogenous enzyme generating a tocolytic is NOS. The fact that NOS is enzymatically active in vitro is evidenced by the demonstration that the NO inhibitor L-NAME stimulated myometrial contractions in vitro, suggesting release from the endogenous inhibitory activity of NO.

Animal studies on the change in endogenous NO synthase activity during pregnancy

The contractility data described above were strongly suggestive that the pregnant uterus generates NO. Subsequently, several studies explored whether NOS activity changes in the uterus with advancing gestation and labor onset. In rabbits, Sladek et al[12] showed that both the decidua and myometrium possessed NOS activity – assessed using the arginine to citrulline conversion assay – at mid–late gestation. Activity was higher in the decidua than the myometrium. In rabbits, NOS activity declined progressively from 27 days of gestation to 30–31 days of gestation (term). Indeed, by the last day of pregnancy, NOS activity was reduced to 20% of the level found at 27 days of gestation. Although the specific isoform of NOS was not formally identified, the fact that it was calcium insensitive suggested that it was iNOS. This decline in NOS activity at the end of pregnancy suggested a role for endogenous NO production in maintaining uterine quiescence during pregnancy, and that at term, as myometrial contractions start, in part, due to release from the suppressive effects of NO. In addition to a role for NO in controlling the timing of parturition in the rabbit pregnancy shown above, a role for increased NO production contributing to uterine quiescence has also been shown in the mouse, rat, guinea pig[13] and in the sheep.[14]

Animal studies on the effect of nitric oxide (NO) inhibition on pregnancy length

If NO production is important in the maintenance of pregnancy, and if a physiological decline in NO contributes to the onset of parturition, one might expect that pharmacological inhibition of NO would initiate preterm delivery. There is good evidence, again from animal studies, that this is the case. For example, pregnant mice were given L-NAME at varying concentrations up to a maximum of 100 mg/kg.[15] Treatments were administered 3–4 days before the end of pregnancy on day 15 and day 16 of gestation. A progressive increase in the proportion of animals delivering preterm was identified with increasing doses of L-NAME. With the larger doses of L-NAME, over 60% of animals delivered preterm (P < 0.01 compared with the control group). Laparotomy of the animals postdelivery showed that preterm delivery was of the entire litter. In a second series of experiments, when the NO donor sodium nitroprusside (10 µg/kg/min) was administered 5 h prior to, and during, the L-NAME infusion (70 mg/kg), preterm delivery was completely abolished. Importantly, there was no evidence of any maternotoxicity of L-NAME. Fetal effects were not described, although other studies have shown that L-NAME can inhibit fetal growth.[16] Together, these data suggest that NO plays a role in regulation of myometrial contractility during pregnancy, and that inhibition of NO production can trigger preterm delivery. Preterm delivery can be prevented in this scenario with exogenously applied NO donors.

ROLE OF NITRIC OXIDE (NO) IN THE MAINTENANCE OF HUMAN PREGNANCY

So what about human pregnancy? We have shown expression of each of the isoforms of NOS in human pregnant uterus by immunohistochemistry. We also quantified NOS activity via the arginine to citrulline conversion assay to determine whether activity levels changed with the onset of labor. We found that although there was NOS activity in each of the myometrium, fetal membranes and the placenta, activity levels were identical comparing levels before and after the onset of labor at term (Table 9.1).[17] Interestingly, on a weight-for-weight basis, there was more NOS activity in placenta than fetal membranes, and more in the fetal membranes than in the myometrium. We later found that eNOS and bNOS protein expression was greater in preterm pregnant myometrium compared with nonpregnant myometrium.[18] Additionally, there was a decline in eNOS but not bNOS protein expression at term. Bansal et al[19] sampled myometrium from nonpregnant women, pregnant women in the early third trimester (both before and after the onset of labor), and pregnant women at term (both before and after labor).[16] Using Western blotting to iNOS, they found greatest expression in the preterm not in labor group compared with all the other groups.

Taken together, these data suggest that the myometrium has the capacity to generate increased amounts of NO during pregnancy, and that this increased production of NO is likely to contribute to uterine quiescence during pregnancy. In contrast to some animal studies, there is no acute change in NO production at the time of the onset of labor at term. Therefore, it seems unlikely that NO regulation plays a role in the timing of the onset of labor. In preterm parturition, it may be that NO levels decline acutely, and this process is likely to contribute to, if not intitiate, the process of parturition.

CONTRACTILITY EXPERIMENTS IN HUMAN MYOMETRIUM

So does NO have a relaxant effect on human myometrium? Following studies in rat myometrium described above, Buhimschi et al[20] showed similar dose-dependent inhibitory effects of NO on contractility of human myometrium.[17] These data support the work of Lees et al,[7] which suggest that exogenously applied

Table 9.1 Nitric oxide synthase (NOS) activity in human uterine tissues before and after the onset of parturition. (Data from Thomson et al, Hum Reprod 1997; 12: 2546–52)

Tissue	Activity before labor onset (fmol/min/mg protein)	Activity after labor onset (fmol/min/mg protein)
Myometrium	<1	<1
Fetal membranes	5	9
Placenta	520	420

NO might be useful as a tocolytic. However, more detailed experiments by the same group also showed that myometrium removed from women in spontaneous labor was in fact less sensitive to the tocolytic effects of NO donors than myometrium removed prior to the onset of labor.[17] Thus, in the very situation where preterm delivery is to be prevented (that of preterm labor) the efficacy of NO donors in causing uterine relaxation is least (Table 9.2).

Whatever the efficacy, the NO donor used by Buhimschi et al[17] is unsuitable for use in vivo. We therefore undertook a study to examine the efficacy of two commonly available NO donor drugs – glyceryl trinitrate and isosorbide mononitrate (IMN) – on contractions of human myometrium.[21] Both agents inhibited the amplitude of contractions of myometrium in a dose-dependent manner, although they were less effective on a molar basis than other potential tocolytic agents such as calcium-channel blockers and potassium-channel openers. So, the NO donors appear to have potential efficacy as tocolytic agents in vivo. One of their attractive features is that NO appears to be an endogenous product of human myometrium and placenta, which is likely to contribute to uterine quiescence. Thus, the use of a NO donor as a tocolytic agent might augment a physiological agent by pharmacological means.

A potential concern about the use of NO donors is their cardiovascular effect in vivo. NO donors are powerful vasodilators, and there is a potential concern that this could be hazardous to both mother and baby during pregnancy. However, available studies have been reassuring on this issue. We gave the NO donor IMN vaginally and measured maternal and fetal heart rate, and maternal blood pressure over the next few hours. Although there was a significant increase in both the maternal and fetal heart rate, and a significant decline in maternal blood pressure, none of these effects were clinically significant, i.e. none of these changes were sufficient to cause concern.[22] There have now been a number of studies looking at the effect of NO donors, administered either in patch or other forms, on uterine, umbilical and fetal middle cerebral arterial blood flow. These studies have largely shown no effect on Doppler parameters of blood flow.[22,23] Indeed, in a small number of studies, normally when fetal blood flow is restricted, e.g. in conditions such as pre-eclampsia, or physiologically in the second trimester, the use of NO donors was associated with a small (10–2.5%) improvement in fetal blood flow.[24]

A potentially more serious concern about the use of NO donors as tocolytic agents (particularly when applied in patch form) is their likely inefficacy on uterine contractions in vivo. In vitro studies have shown that the molar concentration of glyceryl trinitrate required to effect a 10% reduction in myometrial contractions is around 10^{-7} M. When glyceryl trinitrate is applied as a patch, the maximum serum concentration reached is in the order of 200 ng/ml, which is around 10^{-9} M. Thus, assuming the sensitivity of myometrium is similar in vivo and in vitro, around 100 patches would have to be applied simultaneously to effect a 10% reduction in contraction amplitude. In reality, the likely efficacy of NO donor patches may be even less, since the clinical situation in which NO donors are to be applied is one of labor, and, as described above, the sensitivity of myometrium to tocolytic agents is less when in labor than prior to the onset of labor.[17]

So despite the encouraging results of the uncontrolled Lees et al[7] study, in vitro data suggest that the clinical efficacy of NO donors might be poor. Five randomized trials have now been conducted comparing the efficacy of NO donors, either with placebo or with other tocolytic agents, of which four have been published.[24–28] A meta-analysis of these studies was conducted by Duckitt and Thornton.[29] Only one small study is included in the meta-analysis of NO donors

---

Table 9.2 Effect of diethylamine/nitric oxide on in vitro contractions of myometrial strips from nonpregnant, pregnant and laboring women. (Data from Buhimschi et al, Am J Obstet Gynecol 1995; 172: 1577–84)

	Nonpregnant	Pregnant	Labor
Concentration required to inhibit contractility by 10%	5×10^{-7} M	5×10^{-8} M	10^{-6} M
Concentration required to inhibit contractility by 50%	10^{-5} M	10^{-6} M	1.5×10^{-5} M
Concentration required to inhibit contractility by 90%	$>10^{-4}$ M	$>10^{-4}$ M	$>10^{-4}$ M

versus placebo: this shows no difference between the groups in any maternal or fetal outcomes, and indeed shows a trend towards placebo being more effective in prolonging pregnancy for more than 48 h [odds ratio (OR) 3.06 (0.74–12.63)].[28]

Four studies are included in the comparison of NO donors versus alternative tocolytic agents, with the comparators being albuterol (one study),[25] ritodrine (two studies),[27] and magnesium sulfate (one study).[26] In this comparison, NO donors were in fact more effective than the alternative in preventing preterm delivery before 37 weeks of gestation – OR of delivery 0.53 (0.35–0.81).

However, for the more clinically relevant outcomes of delivery before 34 weeks, delivery within 48 h and delivery within 24 h, and for all the fetal outcomes, there was no difference between the two groups. So this meta-analysis does not demonstrate any evidence that NO donors are likely to be clinically useful tocolytic agents (Table 9.3).

Since this meta-analysis was conducted, a further trial of glyceryl trinitrate versus β sympathomimetic agents has been published.[30] The size of this trial (over 230 subjects) is comparable with the biggest single trial in the published meta-analysis. The study was analysed on an intention-to-treat basis, but women in the NO donor group were given rescue therapy if they failed to stop contracting within 24 h. The primary outcome in this study was the interval between treatment and delivery; there were no differences between the treatment groups in this outcome. However, when a survival curve was constructed, comparing the proportion of women in each group who had neither delivered nor needed rescue treatment on each day after recruitment, it became obvious that those in the β sympathomimetic arm fared better than those in the NO donor arm. Thus, the evidence so far, both from in vitro work and from randomized clinical trials, does not support the use of NO donors as tocolytic agents.

NITRIC OXIDE (NO) AND THE CERVIX

Role of NO in the physiology of cervical ripening

In normal labor at term, it is now known that the cervix ripens progressively and slowly over the last 6 weeks or so at the end of pregnancy before labor begins at term.[31] Prostaglandins are known to be crucially important in this process, and indeed are used pharmacologically to ripen the cervix prior to induction of labor at term.

In contrast to effects on the myometrium, where NO may promote pregnancy prolongation, data which has emerged over the last 10 years suggests that NO may promote cervical ripening and delivery.

Nakatsuka et al[32] had previously shown that NO levels were elevated in the amniotic fluid of women with chorioamnionitis. In a subsequent study, they examined levels of nitrate and nitrite, the breakdown product of NO, in vaginal fluid. Women were collected in the presence or absence of preterm labor, and with or without preterm ruptured membranes. Those in preterm labor were then subdivided according to whether or not they subsequently delivered at term.

Table 9.3 Efficacy of nitric oxide donors in preventing preterm delivery. (Data from Duckitt and Thornton, Cochrane Database Syst Rev 2002; CD002860)

Outcome	Comparison	Odds ratio	95% Confidence interval (CI)
Prolongation of pregnancy >48 h	Placebo versus NO donors	3.06	0.74–12.63
Prolongation of pregnancy >48 h	NO donor versus alternative tocolytic	1.43	0.47–4.37
Prevention of delivery before 37 weeks of gestation	NO donor versus alternative tocolytic	0.53	0.35–0.81
Prevention of delivery before 34 weeks of gestation	NO donor versus alternative tocolytic	0.69	0.43–1.13
Use of mechanical ventilation of neonate	NO donor versus alternative tocolytic	0.39	0.1–1.57

Vaginal nitrite and nitrate levels were low in women destined to deliver at term, even if they were sampled in threatened preterm labor. Nitrate and nitrite levels were higher in women who delivered preterm, and highest in those presenting with preterm premature ruptured membranes who subsequently delivered preterm. If we assume that the increase in nitrate/nitrite found in vaginal fluid is a consequence of NO production, these data show that the cervix produces increased amounts of NO in concert with premature cervical ripening leading to preterm delivery.

These data accord with our own data showing a role for endogenous NO production in the cervical ripening which occurs in association with parturition at term. We took cervical biopsies from four cohorts of women: a nonpregnant group at the time of hysterectomy, a group of women in the first trimester of pregnancy undergoing pregnancy termination, a group of women prior to the onset of labor at term, and a group of women in labor at term (both of the latter two groups were delivered by Cesarean section).[33] Each of the isoforms of NOS was localized by immunohistochemistry. Concentration of each of the NOS isoforms was assessed by Western blotting. We found that iNOS activity was higher at the end of pregnancy than either in the first trimester or in the nonpregnant state. There was no further increase in NOS expression after the onset of labor. eNOS was greater in the third trimester (in both laboring and nonlaboring samples) compared with nonpregnant samples. bNOS was greater at all stages of pregnancy compared with nonpregnant samples. These data are in broad agreement with those of Tschugguel et al[34] – who found an increase in iNOS in postpartum compared with nonpregnant samples – and Bao et al[35] – who found an increase in bNOS protein expression in labor. Patterns of NOS expression in term in-labor samples compared to term not-in-labor samples were less consistent, but one isoform (eNOS) was greater in term in-labor samples compared with term not-in-labor samples. Very recent data demonstrates increased endogenous NO production in cervical ripening associated with preterm parturition. Tornblom et al[36] took biopsies from the cervix of women at term (both in labor and not in labor) and from women preterm (again both in labor and not in labor). Each of the three isoforms of NOS was greater in the cervix of women in preterm labor, compared with labor at term.

Taken together, these data imply that increased NO production is involved in the progressive cervical ripening which occurs in the last part of the third trimester of pregnancy. However, increased NO does not appear to occur in the very final process of cervical ripening and cervical dilation that occurs during labor. In preterm labor, the cervix has to change rapidly from a very unripened state to a ripened state, and in this situation NO production is increased.

Use of NO donors to ripen the cervix in the first trimester

In support of these data on endogenous NO synthesis, data from our own group and others suggests that NO applied pharmacologically can induce cervical ripening. Since the method used to assess cervical ripeness clinically, the Bishop score, is relatively subjective with large standard errors, we and others have used the calculation of cervical resistance to further dilation as a marker of cervical ripeness. In a study of the first trimester of pregnancy, we compared cervical resistance to dilation up to 8 mm after treatment with each of the NO donors glyceryl trinitrate and IMN, to gemeprost (a prostaglandin analog), and to a control group who had no treatment.[37] Resistance to dilation was lower in each of the NO donor groups compared to placebo, implying that each agent had induced cervical ripening. Resistance to dilation was least in the gemeprost group, implying that in the formulations and doses used, NO donors were less effective in cervical ripening than prostaglandins. The combination of NO donor and prostaglandin, although superficially attractive to maximize efficacy and minimize side effects, does not in our hands appear to have any advantages over the use of prostaglandin alone,[38] although others have found synergy between the two agents.[39]

Clinical use of NO donors as cervical ripening agents in the third trimester

Paradoxically, the cervical ripening effects of NO donors are a further reason why these agents may be inappropriate and ineffective as tocolytic agents: unless the drug can be delivered to the myometrium without being delivered to the cervix, the tocolytic effects of NO donors on the myometrium may be accompanied by premature cervical ripening, which may itself lead to preterm delivery.

However, the cervical ripening effects of NO donors are potentially useful clinically prior to the induction of labor. Ekerhovd et al[40] assessed the effect of IMN on cervical resistance at term pregnancy, and found that the force required to dilate the cervix was reduced by 60% following its application.[40]

We and others have speculated that NO donors might be the ideal cervical ripening agent.[41,42] The uterine contractile effects of prostaglandins can restrict uterine blood flow during ripening, leading to fetal compromise in vulnerable babies. In contrast, NO donors do not cause uterine contractions, and, as described above, promote rather than reduce uterine blood flow. Thus, the risk of fetal compromise during NO-induced cervical ripening is low, obviating the need for continuous external fetal monitoring.

We undertook a study (the 'PRIM' study) comparing the relative efficacy and side-effect profile of NO donors and prostaglandins for pre-induction cervical ripening at term.[43] The study was designed to test the hypothesis that both agents were equally effective for cervical ripening, but that NO donors would have fewer side effects. Four hundred women were randomized to receive either dinoprostone 2 mg in two doses 16 h apart or IMN 40 mg in two doses given 16 h apart. Each drug was given vaginally. We found that both agents improved the Bishop score over baseline levels. However, prostaglandins were faster than NO donors in improving the Bishop score, so that at 16 and 24 h, respectively, the mean difference in change in modified Bishop scores between the two groups was 0.94 [95% confidence interval (CI) (0.60–1.28)] and 1.45 (95% CI 0.95–1.95), respectively, in favor of dinoprostone. After up to two doses of study treatment, 59% of women in the IMN group and 87% of women in the prostaglandin group did not need any additional ripening agent (Table 9.4).

Regarding adverse effects, there was a significantly greater number of abnormal fetal heart rate tracings in the prostaglandin E_2 (PGE$_2$) group during the ripening phase compared with the IMN group [13 (6.5%) compared with 0 (0%), P = 0.002]. There was one woman who had vaginal bleeding in the PGE$_2$ group, with none in the IMN group. No woman had uterine hypertonus and no woman had hypotension requiring treatment. Headache was the most common side effect in the IMN group (88% compared with 10% in the PGE$_2$ group, P < 0.001), and abdominal/pelvic pain the most common side effect in the PGE$_2$ group (79% compared with 16% in the IMN group, P < 0.0001). Mean maternal satisfaction was significantly greater in the IMN group (P < 0.001). There was no significant difference in mode of delivery or fetal outcome between the two groups.

These data suggest that NO donors are likely to be clinically useful as cervical ripening agents. Whilst not as rapidly effective as prostaglandins in the dose and regimen used here, their side-effect profile is such that they, but probably not prostaglandins, could be used for cervical ripening on an outpatient basis. We are currently conducting a randomized trial comparing IMN with placebo for pre-induction outpatient cervical ripening at term (ISRCTN no. 39772441) to address this issue.[44]

SUMMARY

In summary, it appears that endogenous NO production is important in both human and animal pregnancy in maintaining uterine quiescence and prolonging pregnancy. If NO production is inhibited artificially, preterm labor and delivery ensues. It is not clear whether a decline in endogenous NO production is implicated in the mechanism of the pathophysiological situation of preterm labor.

Initial studies suggested that NO donors such as IMN might be therapeutically useful in the prevention of preterm parturition because of their smooth muscle relaxant effect. However, meta-analyses of randomized trials have failed to show any beneficial effect. In vitro work shows that laboring myometrium is least sensitive to the relaxant effects of NO donors, such that large concentrations would be required to achieve a clinically useful reduction in contractility (Table 9.5). Furthermore, given the effect of NO on the cervix, any beneficial effect of NO donors in inhibiting premature myometrial activation might be offset by their stimulatory role on cervical ripeness.

Regarding the cervix, it appears that an increase in NO production is involved in the physiology of cervical ripening in humans and in animals. NO donors may be useful cervical ripening agents in clinical practice, but further work is required to determine their appropriate place and the optimum regimen for clinical work.

ACKNOWLEDGMENTS

We acknowledge the work of our colleagues and collaborators without whom the work quoted in this paper would not have been possible: Dr Andrew Thomson,

Table 9.4 Efficacy of each of isosorbide mononitrate (IMN) 40 mg (up to two doses) and dinoprostone 2 mg (up to two doses) in ripening the cervix before induction of labor. (Data from Osman et al, Am J Obstet Gynecol 2006; 194)

	IMN group	Dinoprostone group
Ripening achieved with study drug	118/200 (59%)	175/200 (88%)
Ripening achieved with study drug ± a single rescue dose of 1 mg prostaglandin	193/200 (97%)	200/200 (100%)

Table 9.5 Therapeutic uses of nitric oxide (NO) donors in parturition

	Compared with placebo	Compared with alternative agent
Prevention of preterm delivery	Not effective	Some evidence of prevention of late preterm delivery No evidence of prevention of early preterm delivery No evidence of neonatal benefit Effect on cervical ripening further limits use
Cervical ripening	Effective	Less rapidly effective in doses used NO donors may have fewer side effects Further research needed

Dr MarieAnne Ledingham, Dr Joan Telfer, Dr Tony Nicoll, Mrs Anne Young, Mrs Fiona Jordan, Dr Fiona Mackenzie, Mr John Norrie, Professor Ian A Greer, and Professor Iain T Cameron. We also thank the charities and governmental bodies who have funded our work: Wellbeing, SHERT, Tenovus, The Sir Jules Thorn Charitable Trust and the Medical Research Council.

REFERENCES

1. Furchgott RF, Zawadzki JV. The obligatory role of endothelial cells in the relaxation of arterial smooth muscle by acetylcholine. Nature 1980; 288: 373–6.
2. Martin W, Villani GM, Jothianandan D, Furchgott RF. Selective blockade of endothelium-dependent and glyceryl trinitrate-induced relaxation by hemoglobin and by methylene blue in the rabbit aorta. J Pharmacol Exp Ther 1985; 232(3): 708–16.
3. Ignarro LJ, Lippton H, Edwards JC et al. Mechanism of vascular smooth muscle relaxation by organic nitrates, nitrites, nitroprusside and nitric oxide: evidence for the involvement of S-nitrosothiols as active intermediates. J Pharmacol Exp Ther 1981; 218(3): 739–49.
4. Palmer R, Ferrige A, Moncada S. Nitric oxide release accounts for the biological activity of endothelium-derived relaxing factor. Nature 1987; 327: 524–6.
5. Ignarro LJ, Buga GM, Wood KS et al. Endothelium-derived relaxing factor produced and released from artery and vein is nitric oxide. Proc Natl Acad Sci USA 1987; 84: 9265–9.
6. Moncada S, Higgs A. The L-arginine–nitric oxide pathway. New Engl J Med 1993; 329: 2002–12.
7. Norman J. Nitric oxide and the myometrium. Pharmacol Ther 1996; 70: 91–100.
8. Norman J, Cameron I. Nitric oxide in the human uterus. Rev Reprod 1996; 1: 61–8.
9. Ledingham M, Thomson A, Greer I et al. Nitric oxide in pregnancy and parturition. Br J Obstet Gynaecol 2000; 107: 581–93.
10. Lees C, Campbell S, Jauniaux E et al. Arrest of preterm labour and prolongation of gestation with glyceryl trinitrate, a nitric oxide donor. Lancet 1994; 343: 1325–6.
11. Yallampalli C, Izumi H, Byam-Smith M et al. An L-arginine–nitric oxide–cyclic guanosine monophosphate system exists in the uterus and inhibits contractility during pregnancy. Am J Obstet Gynecol 1993; 170: 175–85.
12. Sladek S, Regenstein A, Lykins D et al. Nitric oxide synthase activity in pregnant rabbit uterus decreases on the last day of pregnancy. Am J Obstet Gynecol 1993; 169: 1285–91.
13. Weiner C, Lizasoain I, Baylis S et al. Induction of calcium-dependent nitric oxide synthases by sex hormones. Proc Natl Acad Sci USA 1994; 91: 5212–16.
14. Figueroa J, Massmann G. Estrogen increases nitric oxide synthase activity in the uterus of nonpregnant sheep. Am J Obstet Gynecol 1995; 173: 1539–45.
15. Tiboni G, Giampietro F. Inhibition of nitric oxide synthesis causes preterm delivery in the mouse. Hum Reprod 2001; 15: 1838–43.
16. Tiboni G, Giampietro F, Lamonaca D. The soluble guanylate cyclase inhibitor methylene blue evokes preterm delivery and fetal growth restriction in a mouse model. In vivo 2001; 15: 333–8.
17. Thomson A, Telfer J, Kohnene G et al. Nitric oxide synthase activity and localisation do not change in uterus and placenta during human parturition. Hum Reprod 1997; 12: 2546–52.
18. Norman J, Thomson A, Telfer J et al. Myometrial constitutive nitric oxide synthase expression is increased during human pregnancy. Mol Hum Reprod 1999; 5: 175–81.
19. Bansal R, Goldsmith P, He Y et al. A decline in myometrial nitric oxide synthase expression is associated with labor and delivery. J Clin Invest 1997; 99: 2502–8.
20. Buhimschi I, Yallampalli C, Dong Y-L et al. Involvement of a nitric-oxide guanosine monophosphate pathway in control of human uterine contractility during pregnancy. Am J Obstet Gynecol 1995; 172: 1577–84.
21. Norman J, Ward L, Martin W et al. Effects of cGMP and the nitric oxide donors glyceryl trinitrate and sodium nitroprusside on contractions in vitro of isolated myometrial tissue from pregnant women. J Reprod Fertil 1997; 110: 249–54.
22. Nicoll A, Mackenzie F, Greer I et al. Vaginal application of the nitric oxide donor isosorbide mononitrate for pre-induction cervical ripening: a randomised controlled trial to determine effects on maternal and fetal haemodynamics. Am J Obstet Gynecol 2001; 184: 958–64.
23. Kahler C, Schleussner E, Moller A et al. Nitric oxide donors: effects on fetoplacental blood flow. Eur J Obstet Gynecol Reprod Biol 2004; 115: 10–14.

24. Luzi G, Caserta G, Iammarino G et al. Nitric oxide donors in pregnancy: fetomaternal hemodynamic effects induced in mild pre-eclampsia and threatened preterm labor. Ultrasound Obstet Gynecol 1999; 14: 101–9.

25. Bisits A, Masden G, McLean M et al. Corticotrophin-releasing hormone: a biochemical predictor of preterm delivery in a pilot randomised trial of the treatment of preterm labor. Am J Obstet Gynecol 1998; 178: 862–6.

26. El-Sayed Y, Riley E, Holbrook R et al. Randomised comparison of intravenous nitroglycerin and magnesium sulfate for treatment of preterm labor. Obstet Gynecol 1999; 93: 79–83.

27. Lees CC, Lojacono A, Thompson C et al. Glyceryl trinitrate and ritodrine in tocolysis: an international multicenter randomized study. GTN Preterm Labour Investigation Group. Obstet Gynecol 1999; 94: 403–8.

28. Smith G, Walker M, McGrath M. Randomised, double-blind, placebo controlled pilot study assessing nitroglycerin as a tocolytic. Br J Obstet Gynaecol 1999; 106: 736–9.

29. Duckitt K, Thornton S. Nitric oxide donors for the treatment of preterm labour. Cochrane Database Syst Rev 2002; CD002860.

30. Bisits A, Madsen G, Knox M et al. The Randomized Nitric Oxide Tocolysis Trial (RNOTT) for the treatment of preterm labor. Am J Obstet Gynecol 2004; 191: 683–90.

31. Calder A. The cervix during pregnancy. In: Chard T, Grudzinskas J, eds. The Uterus. Cambridge: Cambridge University Press, 1994; 288–307.

32. Nakatsuka M, Habara T, Kamada Y et al. Elevation of total nitrite and nitrate concentration in vaginal secretions as a predictor of premature delivery. Am J Obstet Gynecol 2000; 182: 644–5.

33. Ledingham M, Thomson A, Macara L et al. Changes in the expression of nitric oxide synthase in the human uterine cervix during pregnancy and parturition. Mol Hum Reprod 2000; 6: 1041–8.

34. Tschugguel W, Schneeberger C, Lass H et al. Human cervical ripening is associated with an increase in cervical inducible nitric oxide synthase expression. Biol Reprod 1999; 60: 1367–72.

35. Bao S, Rai J, Schreiber J. Brain nitric oxide synthase expression is enhanced in the human cervix in labor. J Soc Gynecol Invest 2001; 8: 158–64.

36. Tornblom SA, Maul H, Klimaviciute A et al. mRNA expression and localization of bNOS, eNOS and iNOS in human cervix at preterm and term labour. Reprod Biol Endocrinol 2005; 3: 33.

37. Thomson A, Lunan C, Cameron A et al. Nitric oxide donors induce ripening of the human uterine cervix: a randomised controlled trial. Br J Obstet Gynaecol 1997; 104: 1054–7.

38. Ledingham M, Thomson A, Lunan C et al. A comparison of isosorbide mononitrate, misoprostol and combination therapy for first trimester pre-operative cervical ripening: a randomised controlled trial. Br J Obstet Gynaecol 2000; 108: 276–80.

39. Eppel W, Facchinetti F, Schleussner E et al. Second trimester abortion using isosorbide mononitrate in addition to gemeprost compared with gemeprost alone: a double-blind randomized, placebo-controlled multicenter trial. Am J Obstet Gynecol 2005; 192: 856–61.

40. Ekerhovd E, Bullarbo M, Andersch B et al. Vaginal administration of the nitric oxide donor isosorbide mononitrate for cervical ripening at term: a randomized controlled study. Am J Obstet Gynecol 2003; 189: 1692–7.

41. Norman J, Thomson A, Greer I. Cervical ripening after nitric oxide. Hum Reprod 1998; 13: 251–2.

42. Calder A. Nitric oxide – another factor in cervical ripening. Hum Reprod 1998; 13: 250–1.

43. Osman I, Mackenzie F, Norrie J et al. The 'PRIM' study: a randomised comparison of prostaglandin E2 gel with the nitric oxide donor isosorbide mononitrate for cervical ripening before the induction of labor at term. Am J Obstet Gynecol 2006; 194: 1012–21.

44. Bollapragada S, Mackenzie F, Norrie J et al. IMOP: Randomised placebo controlled trial of outpatient cervical ripening with isosorbide mononitrate (IMN) prior to induction of labour – clinical trial with analyses of efficacy, cost effectiveness and acceptability. BMC Pregnancy Childbirth. 2006; 6(1): 25 [Epub ahead of print].

10

Relaxin-related preterm birth

Gerson Weiss and Laura T Goldsmith

PREMATURITY

The mechanisms involved in normal parturition are not completely understood. Less well understood are the mechanisms responsible for the timing of parturition. The time at which parturition occurs is tightly controlled, to ensure optimal survival of the newborn. There are multiple causes of preterm birth. The proximal causes of preterm birth may be different than the causes of normally timed parturition, even if the final common pathways are similar. By way of example, prematurity due to polyhydramnios, cocaine use, infection or preterm membrane rupture likely have different mechanisms, even though final pathways for uterine contractions and cervical dilation may be similar.

It is now clearly documented that singleton pregnancies that result from assisted reproductive technologies (ART) or superovulation by gonadotropin therapy have double the rate of preterm birth of natural conceptions.[1–3] Figure 10.1 shows the results of a meta-analysis of multiple studies defining the risk of preterm delivery in singleton pregnancies after gonadotropin stimulation.[1] While results in individual studies vary, it can clearly be seen that there is an overall and marked shift to the right, with the relative risk of singleton preterm delivery after gonadotropin stimulation twice that of naturally conceived, singleton pregnancies. In the current report, we summarize the data which demonstrate the relationship between relaxin and preterm delivery due to ovulation induction with gonadotropins. These data show a dramatic increase in circulating relaxin levels throughout ART pregnancies compared to relaxin concentrations in spontaneous ovulation pregnancies. In addition, the data indicate that there is a linear correlation between hyperrelaxinemia and preterm delivery. We herein also discuss some of the mechanisms by which relaxin may contribute to preterm delivery.

RELAXIN

Relaxin is a peptide hormone with structural similarity to insulin. In women, relaxin is produced by many structures, including the corpus luteum, placenta, decidua, brain, cardiac atrium and mammary gland. However, all of the circulating relaxin detected during the late luteal phase and throughout pregnancy is produced by the corpus luteum.[4,5] The corpus luteum is viable, structurally intact and endocrinologically functional for the entire duration of human pregnancy. The human corpus luteum of pregnancy continues to produce relaxin throughout the entire pregnancy.[4,5]

Relaxin has many biological actions. Among these are alterations of connective tissue, vasodilatation and increase in leukocyte infiltration.[6,7] Relaxin aids in maternal accommodation to pregnancy, and results in reproductive tract alterations which facilitate pregnancy and, ultimately, delivery. We have shown that ovulation induction using human menopausal gonadotropin (hMG), as is used in ART, results in a greater than three-fold increase in circulating relaxin.[8,9] This is due to the increased number of corpora lutea induced by exogenous human follicle-stimulating hormone (hFSH). More corpora lutea result in increased relaxin secretion. There is a further increase in circulating relaxin levels in multiple pregnancies,[10,11] since multiple pregnancies result in a greater level of human chorionic gonadotropin (hCG), which is the stimulus for luteal production of relaxin.[12] Of these two factors, hCG and luteal number, the number of corpora lutea is the more significant factor responsible for elevated circulating relaxin levels.[13]

Maternal circulating relaxin is of luteal origin and is present throughout the entire duration of pregnancy, from the end of the luteal phase to the time of delivery.[4,5] In ovum-donation pregnancies, which have no corpora

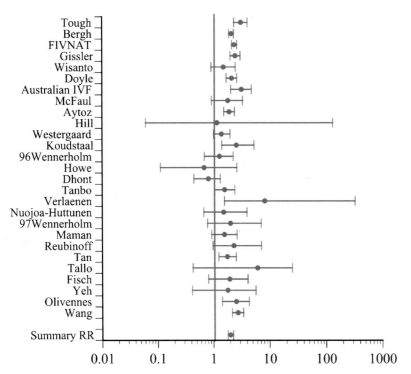

Figure 10.1 Meta-analysis of the relative risk of preterm birth in singleton pregnancies resulting from in vitro fertilization-embryo transfer or gamete intrafallopion transfer. Relative risks (RR) and confidence intervals for each study are shown. (From McGovern et al, Fertil Steril 2004; 82: 1514–20.)

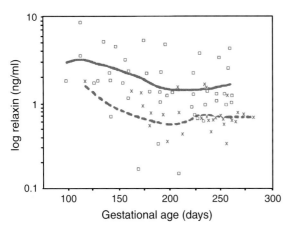

Figure 10.2 Circulating maternal relaxin concentrations throughout singleton pregnancies in women who conceived after gonadotropin stimulation (open squares, solid line) and women who conceived naturally with no stimulation (×s, dashed line). Note: Relaxin is plotted as a log scale. (From Mushayandebvu et al, Obstet Gynecol 1998; 92: 17–20.)

lutea, circulating relaxin is not detectable.[14,15] The only sources of relaxin in ovum-donation pregnancies are local uterine production of relaxin from the decidua and placenta. Lutectomy during mid-pregnancy results in a complete loss of circulating relaxin. Circulating relaxin concentrations peak in the mid–late first trimester, and then stabilize with a slight decrease for the duration of pregnancy.[5] Following this pattern of secretion, levels of relaxin, which are elevated in the first trimester, decline slightly towards the second trimester but remain elevated throughout the remainder of pregnancy, as shown in Figure 10.2.[16]

RELAXIN AND PRETERM BIRTH

To determine whether the marked hyperrelaxinemia seen in ART pregnancies is related to preterm birth, relaxin was measured at 6–12 weeks of pregnancy, and pregnancy outcomes were determined.[17] When there are elevated relaxin levels in the first trimester, relaxin levels remain elevated throughout the duration of pregnancy.[16] Two groups of women were studied, a group achieving pregnancy after ovarian stimulation by hFSH ($n = 114$) and a group achieving pregnancy without treatment ($n = 37$). Fetal number was determined by transvaginal ultrasound. Preterm delivery was determined from the obstetric record. Circulating maternal relaxin concentrations were measured using a specific human relaxin enzyme-linked immunosorbent assay. Hyperrelaxinemia was defined as greater than three standard deviations above the weighted mean of levels in normal, unstimulated singleton pregnancies at 6–12 weeks of gestation. First trimester weighted mean serum relaxin concentrations in unstimulated pregnancies was 1.18 ± 0.69 ng/ml (M $\pm$ SEM), three standard deviations above this mean is 3.25 ng/ml, which we used as the upper limit of normal relaxin levels. The results of this study can be seen in Figure 10.3. Triplets, twins and singleton deliveries are stacked in this 'jitter plot' in which the horizontal axis is relaxin levels, and 3.25 ng/ml is the dotted vertical line. Open circles represent term deliveries and closed circles represent preterm births. The pregnancies with relaxin levels below three standard deviations above the mean are to the left of the vertical line. Most of these pregnancies delivered at term. To the right of the line are relaxin levels in the hyperrelaxinemic pregnancies. The ratio of preterm: term deliveries increased as relaxin levels increased.

Circulating relaxin concentrations >16 ng/ml produced preterm birth in 50% of the women. In multiple gestations, this same level of increase in preterm birth occurs when relaxin concentrations are >7 ng/ml. It can easily be seen that most of the births in the normo-relaxinemia range are at term, whereas an increasing proportion of births are preterm as relaxin levels rise.

Since the relationship is an increasing risk of prematurity with increasing relaxin levels, the association cannot be described adequately by a static evaluation. Logistic regression analysis was therefore used to determine the relationship between singleton pregnancies and increasing relaxin levels. This analysis confirmed the impression derived from perusal of the jitter plot that, in singletons, a greater proportion of pregnancies had preterm birth with increasing relaxin levels. Table 10.1 shows the logistic regression analysis of prematurity risk in the singleton stimulated pregnancies. An increase in relaxin levels of 5 ng/ml results in an increased odds ratio of preterm birth to 2.06. For comparison, an increase in gestation number increases the odds ratio of preterm birth to 3.82. Hence, hyperrelaxinemia is associated with increased risk of preterm birth, but is not as potent a factor as multiple pregnancy.

RELAXIN'S EFFECTS ON TERM PREGNANCY HUMAN CERVIX IN VITRO

We hypothesized that this association of hyperrelaxinemia with prematurity in women is caused by specific effects of relaxin upon the cervix. We studied the effects of relaxin on the human cervix by utilizing human lower uterine segment fibroblasts as an in vitro model of human term pregnancy cervix.[18,19] Our data demonstrate that relaxin is a positive regulator of matrix metalloproteinases (MMP) in human cells isolated

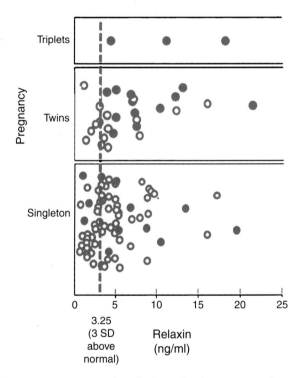

Figure 10.3 Jitter plot of relaxin levels versus number of fetuses. Open circles, uneventful pregnancy; filled circles, preterm delivery or risk. Points were 'jittered' in the vertical direction to allow greater visibility of the density of points at any given relaxin level. The dotted vertical line indicates 3.25 ng/ml, the distinction between normorelaxinemia and hyperrelaxinemia (as described in the text). Note: As relaxin levels increase, the proportion of uneventful to premature increases. SD, Standard deviation. (From Weiss et al, Obstet Gynecol 1993; 82: 821–8.)

Table 10.1 Prematurity risk in singleton stimulated pregnancies (logistic regression model). (From Weiss et al, Obstet Gynecol 1993; 82: 821–8)

Variable	Odds ratio	95% CI for odds ratio	P
Relaxin	2.06*	(1.16–3.67)	0.013
Fetal Number	3.82+	(1.57–9.31)	0.003

*Per 5 ng/ml increase in relaxin.
+Per unit increases in gestation number.

from tissue taken at term pregnancy. The maintenance of connective tissue architecture requires a precise balance between the action of MMP – enzymes which degrade the extracellular matrix – and the endogenous tissue inhibitors of metalloproteinases, which regulate the activity of the metalloproteinases.[20] Since type I collagen is the major collagen type in the human cervix, we studied the effects of relaxin on the expression of interstitial collagenase (MMP-1), stromelysin (MMP-3), which converts procollagenase to its active form, and their endogenous inhibitor tissue inhibitor of metalloproteinase (TIMP) 1. Relaxin significantly increases expression of MMP-1 and MMP-3 at the level of both the protein and mRNA. In addition, relaxin significantly decreases expression of the protein levels of the endogenous inhibitor TIMP-1.[19] Some of these results are seen in Figures 10.4 and 10.5.

Since a hallmark of cervical dilatation at term pregnancy in women is infiltration of leukocytes, we also

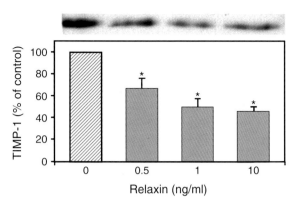

Figure 10.5 Relaxin inhibits levels of tissue inhibitor of metalloproteinase 1 (TIMP-1) protein in an in vitro model of human term pregnancy cervix. *Significant decrease below the control caused by relaxin. (From Palejwala et al, Endocrinology 2001; 142: 3405–13.)

determined the effect of relaxin on gelatinase A (MMP-2), which degrades basement membranes collagens, elastin, laminin and fibronectin. Relaxin significantly increases MMP-2 expression in this in vitro model of human term pregnancy cervix.[19] This action of relaxin may facilitate passage of white blood cells and other cell types through vascular basement membranes into the cervix. This could serve to enhance the direct positive effect of relaxin on MMP expression by increasing the local concentrations of various MMP stimulatory cytokines secreted by these white blood cells.

Our data and those of others suggest that relaxin action upon connective tissue may be unique. Relaxin is clearly a positive regulator of MMP since it stimulates MMP-1 and MMP-3 expression, and inhibits expression of the endogenous inhibitor TIMP-1. Various cytokines such as interleukin (IL) 1α stimulate the production of MMP-1 and MMP-3 in human cervical fibroblasts in vitro.[21] However, unlike relaxin, which inhibits expression of TIMP-1 in our model system, and in dermal fibroblasts, IL-1α increases TIMP-1 production in human cervical fibroblasts and in fibroblasts from other organs.[22–25] Other growth factors and cytokines, such as epidermal growth factor (EGF) and tumor necrosis factor (TNFα), also stimulate production of MMP-1 and MMP-3. However, these agents either stimulate TIMP-1 production in human fibroblasts or have no effect.[26,27] Other factors such as retinoids, interferons and glucocorticoids inhibit TIMP-1 expression, yet they inhibit MMP expression as well.[28] Thus, relaxin may be unique in its ability to cause inhibitory effects upon the endogenous inhibitor of MMP – TIMP-1 – yet stimulate the MMP. This activity of inhibition of TIMP-1 expression by relaxin may account

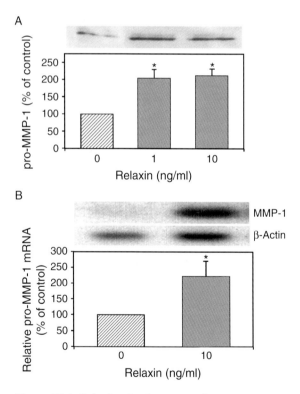

Figure 10.4 Relaxin stimulates procollagenase (pro-MMP-1) protein (A) and mRNA (B) expression in an in vitro model of human term pregnancy cervix. *Significant increase above the control caused by relaxin. (From Palejwala et al, Endocrinology 2001; 142: 3405–13.)

for the more modest stimulatory effects of relaxin upon MMP-1 and MMP-3 expression, as compared with the effects of cytokines such as IL-1α, which also stimulate levels of the inhibitor. This may also have a biological basis – a more modest effect of relaxin may be necessary to allow connective tissue remodeling, yet not cause the kind of connective tissue destruction which may occur in reactions mediated by inflammatory cytokines. Unlike relaxin, MMP stimulatory activities of cytokines such as IL-1 require phorbol-12myristate-13-acetate (PMA)-sensitive protein kinase C in certain cell types, including human cervical fibroblasts.[23] Certain aspects of relaxin signaling which regulate MMP expression in human lower uterine segment fibroblasts may be common to those of other regulators. For example, stromelysin-1 gene induction by platelet derived growth factor (PDGF) is dependent upon Ras, which then directs two distinct pathways, one of which is c-Raf dependent (which may resemble relaxin signaling) and the other of which is c-Raf independent. Cytokines and growth factors have been shown to regulate production of each MMP and endogenous tissue inhibitor using many different pathways in a ligand-, developmental- and tissue-specific manner.

The effects of relaxin upon cervical connective tissue must be considered in relation to the actions of the steroid hormones, estrogen and progesterone. Relaxin and progesterone appear to have opposing influences upon cervical MMP expression. Relaxin is a positive regulator of MMP, whereas progesterone is a negative regulator of MMP expression. Progesterone significantly decreases MMP-1 and MMP-3 protein expression, and has no effect upon TIMP-1 protein levels in the in vitro model of the human term pregnancy cervix.[19] The opposing actions of relaxin and progesterone may be required to maintain a balance resulting in a net effect of maintaining cervical connective tissue integrity during pregnancy. At term pregnancy in women, or during premature labor, alterations in progesterone metabolism or progesterone action, such as those which have been proposed to be involved in functional progesterone withdrawal,[29] may allow the balance to be shifted to a more pronounced effect of relaxin in concert with a lesser effect of progesterone. This may result in the rearrangement of connective tissue caused by the relative increase in MMP activity and decrease in TIMP-1 activity. The data allow for the hypothesis that progesterone may, to some extent, block or prevent the effects of relaxin upon the cervix. A greater effect of relaxin may occur when the action(s) of progesterone is suppressed. Thus, in women, relaxin action upon the cervix may be more robust at term pregnancy when progesterone biological activity may be decreased. Also, when relaxin concentrations are elevated, the blockage of relaxin action by progesterone may be overcome causing an increase in prematurity.

The mechanisms utilized to accomplish cervical ripening during human pregnancy are extremely complex, and require the actions of multiple interacting peptide and steroid hormones, and other factors and cellular responses. The evidence that relaxin is a positive regulator of MMP which affect type I collagen – in contrast to the negative effects of progesterone – and that relaxin stimulates gelatinase expression (which degrades basement membranes), provide a potential explanation for the relationship between increased circulating maternal levels of relaxin and the increased risk of prematurity.

A RHESUS MONKEY MODEL OF RELAXIN'S PREGNANCY EFFECTS

To determine the effects of relaxin in an in vivo primate model, we established a rhesus monkey (*Macaca mulatta*) model of early human pregnancy.[7] Ovariectomized rhesus monkeys were given exogenous estradiol and progesterone in a manner which achieves levels similar to those of the menstrual cycle. Animals were then randomized to two groups. One group was given exogenous human relaxin in amounts that achieved physiologic circulating levels, equivalent to those detected in early human pregnancy. The other group was given vehicle only and served as controls. This model thus ensured that relaxin was the only independent variable. Various structural and biochemical features of the uteri of these animals were studied.

The first assessment was the effect of relaxin upon uterine weight. A pronounced increase in uterine weight was demonstrated in the relaxin-treated animals, while there was no effect of relaxin on body weight (see Table 10.2).

The cervix is an elastic organ primarily composed of connective tissue, which consists of fibrillar collagens, elastin,[30] and proteoglycans.[31,32] Connective tissue remodeling, such as that which occurs in the cervix during pregnancy, requires changes in collagen fibrils, including destruction of collagen and changes in the proteoglycan ground substance which maintain the fibrillar arrangement. The family of small leucine-rich proteoglycans, which includes lumican and decorin, are important in the regulation of collagen fibrinogenesis in the uterus. Lumican promotes collagen fibril formation.[33] We utilized the rhesus monkey model to determine the effects of relaxin upon the cervix by assessing the abundance of collagen expression, the abundance of elastin, the orientation of elastin fibers and MMP, and proteoglycan levels. Quantitative morphometric determination of collagen abundance in trichrome-stained

Table 10.2 Body and uterine weights in rhesus monkey model of early pregnancy. (From Goldsmith et al, Proc Natl Acad Sci USA 2004; 101: 4685–9)

	Control group				Mean (±SEM)	Relaxin-treated group				Mean (±SEM)
Animal	1	2	3	4		5	6	7	8	
Body weight (kg)	5.8	4.9	7.4	5.6	5.9 (0.53)	9.1	6.5	5.7	4.6	6.5 (0.95)
Uterine weight (g)	12.36	12.81	9.87	12.86	11.98 (0.7)	27.21	19.13	14.93	12.95	18.56 (3.15)

Body weight, P = 0.79; uterine weight, P = 0.014.

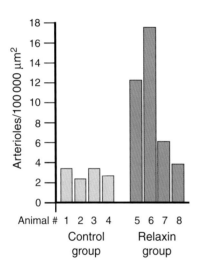

Figure 10.6 Relaxin significantly increases endometrial arteriole number in a rhesus monkey model of early pregnancy. (From Goldsmith et al, Proc Natl Acad Sci USA 2004; 101: 4685–9.)

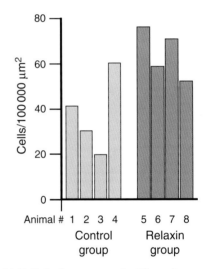

Figure 10.7 Relaxin causes a significant increase in the number of resident endometrial lymphocytes in a rhesus monkey model of early pregnancy. (From Goldsmith et al, Proc Natl Acad Sci USA 2004; 101: 4865–9.)

sections revealed a significantly decreased cervical collagen content in the relaxin-treated group of monkeys, and significantly decreased cervical expression of elastin. Relaxin also caused distinct fragmentation of cervical elastin fibers. Relaxin significantly elevated cervical levels of matrilysin (MMP-7), which can degrade a wide range of matrix proteins and can activate several other MMP, including MMP-1.[34] Relaxin had no effect upon cervical decorin expression but significantly inhibited cervical lumican protein expression. These dramatic biochemical effects of relaxin in the cervix in a monkey model of early human pregnancy provide strong evidence that relaxin contributes to the structural changes which occur in the cervix during pregnancy.

The endometria of control animals had a histology similar to a secretory phase endometrium. The addition of relaxin to estradiol and progesterone resulted in histology which showed greater decidualization. There were no differences between the two groups of monkeys in the number of epithelial cells per unit area or the

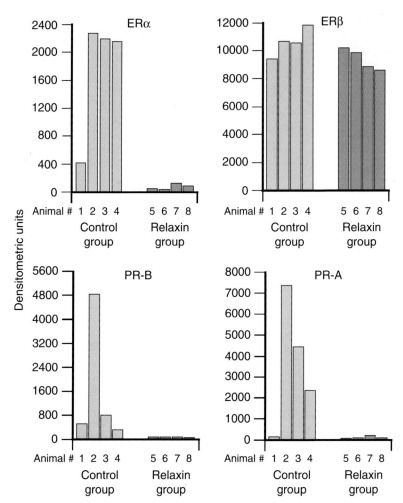

Figure 10.8 Relaxin significantly decreases levels of endometrial estrogen receptor alpha (ERα) protein (upper left) and progesterone receptor (PR) protein isoforms B and A (lower left and right) in a rhesus monkey model of early pregnancy. No effect was observed upon estrogen receptor beta (ERβ) (upper right) protein levels. (From Goldsmith et al, Proc Natl Acad Sci USA 2004; 101: 4865–9.)

stromal area. There were also no differences in endometrial collagen expression between relaxin-treated and control animals, in contradistinction to the finding in the monkey cervix, in which relaxin significantly decreases collagen abundance. However, relaxin caused marked affects upon endometrial vasculature. Relaxin significantly increased the arteriolar number compared to controls, as shown in Figure 10.6. Quantitative assessment revealed that the mean ($\pm$ SEM) number of endometrial arterioles in the relaxin-treated animals was significantly higher than that for the control animals (9.9 ± 3.1 versus 2.9 ± 0.3 cells/100 000 μm^2, $P = 0.014$). In addition, the endometria of relaxin-treated animals had a significantly greater number of lymphocytes, as shown in Figure 10.7. The number of endometrial lymphocytes for the relaxin-treated animals was significantly higher than that for the control animals (64.1 ± 5.5 versus 37.4 ± 8.6 cells/100 000 μm^2, $P = 0.03$). In a similar fashion, relaxin significantly increased

endometrial macrophage number ($P = 0.001$) and endometrial uterine natural killer (NK) cell number ($P = 0.0009$). These increases are remarkably similar to the increased number detected during decidualization of the endometrium in natural pregnancies in rhesus monkeys and women.[35]

Our prior studies[36] and those of Unemori et al[37] have demonstrated that relaxin stimulates expression of endometrial vascular endothelial growth factor (VEGF), which suggested a role for relaxin in endometrial angiogenesis. This is supported by demonstration of an increase in endometrial arteriolar number. Relaxin increases the number of endometrial lymphocytes, macrophages and uterine NK cells, which are sources of stimulatory cytokines such as IL-1, IL-8 and TNF-β. These biochemical mediators may accelerate the processes which ultimately result in uterine contractility and delivery. This may be a mechanism by which hyperrelaxinemia is related to preterm delivery.

Since the significance of the actions of estrogen and progesterone to establishment of pregnancy, and its maintenance, is well documented, we determined whether relaxin alters endometrial steroid hormone action in the rhesus monkey model. As can be seen in Figure 10.8, the relaxin-treated group of monkeys had significantly decreased endometrial expression of estrogen receptor alpha (ERα) protein compared to the control group (P = 0.01). There were no differences in endometrial ERβ protein levels between the two groups. In addition, both progesterone receptor (PR) B (PR-B) and PR-A were significantly decreased by relaxin treatment (P = 0.01 and 0.03, respectively). The net result of these alterations could produce an estrogen-dominant endometrium which would be more conducive to the onset of labor.

SUMMARY

In summary, marked hyperrelaxinemia correlates with preterm birth, even in singleton pregnancies. Results of studies in both an in vitro term pregnancy human model and an in vivo rhesus monkey model provide mechanisms responsible for the relationship between elevated maternal relaxin concentrations and preterm birth. Relaxin has actions which both facilitate cervical ripening and uterine contractibility. It is thus likely that the hyperrelaxinemia of ART is the cause of preterm birth associated with ART.

ACKNOWLEDGMENTS

The studies were supported by NIH Grant HD 22338. We thank Donna Cole for assistance in preparation of the manuscript.

REFERENCES

1. McGovern PG, Llorens AL, Skurnick JH et al. Increased risk of preterm birth in singleton pregnancies resulting from in vitro fertilization-embryo transfer or gamete intrafallopian transfer: a meta-analysis. Fertil Steril 2004; 82: 1514–20.
2. Jackson RA, Gibson KA, Wu YW et al. Perinatal outcomes in singletons following in vitro fertilization: a meta-analysis. Obstet Gynecol 2004; 103: 551–63.
3. Helmerhorst FM, Perquin DAM, Donker D et al. Perinatal outcome of singletons and twins after assisted conception: a systematic review of controlled studies. Br Med J 2004; 328: 261–5.
4. Weiss G, O'Byrne EM, Steinetz BG. Relaxin: a product of the human corpus luteum of pregnancy. Science 1976; 194: 948–9.
5. Goldsmith LT, Weiss G, Steinetz BG. Relaxin and its role in pregnancy. In: Jovanovic-Peterson L, Peterson CM, eds. Endocrinology and Metabolism Clinics of North America: Endocrine Diseases in Pregnancy. Philadelphia: WB Saunders Co, 1995; 171–86.
6. Sherwood OD. Relaxin's physiological roles and other diverse actions. Endocrinol Rev 2004; 25: 205–34.
7. Goldsmith LT, Weiss G, Palejwala S et al. Relaxin regulation of endometrial function in the rhesus monkey. Proc Natl Acad Sci USA 2004; 101: 4685–9.
8. Garcia A, Skurnick JH, Goldsmith LT et al. Human chorionic gonadotropin and relaxin concentrations in early ectopic and normal pregnancies. Obstet Gynecol 1990; 75: 779–83.
9. Haning RV, Canick JA, Goldsmith LT et al. The effect of ovulation induction on the concentration of maternal serum relaxin in twin pregnancies. Am J Obstet Gynecol 1996; 174: 227–32.
10. Haning Jr RV, Steinetz BG, Weiss G. Elevated serum relaxin levels in multiple pregnancy after menotropin treatment. Obstet Gynecol 1985; 66: 42–5.
11. Haning RV, Goldsmith LT, Seifer DB et al. Relaxin secretion in in vitro fertilization pregnancies. Am J Obstet Gynecol 1996; 174: 227–32.
12. Quagliarello J, Goldsmith L, Steinetz B et al. Induction of relaxin secretion in nonpregnant women by human chorionic gonadotropin. J Clin Endocrinol Metabol 1980; 51: 74–7.
13. Seki K, Kato K. Evidence of luteal source of circulating relaxin in molar pregnancy. Acta Obstet Gynecol Scand 1987; 66: 319–20.
14. Emmi AM, Skurnick J, Goldsmith LT et al. Ovarian control of pituitary hormone secretion in early human pregnancy. J Clin Endocrinol Metabol 1991; 72: 1359–63.
15. Johnson MR, Wren ME, Abdulla H et al. Relaxin levels in ovum donation pregnancies. Fertil Steril 1991; 56: 59–61.
16. Mushayandebvu T, Goldsmith LT, Von Hagen S et al. Elevated maternal serum relaxin concentrations throughout pregnancy in singleton gestations following superovulation. Obstet Gynecol 1998; 92: 17–20.
17. Weiss G, Goldsmith LT, Sachdev R et al. Elevated first trimester serum relaxin concentrations in pregnant women following ovarian stimulation predict prematurity risk and preterm labor. Obstet Gynecol 1993; 82: 821–8.
18. Palejwala S, Stein D, Wojtczuk A et al. Demonstration of a relaxin receptor and relaxin stimulated tyrosine phosphorylation in human lower uterine segment fibroblasts. Endocrinology 1998; 139: 1208–12.
19. Palejwala S, Stein DE, Weiss G et al. Relaxin positively regulates matrix metalloproteinase expression in human lower uterine segment fibroblasts using a tyrosine kinase signalling pathway. Endocrinology 2001; 142: 3405–13.
20. Nagase H, Woessner JF. Matrix metalloproteinases. J Biol Chem 1999 ; 274: 21 491–4.
21. Takahashi S, Sato T, Ito A et al. Involvement of protein kinase C in the interleukin 1α-induced gene expression of matrix metalloproteinases and tissue inhibitor-1 of metalloproteinases (TIMP-1) in human uterine cervical fibroblasts. Biochim Biophys Acta 1993; 1220: 57–65.
22. Unemori EN, Amento EP. Relaxin modulates synthesis and secretion of procollagenase and collagen by human dermal fibroblasts. J Biol Chem 1990; 265: 10 681–5.
23. Takahashi S, Ito A, Nagano M et al. Cyclic adenosine 3′,5′-monophosphate suppresses interleukin 1-induced synthesis of matrix metalloproteinases but not of tissue inhibitor of metalloproteinases in human uterine cervical fibroblasts. J Biol Chem 1991; 266: 19 894–9.
24. Murphy G, Reynolds JJ, Werb Z. Biosynthesis of tissue inhibitor of metalloproteinases by human fibroblasts in culture. Stimulation by 12-O-tetradecanoylphorbol 13-acetate and interleukin 1 in parallel with collagenase. J Biol Chem 1985; 260: 3079–83.
25. Sato T, Ito A, Mori Y. Interleukin 6 enhances the production of tissue inhibitor of metalloproteinases (TIMP) but not that of matrix metalloproteinases by human fibroblasts. Biochem Biophys Res Commun 1990; 170: 824–9.

26. Hosono T, Ito A, Sato T et al. Translational augmentation of pro-matrix metalloproteinase 3 (prostromelysin 1) and tissue inhibitor of metalloproteinases (TIMP)-1 mRNAs induced by epidermal growth factor in human uterine cervical fibroblasts. FEBS Lett 1996; 381: 115–18.

27. Chua CC, Chua BHL. Tumor necrosis factor-α induces mRNA for collagenase and TIMP in human skin fibroblasts. Connect Tissue Res 1990; 25: 161–70.

28. Brinckerhoff CE, Auble D. Regulation of collagenase gene expression in synovial fibroblasts. Ann NY Acad Sci 1990; 580: 355–74.

29. Messiano S. Roles of estrogen and progesterone in human parturition. In: Smith R, ed. The Endocrinology of Parturition, Basic Science and Clinical Application. Front Horm Res. Basel, Karger, 2001; 27: 86–104.

30. Leppert PC, Keller S, Cerreta J et al. Conclusive evidence for the presence of elastin in human and monkey cervix. Am J Obstet Gynecol 1982; 142: 179–82.

31. Danforth DN, Veis A, Breen M et al. The effects of pregnancy and labor on the human cervix: changes in collagen, glycoproteins and glycosaminoglycans. Am J Obstet Gynecol 1974; 120: 641–9.

32. Uldbjerg N, Ekman G, Malmstrom AK et al. Ripening of the human uterine cervix related to changes in collagen, glycosaminoglycans and collagenolytic activity. Am J Obstet Gynecol 1983; 147: 662–6.

33. Chakravarti S, Magnuson T, Las JH et al. Lumican regulates collagen fibril assembly: skin fragility and corneal opacity in the absence of lumican. J Cell Biol 1998; 141: 1277–86.

34. Woessner JF. Regulation of matrilysin in the rat uterus. Biochem Cell Biol 1996; 74: 777–84.

35. Slukvin II, Brebruda EE, Golos TG. Dynamic changes in primate endometrial leukocyte populations: differential distribution of macrophages and natural killer cells at the rhesus monkey implantation site and in early pregnancy. Placenta 2004; 25: 297–307.

36. Palejwala S, Tseng L, Wojtczuk A et al. Relaxin gene and protein expression and its regulation of procollagenase and vascular endothelial growth factor in human endometrial cells. Biol Reprod 2002; 66: 1743–8.

37. Unemori EN. Erikson MD, Rocco SE et al. Relaxin stimulates expression of vascular endothelial growth factor in normal human endometrial cells in vitro and is associated with menometrorrhagia in women. Hum Reprod 1999; 14: 800–6.

SECTION III

METHODS OF PREDICTION AND PREVENTION

11

Biochemical markers of preterm delivery

Charles J Lockwood

INTRODUCTION

The delivery of infants prior to 37 weeks of gestation complicated 12.3% of births in the United States (US) in 2003, and was the leading cause of neonatal morbidity and mortality.[1] The US preterm delivery (PTD) rate has climbed 14% during the past 15 years, reflecting both a 40% rise in multifetal pregnancies and an increase in prematurity among women with singleton gestations from 9.7 to 10.4%.[2] Racial and ethnic disparities exist in the US PTD rate with 11% of non-Hispanic white births and 17.7% of non-Hispanic black births occurring preterm.[2] Comparable increases in PTD rates have been observed in Europe, though overall rates tend to be lower than in the US (e.g. 6.9% in Denmark).[3] Antecedents to PTD include those indicated by deteriorating maternal or fetal health, which account for about 25% (range 18.7–35.2%) of cases, and spontaneous PTD, which either follow preterm premature rupture of membranes (PPROM) (30%; range 7.1–51.2% of cases), or spontaneous preterm labor with intact fetal membranes (PTL) (45%; 23.2–64.1% of cases).[4] This review will focus on the latter two categories.

PATHOGENESIS OF PRETERM DELIVERY (PTD)

Final common pathway

Four distinct pathogenic pathways appear to mediate spontaneous PTD: premature activation of the fetal hypothalamic–pituitary–adrenal (HPA) axis, decidual-chorio-amnionic inflammation, decidual hemorrhage, and uterine overdistention. Each has a distinct set of genetic and/or epidemiological risk factors, and each exploits a unique set of biochemical triggers. However, in all four pathways PTD is ultimately mediated by prostaglandin (PG) and protease production (see Figure 11.1). Concentrations of PG in maternal plasma and amniotic fluid are increased just prior to and during parturition,[5–7] while expression of myometrial PG receptors increases with the onset of labor.[8] PG mediate contractions through enhancement of sarcoplasmic and transmembrane calcium fluxes, as well as by stimulating transcription of myometrial contractile protein genes including oxytocin receptor, connexin 43 (gap junctions), the PG receptors EP1-4 and FP, as well as the crucial mediator of PG synthesis, cyclooxygenase (COX) 2.[9,10] PG also promote membrane rupture and cervical change by enhancing the synthesis of interstitial collagenase, also known as matrix metalloproteinase (MMP) 1, in the fetal membranes and cervix, and by increasing cervical expression of interleukin (IL) 8, which recruits and activates neutrophils, releasing additional MMP.[9,11,12] Moreover, in vitro studies in human myometrial cells suggest that both PGE_2, and $PGF_{2\alpha}$, acting via the protein kinase C pathway increase the ratio of progesterone receptor (PR) isoforms A and B.[13] Since PR-A can antagonize the classical PR-mediated genome effects of PR-B, these findings suggest that PG can induce functional progesterone withdrawal.

Premature activation of the fetal HPA axis

There is evidence that both maternal and fetal stress is associated with PTD. The Maternal–Fetal Medicine Unit Network (MFMN) observed that objective measures of maternal aggregate stress were modestly associated with spontaneous PTD with an odds ratio (OR) of 1.16 [95% confidence interval (CI) 1.05–1.29].[14] Placental pathology provides indirect evidence of a link between fetal physiological stress and PTD, since 28.3% of patients with spontaneous PTD display placental ischemic changes compared with 3.7% of term controls, and 77.1% of such patients have abnormal

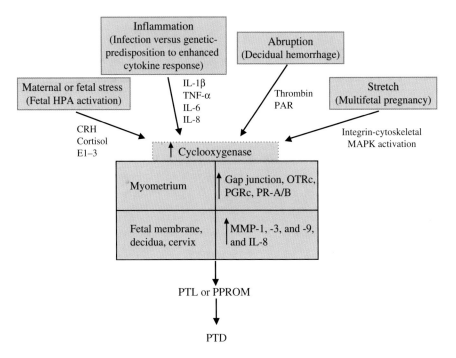

Figure 11.1 Pathogenic pathways: Each of these four preterm delivery (PTD) pathogenic mechanisms – maternal and fetal stress-induced premature activation of the fetal HPA axis, amnio-chorionic-decidual inflammation, abruption-decidual hemorrhage and mechanical stretch, has a distinct biochemical or biophysical/biochemical profile involving discrete mediators. However, each pathway converges into a final common pathway involving increased PG, MMP and IL-8 production, as well as activation of the myometrium. Prior to 20 weeks, myometrial quiescence is likely to maintain despite these stimuli due to low levels of circulating estrogen and its receptor, high levels of PR-B and reduced basal expression of oxytocin receptors, gap junctions, etc. Thus, the most likely presentation of inflammation, abruption and excess stretch prior to 20–24 weeks would be 'incompetent cervix' with or without PPROM and not PTL. After this point PTL, PPROM or both will occur.

uterine artery Doppler waveforms versus 47.1% of controls.[15] Arias et al[16] identified maternal placental vascular lesions in 34.1% patients with PTL, and 35.1% of patients with PPROM versus 11.8% of term control patients (OR 3.8 and 4.0, and 95% CI 1.3–11.1 and 1.5–10.8, respectively).[16] Thus, about one-third of spontaneous PTD are associated with evidence of uteroplacental insufficiency. There is evidence that these placental lesions are associated with elevated umbilical cord cortisol, and acceleration of maturity of fetal lungs and other organ systems.[17]

A critical mediator of stress-induced prematurity appears to be corticotropin-releasing hormone (CRH), a 41 amino acid peptide initially localized to the hypothalamus but also expressed by cells in the placenta, chorion, amnion and decidua.[18] Placental-derived maternal plasma CRH concentrations rise during the second

half of pregnancy and peak during labor, while levels of the CRH-inactivating binding protein decline across the third trimester.[19] In vitro, CRH enhances synthesis of PGE_2 output by amnionic, chorionic and placental cells but not by decidua, while it enhanced expression of $PGF_{2\alpha}$ in amnionic, decidual and placental cells but not chorion.[18] The production of placental PG by CRH appears to be mediated through production of placental adrenocorticotropin (ACTH).[20] As noted above, PG can, in turn, induce uterine contractions, reproductive tract MMP production and functional progesterone withdrawal to mediate PTD.

Whereas glucocorticoids inhibit the hypothalamic release of CRH, increases in fetal or maternal cortisol enhance placental production of CRH.[18,20] Placental CRH production stimulates the release of ACTH from the fetal pituitary gland, which, in turn, stimulates fetal adrenal cortisol production.[21] Fetal cortisol directly increases the production of CRH by the placenta and fetal membranes to create a feed-forward cycle driving parturition.[18] Rising fetal plasma and amniotic fluid cortisol can also act directly on the fetal membranes to induce PG production. For example, cortisol increases amnion COX-2 and inhibits chorionic 15-hydroxy-prostaglandin dehydrogenase (PGDH), a PG-metabolizing enzyme, to enhance net synthesis of PGE_2.[22,23] Moreover, decidual $PGF_{2\alpha}$ enhances chorionic 11-β-hydroxysteroid dehydrogenase to convert cortisone to cortisol, further impeding chorionic PDGH and increasing net amnion and decidual PG output.[24]

Dehydroepiandrosterone sulfate (DHEAS) is the major steroid produced by the fetal adrenal zone.[25] Greatly enhanced DHEAS synthesis accompanies increases in fetal adrenal cortisol production.[25] Moreover, CRH can directly augment fetal adrenal androgen production.[26] In the placenta, sulfatases cleave the sulfate conjugates of DHEAS allowing their conversion to estradiol (E2) and estrone (E1), while conversion of the 16-hydroxy-DHEAS derivative produces estriol (E3).[26] These placental-derived estrogens working in concert with rising estrogen receptor-α levels, induced by the falling PR-β levels, activate the myometrium by enhancing expression of the oxytocin receptor, connexin 43, PG receptors, and COX-2.[27–30] Studies of salivary estriol levels strongly suggest that this stress-associated PTD pathway is not present until after 31 weeks, suggesting that maturation of the fetal HPA axis and development of the fetal adrenal zone are prerequisites to this subset of PTD.[31]

Decidual-Amnion-Chorion Inflammation

The relationship between PTD and intrauterine infection and inflammation is supported by considerable epidemiological, clinical, microbial and placental pathological studies (see ref 32 for review). These studies indicate that inflammation is the most common cause of PTD occurring prior to 32 weeks, and likely account for half of all PTDs.[33,34] Vaginal organisms either reside in, or ascend to, the choriodecidual space, then migrate into the amnion, followed by the umbilical cord and amniotic fluid, and ultimately into the fetus.[32] Such infections may occur quite early in pregnancy and remain indolent for many weeks.[35]

Decidual-chorionic, chorio-amnionic and intra-amniotic infections are associated with the activation of IL-1β and tumor necrosis factor (TNF) α in the genital tract.[32] These cytokines directly and indirectly stimulate COX-2 synthesis in the fetal membranes and decidua, and inhibit chorionic PGDH to increase net

PG output.[32,36,37] Similarly, PGE_2, IL-1β and/or TNF directly enhance the expression of urokinase-type plasminogen activator and/or MMP-1, -3 and/or -9, as well as IL-8 in the amnio-chorion, decidua, and cervix to degrade the extracellular matrix of the fetal membranes and cervix.[38–43] Both TNF and MMP-9 promote programmed death (apoptosis) of amnionic epithelial cells.[39] The combined effect of these mechanisms is to promote PTL and/or PPROM.

The pro-parturition effects of TNF and IL-1β on PG and protease production are amplified by induction of IL-6 production by bacterial-derived lipopolysaccharide, TNF and/or IL-1β in amniochorion and decidua.[44,45] Elevated amniotic fluid IL-6 concentrations and increased placental IL-6 expression as early as 16 weeks of gestation are associated with subsequent PTD, intra-amniotic infection and the development of cerebral palsy in neonates.[46,47] Moreover, the quantity of IL-6 produced in these tissues exceeds that of IL-1 by approximately 1000-fold.[44,45] Amnionic and decidual PG production is increased by IL-6 to potentiate the PTD process.[48]

Parturition in humans is associated with increases in IL-8 expression in the myometrium, decidua, cervix and fetal membranes.[49–51] As noted above, this potent neutrophil chemoattractant and activator causes the release of neutrophil-derived MMP-8 and -9.[49] We have demonstrated that compared to term decidual cell cultures maintained in a progestin alone, the addition of IL-1β and TNF enhance decidual cell immunoreactive IL-8 expression 562- and 154-fold, respectively.[52] Comparable results were obtained for the corresponding mRNA species. Moreover, IL-1β and TNF induced IL-8 production in the fetal membranes and cervix, and these effects are potentiated by IL-6.[45,53] Given that IL-8 causes recruitment and activation of neutrophils that release additional MMP and elastases, its expression serves to further exacerbate the PTD-enhancing effects of genital tract inflammation.

Interestingly, the most common micro-organisms (e.g. *Ureaplamsa urealyticum*, *Mycoplasma hominis*, *Gardnerella vaginalis*, and bacteroides species) isolated from the amniotic fluid and fetal membranes of PTD patients are of relatively low virulence.[54–56] Moreover, only about half of patients with U urealyticum incidentally detected in their amniotic fluid at the time of genetic amniocentesis have adverse outcomes.[57] These findings suggest that it is the maternal and/or fetal inflammatory response to such organisms rather than their presence per se that triggers PTD. There is, in fact, growing evidence of a genetic etiology for PTD. For example, woman with prior PTD have higher rates of recurrence, and the earlier their PTD and the greater the number of prior PTD, the higher the rate of recurrence.[58]

Women and their sister(s) who deliver preterm have higher rates of PTD in their own pregnancies.[59] African-American women have higher rates of PTD even after controlling for social and economic confounders.[60]

That this genetic link may be tied to an altered inflammatory response is suggested by the growing body of evidence that specific polymorphisms in mediators of the adaptive and innate immune system are linked to spontaneous PTD. For example, homozygosity for the IL-1β+3953 allele 1 by fetuses of African descent is associated with an increased risk of PTD, while Hispanic fetuses carrying the IL-1RN allele 2 have an increased risk for PPROM (OR 6.5; 95% CI 1.25–37.7).[61] African-American mothers who carry the TNF-308 polymorphism are at higher risk of PPROM (OR 3.18; 95% CI 1.33–7.83),[62] while African-American's harboring both the TNF-308 polymorphism and having bacterial vaginosis (BV) are at synergistically increased risk of PTD (OR 6.1; 95% CI 1.9–21.0).[63] In contrast, the presence of this mutation in white women did not confer increased PTD risk.[64] Moreover, Simhan et al[65] reported the association between the IL-6-174 promoter polymorphism and a decreased risk of PTD among white women.[65] These findings may help account for the persistence of racial disparities in PTD rates after adjusting for sociodemographic confounders. Lorenz et al[66] observed an increased frequency of two polymorphisms (Asp299Gly and Thr399Ile) for toll-like receptor (TLR) 4 – the major endotoxin-signaling receptor of the innate immune system – in a population of white infants delivering preterm.[66] Among singleton gestations, 23.8% of premature infants and 24.2% of their mothers had the 299Gly allele compared with 15.9% of term infants and 15.0% of term mothers. Thus, a genetic predisposition to exaggerated immune responses may also underlie a substantial proportion of PTD among white women.

Decidual hemorrhage (abruption)-associated PTD

Placental abruption (i.e. decidual hemorrhage) is strongly associated with PTD. Women experiencing vaginal bleeding in the first trimester have twice the risk of PTD of those experiencing no bleeding (adjusted risk ratio (RR) 2.0; 95% CI 1.6–2.5).[67] Moreover, vaginal bleeding occurring in more than one trimester is associated with a greater than seven-fold increased risk of PPROM (OR 7.4; 95% CI 2.2–25.6).[68] Virtually all such vaginal bleeding derives from hemorrhage into the decidua basalis (i.e. an abruption) or between the decidua parietalis and chorion (i.e. retrochorionic hematoma). Moreover, occult decidual hemorrhage,

as manifested by hemosiderin deposition and retrochorionic hematoma formation is present in 38% of patients with PTD between 22 and 32 weeks of gestation due to PPROM, and 36% of patients experiencing PTD after PTL compared with only 0.8% following term delivery (P < 0.01).[69] Placental lesions associated with abruption include uteroplacental/spiral artery vascular thrombosis and failed physiological transformation of uteroplacental vessels.[69] Such vascular disease can result from environmental exposures such as heavy cigarette smoking, cocaine abuse and trauma, as well as intrinsic factors such as maternal thrombophilias and age-related intrinsic vascular disease.[70–72] Sclerotic lesions in myometrial spiral arteries increase from 11% at age 17–19 years to 83% after age 39.[73] Consistent with these vascular etiologies, abruption-associated PTD is more common in older, married, parous, college-educated patients, which comprise a distinct epidemiological cohort than that associated with inflammation-derived PTD.[74]

Stromelysin-1 (MMP-3) is a protease capable of degrading the extracellular matrix of the decidua and activating MMP-1 and -9, which can target amniochoirion and cervical extracellular matrices.[75] While basal MMP-3 protein and mRNA output by cultured term decidual cells is significantly inhibited by progestin, thrombin reverses this progestin inhibition by interacting with its type-1 protease-activated receptor (PAR-1).[76] Thrombin binding to PAR receptors also greatly augments interstitial collagenase (MMP-1) protein and mRNA expression in term decidual cells.[77] Abruption-associated PPROM is accompanied by dense decidual neutrophil infiltration in the absence of infection, and these neutrophils co-localize with areas of thrombin-induced fibrin deposition.[78] Consistent with these in vivo observations, thrombin acting through PAR receptors markedly enhances mRNA and protein expression of IL-8 in cultured term decidual cells.[78] As noted, neutrophils are a rich source of elastase and MMP-9[79] which can mediate the decidual-amnion-chorion extracellular matrix degradation observed in abruption-associated PPROM. We have also now demonstrated that thrombin also upregulates immunoreactive IL-6 production seven-fold in term decidual cells (Figure 11.2), as well as IL-6 mRNA (not shown). While these studies suggest a mechanism linking abruption and decidual thrombin/PAR interactions with PPROM, thrombin can also stimulate myometrial contractions via PAR receptors, further implicating it in the genesis of PTL.[80]

Multifetal gestations and stretching of the myometrium, cervix and fetal membranes

Approximately 16% of all PTD are due to multifetal gestations, and the mean gestational age at delivery

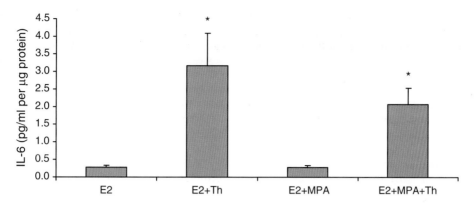

Figure 11.2 Effects of thrombin on decidual cell interleukin (IL) 6 production. Term decdiual cells isolated and cultured as described by Mackenzie et al (Am J Obstet Gynecol 2004; 191; 1996–2001) were incubated for 7 days in 10^{-8} M estradiol E2 or $E2+10^{-7}$ M medoxyprogesterone acetate (MPA) then switched to a defined medium with the corresponding steroid(s) ±2.5U thrombin (American Diagnostica, Greenwich, CT). IL-6 measured by ELISA from R&D Systems, Minneapolis, MN. Thrombin effects on IL-6 for term decidua (n = 9 + SEM). *Versus E2 and E2+MPA. Kruskal–Wallis and then Student–Neuman–Keuls post-test (P < 0.05).

decreases with increasing numbers of fetuses.[81] These findings suggest that mechanical stretch, resulting from the rapid increase in intrauterine contents accompanying multiple gestations, may play a pivotal role in such PTD. Indeed, mechanical dilation with a Foley balloon catheter is a well-established method of promoting cervical ripening through the induction of endogenous PG. Moreover, the greater the mechanical stretch, the more successful the cervical ripening.[82] Both PG application and mechanical stretch can induce MMP-1 expression in cervical fibroblasts.[83] The fetal membranes and myometrium appear to respond to mechanical stretch in a similar fashion. Amnion COX-2 expression and PG production is induced by polyhydramnios or multifetral gestation-induced mechanical stretch.[84,85] Mechanical stretch induces myometrial oxytocin receptor, COX-2, and IL-8 expression, possibly through integrin-cellular cytoskeleton activation of a mitogen-activated protein kinase (MAPK) pathway.[86–88]

BIOCHEMICAL MARKERS OF PRETERM DELIVERY (PTD)

Each of the four PTD pathogenic processes presents a unique biochemical or biophysical signature (Figure 11.1) which can be used with varying degrees of efficiency to identify patients at risk. As noted, each also shares a final common pathway that leads to proteolytic disruption of the fetal membrane–uterine interface, and cervical shortening that can be discerned by assessment of various peptides in the cervico-vaginal secretions, e.g. fetal fibronectin and/or by sonographic cervical length

determination, respectively. Unfortunately, the literature examining the efficacy of these markers is compromised by heterogeneous patient populations with a varying prevalence of PTD, relative contributions of the individual pathways, degrees of symptoms and risk, definitions of PTD, and biochemical cut-off values. Therefore, the following sections will present the utility of these markers in terms of their positive and negative likelihood ratios (LR). The LR is a measure of the predictive accuracy of a diagnostic test independent of disease prevalence. It also allows comparisons of different tests across heterogeneous populations and amongst studies of differing design (e.g. case-control versus cohort), and differing sample sizes. A positive likelihood ratio (LR+) is calculated by dividing the sensitivity by the false-positive rate, and describes how much a given positive test result raises the a priori odds of, in this case, PTD. Conversely, a negative likelihood ratio (LR−) is calculated by dividing the false-negative rate by the specificity, and demonstrates how a given negative test result lowers the odds of PTD. The ratio of the LR+: LR− provides an overall measure of test performance, with a LR+:LR− ratio >50 indicating that a test is performing well.

Markers of maternal and/or fetal stress/premature fetal HPA axis activation

CRH

Maternal circulating CRH levels are primarily placental-derived and reflect activation of the fetal HPA axis.[89] Since CRH enhances placental, fetal membrane, and decidual PG production, this observation links fetal HPA axis activation caused by maternal and fetal stress with the onset of parturition.[19] In addition, this pre-parturitional increase in CRH is accompanied by a fall in CRH binding protein, leading to a rapid increase in circulating concentrations of bioactive CRH at term.[19] In addition, there is a relationship between maternal CRH values and both PTD and psychological stress,[90] and between both maternal and fetal CRH levels and intrauterine growth restriction (IUGR).[91,92] These findings suggest that CRH is a marker of PTD due to maternal or fetal stress-induced fetal HPA axis activation. Unfortunately, elevated maternal serum CRH concentrations obtained in asymptomatic women in the second trimester predict subsequent PTD with only modest efficiency (see Table 11.1). The test performs no better among symptomatic patients with a LR+ of 3.9 and a LR− of 0.67.[93]

Explanations for these variable, and generally disappointing, results include the absence of a highly reliable immunoassay, difficulty in distinguishing free from bound CRH, and the intrinsically high inter- and intraassay coefficients of variation. The modest improvement in screening efficacy reported in the later studies may be an indication of improved assay performance. However, an equally important source of testing variability is the variable contribution of stress to PTD across differing populations. For example, we were unable to confirm any difference in CRH levels between cases and controls in an indigent population at very high risk of infection associated PTD.[94] Moreover, heterogeneity in gestational age definitions of PTD may contribute to variable results as it is likely that CRH is most predictive of stress associated PTD occurring after 32 weeks. Thus, it is not surprising that the best results were obtained with relatively late patient sampling (i.e. 26 weeks) for PTD occurring late at 30–37 weeks of gestation.[95]

Estradiol (E2) and estriol (E3)

As noted, maternal serum estrogens are primarily derived from placental conversion of the fetal adrenal-derived androgens, DHEAS and its 16-hydroxylated metabolite. These androgens reflect fetal HPA axis activation. Amniotic fluid E2 is significantly elevated in women with preterm contractions who deliver prematurely compared to those with Braxton-Hicks contractions.[99] The detection of E3 levels >2.1 ng/ml in the saliva has been shown to be predictive within 72 h of spontaneous PTD between 32 and 37 weeks with a LR+ of 2.37 and a LR− of 0.61.[100,101] Given that administration of glucocorticoids to the mother suppresses fetal adrenal DHEAS production, and hence placental estrogen synthesis, the test is not predictive of PTD in women who have been treated with glucocorticoid therapy.

Markers of uteroplacental insufficiency including maternal serum alpha-fetoprotein (MSAFP) and human chorionic gonadotropin (hCG)

As noted, uteroplacental vascular abnormalities with or without associated fetal growth abnormalities are associated with spontaneous PTD. Elevated levels of MSAFP and hCG, obtained during the second trimester to screen for fetal aneuploidy, have been linked with uteroplacental abnormalities including IUGR, abruption, stillbirth and pre-eclampsia.[102] Predictably, abnormal values of these two analytes are also associated with PTD. Hurley et al[103] observed that patients with elevated MSAFP values who also had abnormal hCG levels [<0.5 or >2.5 multiples of the median (MOM)] had a LR+ of 5.0 and a LR− of 0.47 for PTD.[103] Patients with elevated levels of both MSAFP and hCG

Table 11.1 The predictive accuracy of corticotrophin-releasing hormone (CRH) for asymptomatic screening

Ref	Population (gestational age at sampling [weeks])	Cut-off	Definition of PTD (weeks)	LR+	LR−	LR+:LR−
96	Asymptomatic white (15–19)	1.5 MOM	<35	1.8	0.73	2.5
96	Asymptomatic black (15–19)	1.5 MOM	<35	2.05	0.74	2.8
97	Asymptomatic (17–30)	3.5 MOM	<37	4.0	0.77	5.2
98	Asymptomatic (15–20)	1.9 MOM	<34	3.3	0.47	7.0
95	Asymptomatic (26)	90pM	<37	7.5	0.59	12.7

LR, Likelihood ratio; MOM, multiple of the median; PTD, preterm delivery.

have about a 50% risk of PTD.[104] Isolated elevations of hCG concentrations >4 MOM were also associated with an increased risk of PTD (OR 3.3),[105] whereas there are conflicting reports of the link between lesser elevations of hCG (>2.0–2.5 MOM) and PTD.[104,106–108] While these findings buttress the link between fetal stress and PTD, since concomitant and/or substantial elevations of hCG and MSAFP are uncommon, the utility of these markers for use in screening for patients appears low. Moreover, it is unclear what percentage of these PTD cases were truly spontaneous.

The association between increased placental production of hCG and PTD prompted a number of investigators to assess the utility of cervicovaginal hCG determinations in the prediction of spontaneous PTD. In a case-control study involving a PTL group and a normal pregnancy group, Guvenal et al[109] observed that the optimal cut-off value for cervicovaginal hCG (27.1 mIU/ml) gave a LR+ of 2.77 and a LR− of 0.18. In contrast, Garshasbi et al[110] conducted a cohort study in asymptomatic high-risk patients in whom cervicovaginal samples were collected between 20 and 28 weeks. They observed a 3.2-fold increase in hCG levels among PTD patients with a single hCG value >77.8 mIU/ml associated with a LR+ of 29.0 and a LR− of 0.13.[110] These interesting findings await confirmation.

Markers of inflammation and infection

Microbiological markers

Leitich et al[111] conducted a meta-analysis of the association between BV and the risk of PTD in 18 studies enrolling 20 232 patients, and noted a pooled OR of 2.19 (95% CI 1.54–3.12). The PTD risk increased with diagnoses of BV prior to 16 weeks (OR 7.55; 95% CI 1.80–31.65). A large multicenter study reported a BV-associated OR for PTD of 1.84 when BV was detected at 28 weeks.[112] Hillier et al[113] found a similar modest association between BV detected at 23–26 weeks of gestation and PTD (OR 1.4; 95% CI 1.1–1.8). Moreover, a significant reduction in PTD was observed in 338 high-risk patients who received oral antibiotic regimens with treatment durations of ≥1 week (OR 0.42; 95% CI 0.27–0.67).[114]

Meta-analysis of cohort studies showed that untreated asymptomatic bacteriuria is associated with an increased PTD rate. Conversely, nonbacteriuric patients had half the risk of PTD (RR 0.50; 95% CI 0.36–0.70) of patients with untreated asymptomatic bacteriuria.[115] A second meta-analysis indicates that treatment of asymptomatic bacteriuria reduces PTD risk (RR 0.53, 95% CI 0.33–0.86).[116] While vaginal *E coli* colonization was

associated with a modest increased risk of PTD <34 weeks (RR 1.7; 95% CI 1.3–2.3),[117] there is no evidence that attempted eradication of such colonization with antibiotics reduces PTD risk. Thus, screening all pregnant women for asymptomatic bacteriuria and treating positives, and screening all high-risk patients for BV prior to 20 weeks and treating positives with at least 1 week of oral antibiotics would appear to be a reasonable and prudent approach.

Cytokine markers

Meta-analysis suggests that the association between elevated amniotic fluid (AF) IL-6 and PTD is greater than that for intra-amniotic infection detected by culture or polymerase chain reaction (PCR) and that 33–70% of women without evidence of microbial invasion of the amniotic cavity, but with elevated AF IL-6 levels deliver preterm.[118] However, this invasive approach is not suitable for screening. By contrast, detection of elevated levels of immunoreactive IL-6 in cervical secretions appears to have modest predictive value in both high-risk asymptomatic and symptomatic patients (see Table 11.2). However, the wide variation in results reflect variability in cut-off values chosen, inter- and intra-assay variability, variations in the gestational age definition of PTD, and variation in the prevalence of inflammation-induced PTD amongst studies. For example, even if an elevated cervical IL-6 detects all patients with inflammation its sensitivity would be consistently less than 50% for PTD <37 weeks. Detection of elevated cervical IL-6 mRNA levels may provide an alternative approach (Table 11.2).

Holst et al[123] observed elevated levels of IL-8 in cervical fluid among women who subsequently delivered preterm (median 11.3 ng/ml, range 0.15–98.1 versus 4.9 ng/ml, range 0.15–41.0 ng/ml, P = 0.002). The presence of cervical IL-8 values >7.7 ng/ml predicted PTD ≤7 days with a LR+ of 2.38 and a LR− of 0.51. Kurkinen-Raty et al[120] observed a LR+ of 1.4 (95% CI 0.9–2.4) for a cervical IL-8 value >3.7 μg/l among symptomatic patients sampled between 22 and 32 weeks. Rizzo et al[125] observed that cervical IL-8 values >450 pg/ml were comparable to that of a fetal fibronectin (FFN) value >50 ng/ml in predicting PTD, and that a cervical IL-8 level >860 pg/ml predicted a positive amniotic fluid culture with a LR+ of 2.4 and a LR− of 0.28. In contrast, Coleman et al[122] were not able to ascribe any PTD predictive value to cervical IL-8 determinations. These results are surprising given the central role that IL-8 generally plays in all four pathogenic pathways, and may reflect a relative paucity of secretion into cervicovaginal secretion or prompt degradation in that milieu. Elevated (greater than 75th percentile) plasma granulocyte colony-stimulating factor

Table 11.2 The predictive accuracy of cervical interleukin (IL) 6 in asymptomatic and symptomatic patients at risk for preterm delivery (PTD)

Ref	Population ([gestational age at sampling [weeks])	Cut-off	Definition of PTD	LR+	LR−	LR+:LR−
119	Asymptomatic every 3–4 weeks (24–36)	250 pg/ml	<37 weeks	3.33	0.59	5.6
120	Symptomatic (22–32)	61 ng/L	<37 weeks	1.87	0.44	4.25
121	Symptomatic (<34)	20 pg/ml	<34 weeks	3.03	NA	NA
122	Symptomatic (24–34)	35 pg/ml	<7 days	1.82	0.52	3.5
123	Symptomatic at (<34)	1.7 ng/ml	<7 days	3.62	0.30	12.1
124	Symptomatic	Presence of mRNA	<34 weeks	2.81	0.80	3.5

LR, Likelihood ratio; NA, not applicable.

(GCSF) concentrations at 28 weeks are associated with PTD <32 weeks with a LR+ of 6.9 and a LR− of 0.67.[126] Not surprisingly, given the preponderance of early PTD among patients with genital tract inflammation, GCSF did not predict PTD at later gestational ages.

Non-specific markers of inflammation

Levels of lactoferrin, an iron-binding protein with bacteriostatic effects released by activated neutrophils, correlated with high cervical IL-6 levels and sialidase activity, as well as the presence of BV, but proved a very insensitive predictor of PTD (<5%) among asymptomatic patients screened between 22 and 24 weeks.[127] Similarly, levels of the acute phase reactant ferritin present in cervical secretions greater than the 75th percentile at 22–24 weeks predicted subsequent PTD <32 weeks with a LR+ of 4.0 and a LR− of 0.63 in a nested case-control study in asymptomatic patients.[128] Vogel et al[129] evaluated the predictive value of the activated macrophage product, soluble CD163 (sCD163), and C-reactive protein (CRP), among 93 symptomatic patients. They noted that serum sCD163 values >5 mg/l and CRP values >47 mg/l were associated with an increased risk of PTD <34 weeks, with a LR+ for PTD <34 weeks of 8.6 (95% CI 2.8–14) and 2.8 (0–6.2), respectively.[129] Other markers of lower genital tract infection, including cervical sialidase, defensins, follistatin-free activin, serum β-2-microglobulin, latex CRP, intracellular adhesion molecule-1, elevated vaginal pH and neutrophils, were not predictive of PTD.[130–132]

Markers of decidual hemorrhage/abruption

The decidua, the site of hemorrhage in abruption, is richly endowed in tissue factor, which mediates hemostasis by facilitating the generation of thrombin. In addition to its role in clotting, thrombin binds to PAR receptors to promote decidual protease production and myometrial contractions.[75–78,80] Thus, thrombin would appear to be an ideal target for the detection of abruption-associated PTD. Table 11.3 lists the results of studies of the predictive value of thrombin–antithrombin complexes (TAT), which serve as a surrogate for thrombin generation. Since the majority of these patients exhibited no signs of abruption,[135] or overt abruption, and maternal thrombophilia were exclusion criteria,[136] these findings suggest that occult abruption is far more common than clinically suspected, in line with placental histology studies.[69]

Markers of uterine distention

Pathologic uterine distention or stretch is caused by conditions that abnormally increase intrauterine volume (e.g. multifetal gestations and polyhydramnios), and perhaps by conditions that limit potential uterine expansion (e.g. Müllerian duct anomalies). Both clinical settings are strongly associated with the occurrence of PTD. While there are no current biochemical markers of excess myometrial, cervical, decidual or fetal membrane stretch, the mere presence of multiple gestations or polyhydramnios, or known uterine anomalies, represent a significant risk factor.

Markers of the final common pathway

As noted above, each pathogenic pathway – premature activation of the fetal HPA axis, decidual-chorio-amnionic inflammation, decidual hemorrhage and uterine over-distention, has a unique set of biochemical initiators (Figure 11.1). However, each ultimately results in

Table 11.3 The predictive accuracy of plasma thrombin–antithrombin complex (TAT) levels in asymptomatic and symptomatic patients at risk for preterm delivery (PTD)

Ref	Population (gestational age at sampling [weeks])	Cut-off	Definition of PTD	LR+	LR−	LR+:LR−
134	Asymptomatic (22–34)	3.9 μg/l	Subsequent PPROM <37 weeks	2.75	0.18	15.3
135	Symptomatic (24–33)	6.3 ng/ml	PTD within 3 weeks	5.5	0.55	10
136	Symptomatic (<37)	20 μg/l	<37 weeks	2.94	0.6	4.9

LR, Likelihood ratio.

increased genital tract MMP, PG and IL-8 production. These effectors promote cervical change, which can be detected by transvaginal ultrasound and proteolytic degradation of the decidua and fetal membranes. The latter causes the release of fetal membrane-specific protein such as fetal fibronectin (FFN) or decidual-derived proteins such as prolactin, type 1 insulin-like growth factor binding protein (IGFBP-1). All three of these PTD markers also concentrate in the amniotic fluid and may leech out into cervicovaginal secretions through damaged membranes with occult or overt PPROM.

FFN

Fibronectins are large molecular weight (450 kDa) glycoproteins present in both the plasma and tissue extracellular matrices. Fibronectin present in the amniotic fluid, extracts of placental tissue, and malignant cell lines contains a heavily glycosylated oncofetal epitope, termed FFN.[138] The FFN molecule is produced by extravillous cytotrophoblasts in the placenta and chorion, and is thought to promote cellular adhesion at uterine–placental and decidual–fetal membrane interfaces; it is released when the extracellular matrix of the chorionic–decidual interface is disrupted prior to labor.[139] Interestingly, the content and size of FFN carbohydrate side chains increase across gestation, resulting in decreased binding affinity for other extracellular matrices.[140] Since FFN is also present at points of cleavage of the placenta and chorion from the decidua, after delivery of the fetus heavily glycosylated FFN may serve to facilitate a successful third stage of labor.

The presence of cervicovaginal FFN (>50 ng/ml) between 22 and 37 weeks of gestation is associated with an increased risk of PTD among symptomatic patients with a LR+ of 4.67 and a LR− of 0.22 and a LR+:LR− of 21.2.[138] Cognizant that the FFN test was only predictive for 2–3 weeks, Peaceman et al[141] evaluated the predictive value of FFN for predicting PTD within 7 and 14 days, and noted LR+ of 4.9 and 4.9, respectively, and LR− of 0.15 and 0.21, respectively. Of note, the corresponding negative predictive values in this population-based study were 99.5 and 99.2%, respectively. Lockwood et al[142] also reported the utility of cervicovaginal FFN in the prediction of subsequent PTD amongst asymptomatic patients sampled every 2–4 weeks between 24 and 37 weeks of gestation. The population had a spontaneous PTD rate of 11% (49/429), and a cervical FFN value >60 ng/ml was noted to predict PTD with a LR+ of 2.6 and a LR− of 0.38. The comparable results for a vaginal FFN value of >50 ng/ml were a LR+ of 3.4 and a LR− of 0.4. The authors noted that cervical and vaginal FFN predicted PTD due to PTL and PPROM with equal efficiency. The MFMN assessed the value of cervicovaginal FFN obtained at 22–24 weeks among 2929 asymptomatic women, and found a LR+ of 6.3 and a LR− of 0.84 with a LR+:LR− of 7.5.[143] Meta-analysis of 41 studies examining the accuracy of FFN in predicting PTD in both symptomatic and high-risk asymptomatic patients are presented in Table 11.4.[144]

Recent studies suggest that the test is equally valid in patients with twins, cerclage and prior multifetal reduction procedures, and that a speculum need not be used to obtain a vaginal specimen.[145–148] While the principal utility of the FFN lies in its very high negative predictive value (>99% for delivery within 2 weeks), most studies suggest a positive predictive value for PTD around >50%, suggesting that FFN positive patients beyond 23 completed weeks of gestation should receive corticosteroids.

Table 11.4 The predictive accuracy of fetal fibronectin (FFN) in asymptomatic and symptomatic patients at risk for preterm delivery (PTD)

Prediction target	Number of studies	Pooled LR+ (95% CI)	Pooled LR− (95% CI)	LR+:LR−
Symptomatic patients				
PTD <7–10 days	14	5.43 (4.36–6.74)	0.25 (0.2–0.31)	21.7
PTD <34 weeks	8	3.64 (3.32–5.73)	0.32 (0.16–0.66)	11.4
PTD <37 weeks	27	3.27 (2.74–3.92)	0.48 (0.41–0.56)	6.8
Asymptomatic patients				
PTD <34 weeks	12	4.01 (2.93–5.49)	0.78 (0.72–0.84)	5.1
PTD <37 weeks	23	2.94 (2.47–3.50)	0.52 (0.44–0.62)	5.6

CI, Confidence interval; LR, Likelihood ratio.

Table 11.5 The predictive accuracy of cervicovaginal prolactin in symptomatic patients at risk for preterm delivery (PTD)

Ref	Population (gestational age at sampling [weeks])	Cut-off (ng/ml)	Definition of PTD	LR+	LR−	LR+:LR−
151	Symptomatic (<32)	2	<37 weeks	2.44	0.52	4.7
152	Symptomatic (21–34)	2	<34 weeks	4.75	0.49	9.7
153	Symptomatic (29–36)	50	PTD <12 days	13.0	0.37	35.1
154	Symptomatic (24–36)	1.8	<37 weeks	12.5	0.52	23.1

LR, Likelihood ratio.

Cervicovaginal prolactin

Prolactin is produced by decidualized endometrial stromal cells in response to progesterone.[149] Prolactin accumulates in the amniotic fluid and its presence is a marker of PPROM.[150] Given that disruption of the chorionic decidual interface and/or increased fetal membrane permeability likely precede most cases of PTD, cervicovaginal prolactin has been assessed as a marker of PTD (Table 11.5). Preliminary studies suggest that it appears to have predictive efficacy analogous to FFN.

Cervicovaginal IGFBP-1

IGFBP-1 is a major secretory protein of decidualized endometrium, and like prolactin accumulates in high concentrations in the amniotic fluid where it serves as a marker of PPROM.[155] Vogel et al[156] examined vaginal IGFBP-1 as a marker of PTD in symptomatic patients, and observed that elevated values predicted PTD poorly with a sensitivity of only 13% (a LR+ of 3.0 and a LR− of 0.88). Since the nonphosphorylated form of IGFBP-1 is mainly found in the amniotic fluid, and the phosphorylated form is predominantly secreted by decidual cells, the presence of the former in cervicovaginal secretions is a better diagnostic test for overt PROM. Presence of the latter could reflect increased proteolytic activity of the chorionic–decidual interface that precedes PTD.[157] Thus, a number of investigators have examined the predictive value of phosphorylated IGFBP-1, and these results are presented in Table 11.6.

Multiple marker testing

Given that no single test, with the exception of FFN, in the largest study consistently yields LR+:LR− >25–50,

Table 11.6 The predictive accuracy of cervicovaginal insulin-like growth factor binding protein (IGFBP) 1 in symptomatic patients at risk for preterm delivery (PTD)

Ref	Population (gestational age at sampling [weeks])	Cut-off (μg/L)	Definition of PTD (weeks)	LR+	LR−	LR+:LR−
158	Symptomatic (22–37)	10	<37	3.68	0.37	9.9
120	Symptomatic (22–32)	6.4	<37	1.8	NA	NA
159	Symptomatic (20–36)	10	<37	15.2	0.11	138.2
160	Symptomatic (23–33)	10	<37	4.24	0.32	13.2

LR, Likelihood ratio; NA, not applicable.

and since pathway-specific tests will vary in efficacy with the relative contribution of that specific pathway to the total universe of PTD cases, attention has focused on the value of using multiple individual and/or common pathway markers. For example, asymptomatic women assessed once at 24–28 weeks and found to have both a positive FFN and a short cervix on transvaginal ultrasound are at relatively high risk of spontaneous PTD (33.3%), while the absence of either marker places them at very low risk of PTD <34 weeks (1.3%).[161] The MFMN evaluated 28 putative biologic markers for spontaneous PTD in asymptomatic women at 23–24 weeks using a nested case-control design and noted that 93% of cases had at least one positive test result versus 34% of control subjects (OR 24.0; 95% CI 6.4–93.4).[161] However, it remains to be seen whether serial multimarker screening will yield more satisfying results.

SUMMARY

While our understanding of the pathogenesis of PTD has never been more refined we have not been able to translate these advances into well-performing diagnostic or screening tests in either symptomatic or asymptomatic patients. Recent attention has focused on leveraging the new science of proteomics toward this end, but thus far the complex nature of the accessible media – blood and cervicovaginal secretions – has stymied such efforts. A growing awareness of the genetic predisposition to PTD may offer a complimentary pathway to predictive tests, but this promise has yet to be realized. Finally, the absence of truly effective therapies undermines our efforts at developing efficient diagnostic and screening tests. Current practice generally exploits the high negative predictive value of a long cervix and/or negative FFN to avoid introduction of costly, and potentially dangerous, interventions of unproven efficacy.

REFERENCES

1. www.cdc.gov/nchs/pressroom/04facts/birthrates.htm; National Vital Statistics Reports 2003; 52: 1–116.
2. National Vital Statistics Reports 2003; 52: 1–116.
3. Vogel I, Thorsen P, Curry A, Sandager P, Uldbjerg N. Biomarkers for the prediction of preterm delivery. Acta Obstet Gynecol Scand 2005; 84: 516–25.
4. Parry S, Strauss 3rd JF. Premature rupture of the fetal membranes. N Engl J Med 1998; 338: 663–70.
5. Husslein P, Sinzinger H. Concentration of 13,14-dihydro-15-keto-prostaglandin E2 in the maternal peripheral plasma during labour of spontaneous onset. Br J Obstet Gynaecol 1984; 91: 228–31.
6. Sellers SM, Hodgson HT, Mitchell MD, Anderson AB, Turnbull AC. Raised prostaglandin levels in the third stage of labor. Am J Obstet Gynecol 1982; 144: 209–12.
7. Keirse MJNC, Turnbull AC. Prostaglandins in amniotic fluid during late pregnancy and labour. J Obstet Gynaecol Br Commonw 1973; 80: 970–3.
8. Brodt-Eppley J, Myatt L. Prostaglandin receptors in lower uterine segment myometrium during gestation and labor. Obstet Gynecol 1999; 93: 89–93.
9. Olson DM. The role of prostaglandins in the initiation of parturition. Best Pract Res Clin Obstet Gynaecol 2003; 17: 717–30.
10. Lye SJ, Challis JRG. Paracrine and endocrine control of myometrial activity. In Gluckman PD, Johnson BM, Nathanielsz PW, eds. Advances in Fetal Physiology: Reviews in Honour of G.C. Liggins. Advances in Perinatal Medicine (VII). Ithaca, NY: Perinatology Press, 1989, 361–75.
11. Yoshida M, Sagawa N, Itoh H et al. Prostaglandin F(2alpha), cytokines and cyclic mechanical stretch augment matrix metalloproteinase-1 secretion from cultured human uterine cervical fibroblast cells. Mol Hum Reprod 2002; 8: 681–7.
12. Denison FC, Calder AA, Kelly RW. The action of prostaglandin E2 on the human cervix: stimulation of interleukin 8 and inhibition of secretory leukocyte protease inhibitor. Am J Obstet Gynecol 1999; 180: 614–20.
13. Madsen G, Zakar T, Ku CY et al. Prostaglandins differentially modulate progesterone receptor-A and -B expression in human

myometrial cells: evidence for prostaglandin-induced functional progesterone withdrawal. J Clin Endocrinol Metab 2004; 89: 1010–13.

14. Copper RL, Goldenberg RL, Das A et al. The preterm prediction study: maternal stress is associated with spontaneous preterm birth at less than thirty-five weeks' gestation. National Institute of Child Health and Human Development Maternal–Fetal Medicine Units Network. Am J Obstet Gynecol 1996; 175: 1286–92.

15. Germain AM, Carvajal J, Sanchez M et al. Preterm labor: placental pathology and clinical correlation. Obstet Gynecol 1999; 94: 284–9.

16. Arias F, Rodriquez L, Rayne SC, Kraus FT. Maternal placental vasculopathy and infection: two distinct subgroups among patients with preterm labor and preterm ruptured membranes. Am J Obstet Gynecol 1993; 168: 585–91.

17. Amiel-Tison C, Cabrol D, Denver R et al. Fetal adaptation to stress. Part I: acceleration of fetal maturation and earlier birth triggered by placental insufficiency in humans. Early Hum Dev 2004; 78: 15–27.

18. Challis JR, Lye SJ, Gibb W et al. Understanding preterm labor. Ann NY Acad Sci 2001; 943: 225–34.

19. McLean M, Bisits A, Davies J et al. A placental clock controlling the length of human pregnancy. Nat Med 1995; 1: 460–3.

20. Jones SA, Challis JR. Steroid, corticotrophin-releasing hormone, ACTH and prostaglandin interactions in the amnion and placenta of early pregnancy in man. J Endocrinol 1990; 125: 153–9.

21. Lockwood CJ, Radunovic N, Nastic D et al. Corticotropin-releasing hormone and related pituitary-adrenal axis hormones in fetal and maternal blood during the second half of pregnancy. J Perinat Med 1996; 24: 243–51.

22. Zakar T, Hirst JJ, Mijovic JE, Olson DM. Glucocorticoids stimulate the expression of prostaglandin endoperoxide H synthase-2 in amnion cells. Endocrinology 1995; 136: 1610–19.

23. Patel FA, Clifton VL, Chwalisz K, Challis JR. Steroid regulation of prostaglandin dehydrogenase activity and expression in human term placenta and chorio-decidua in relation to labor. J Clin Endocrinol Metab 1999; 84: 291–9.

24. Alfaidy N, Xiong ZG, Myatt L et al. Prostaglandin F2alpha potentiates cortisol production by stimulating 11beta-hydroxysteroid dehydrogenase 1: a novel feedback loop that may contribute to human labor. J Clin Endocrinol Metab 2001; 86: 5585–92.

25. Mastorakos G, Ilias I. Maternal and fetal hypothalamic-pituitary-adrenal axes during pregnancy and postpartum. Ann NY Acad Sci 2003; 997: 136–49.

26. Chakravorty A, Mesiano S, Jaffe RB. Corticotropin-releasing hormone stimulates P450 17alpha-hydroxylase/17,20-lyase in human fetal adrenal cells via protein kinase C. J Clin Endocrinol Metab 1999; 84: 3732–8.

27. Di WL, Lachelin GC, McGarrigle HH, Thomas NS, Becker DL. Oestriol and oestradiol increase cell to cell communication and connexin43 protein expression in human myometrium. Mol Hum Reprod 2001; 7: 671–9.

28. Richter ON, Kubler K, Schmolling J et al. Oxytocin receptor gene expression of estrogen-stimulated human myometrium in extracorporeally perfused non-pregnant uteri. Mol Hum Reprod 2004; 10: 339–46.

29. Matsui K, Higashi K, Fukunaga K et al. Hormone treatments and pregnancy alter myosin light chain kinase and calmodulin levels in rabbit myometrium. J Endocrinol 1983; 97: 11–19.

30. Fuchs AR, Fuchs F. Endocrinology of human parturition: a review. Br J Obstet Gynaecol 1984; 91: 948–67.

31. Heine RP, McGregor JA, Goodwin TM et al. Serial salivary estriol to detect an increased risk of preterm birth. Obstet Gynecol 2000; 96: 490–7.

32. Goldenberg RL, Hauth JC, Andrews WW. Intrauterine infection and preterm delivery. N Engl J Med 2000; 342: 1500–7.

33. Mueller-Heubach E, Rubinstein DN, Schwarz SS. Histologic chorioamnionitis and preterm delivery in different patient populations. Obstet Gynecol 1990; 75: 622–6.

34. Cassell G, Hauth J, Andrews W, Cutter G, Goldenberg R. Chorioamnion colonization: correlation with gestational age in women delivered following spontaneous labor versus indicated delivery. Am J Obstet Gynecol 1993;168: 425.

35. Gray DJ, Robinson HB, Malone J, Thomson RB Jr. Adverse outcome in pregnancy following amniotic fluid isolation of Ureaplasma urealyticum. Prenat Diagn 1992; 12: 111–17.

36. Goldenberg RL, Van Meir CA, Sangha RK et al. Immunoreactive 15-hydroxyprostaglandin dehydrogenase (PGDH) is reduced in fetal membranes from patients at preterm delivery in the presence of infection. Placenta 1996; 17: 291–7.

37. Challis JR, Lye SJ, Gibb W et al. Understanding preterm labor. Ann NY Acad Sci 2001; 943: 225–34.

38. McLaren J, Taylor DJ, Bell SC. Prostaglandin E(2)-dependent production of latent matrix metalloproteinase-9 in cultures of human fetal membranes. Mol Hum Reprod 2000; 6: 1033–40.

39. Lei H, Furth EE, Kalluri R et al. A program of cell death and extracellular matrix degradation is activated in the amnion before the onset of labor. J Clin Invest 1996; 98: 1971–8.

40. Ito A, Nakamura T, Uchiyama T et al. Stimulation of the biosynthesis of interleukin 8 by interleukin 1 and tumor necrosis factor alpha in cultured human chorionic cells. Biol Pharm Bull 1994; 17: 1463–7.

41. Arechavaleta-Velasco F, Ogando D, Parry S, Vadillo-Ortega F. Production of matrix metalloproteinase-9 in lipopolysaccharide-stimulated human amnion occurs through an autocrine and paracrine proinflammatory cytokine-dependent system. Biol Reprod 2002; 67: 1952–8.

42. So T, Ito A, Sato T, Mori Y, Hirakawa S. Tumor necrosis factor-alpha stimulates the biosynthesis of matrix metalloproteinases and plasminogen activator in cultured human chorionic cells. Biol Reprod 1992; 46: 772–8.

43. Fortunato SJ, Menon R, Lombardi SJ. Role of tumor necrosis factor-alpha in the premature rupture of membranes and preterm labor pathways. Am J Obstet Gynecol 2002; 187: 1159–62.

44. Dudley DJ, Trautman MS, Araneo BA, Edwin SS, Mitchell MD. Decidual cell biosynthesis of interleukin-6: regulation by inflammatory cytokines. J Clin Endocrinol Metab 1992; 74: 884–9.

45. Fortunato SJ, Menon RP, Swan KF, Menon R. Inflammatory cytokine (interleukins 1, 6 and 8 and tumor necrosis factor-alpha) release from cultured human fetal membranes in response to endotoxic lipopolysaccharide mirrors amniotic fluid concentrations. Am J Obstet Gynecol 1996; 174: 1855–61.

46. Yoon BH, Jun JK, Romero R et al. Amniotic fluid inflammatory cytokines (interleukin-6, interleukin-1beta, and tumor necrosis factor-alpha), neonatal brain white matter lesions, and cerebral palsy. Am J Obstet Gynecol 1997; 177: 19–26.

47. Romero R, Avila C, Santhanam U, Sehgal PB. Amniotic fluid interleukin 6 in preterm labor. Association with infection. J Clin Invest 1990; 85: 1392–400.

48. Mitchell MD, Dudley DJ, Edwin SS, Schiller SL. Interleukin-6 stimulates prostaglandin production by human amnion and decidual cells. Eur J Pharmacol 1991; 192: 189–91.

49. Osmers RG, Blaser J, Kuhn W, Tschesche H. Interleukin-8 synthesis and the onset of labor. Obstet Gynecol 1995; 86: 223–9.

50. Barclay CG, Brennand JE, Kelly RW, Calder AA. Interleukin 8 production by the human cervix. Am J Obstet Gynecol 1993; 169: 625–32.

51. Kelly RW, Leask R, Calder AA. Choriodecidual production of interleukin-8 and mechanism of parturition. Lancet 1992; 339: 776–7.

52. Lockwood CJ, Arcuri F, Toti P, et al. Tumor necrosis factor-alpha and interleukin-1-beta regulate interleukin-8 expression in third trimester decidual cells: inplications for the genesis of chorioamnionitis. Am J Pathol 2006; 169(4): 1294–302.

53. Holst RM, Mattsby-Baltzer I, Wennerholm UB, Hagberg H, Jacobsson B. Interleukin-6 and interleukin-8 in cervical fluid in a population of Swedish women in preterm labor: relationship to microbial invasion of the amniotic fluid, intra-amniotic inflammation, and preterm delivery. Acta Obstet Gynecol Scand 2005; 84: 551–7.

54. Hillier SL, Martins J, Krohn M et al. A case-control study of chorioamnionic infection and histologic chorioamnionitis in prematurity. N Engl J Med 1988; 319: 972–8.

55. Andrews WW, Goldenberg RL, Hauth JC. Preterm labor: emerging role of genital tract infections. Infect Agents Dis 1995; 4: 196–211.

56. Gibbs RS, Romero R, Hillier SL, Eschenbach DA, Sweet RL. A review of premature birth and subclinical infection. Am J Obstet Gynecol 1992; 166: 1515–28.

57. Horowitz S, Mazor M, Romero R, Horowitz J, Glezerman M. Infection of the amniotic cavity with Ureaplasma urealyticum in the midtrimester of pregnancy. J Reprod Med 1995; 40: 375–9.

58. Bakketeig LS, Hoffman HJ. Epidemiology of preterm birth: results from a longitudinal study of births in Norway. In: Elder LS, Hendricks CH, eds. Preterm Labor. London/Boston: Butterworth, 1981: 174.

59. Porter TF, Fraser A, Hunter CY, Ward R, Varner MW. The intergenerational predisposition to preterm birth. Obstet Gynecol 1997; 90: 63–7.

60. Adams MM, Elam-Evans LD, Wilson HG, Gilbertz DA. Rates of and factors associated with recurrence of preterm delivery. JAMA 2000; 283: 1591–6.

61. Genc MR, Gerber S, Nesin M, Witkin SS. Polymorphism in the interleukin-1 gene complex and spontaneous preterm delivery. Am J Obstet Gynecol 2002; 187: 157–63.

62. Roberts AK, Monzon-Barbonaba F, Van Deerlin PG et al. Association of polymorphism with the promoter of the tumor necrosis factor gene with increased risk of preterm premature rupture of the fetal membranes. Am J Obstet Gynecol 1999; 180: 1297–302.

63. Macones GA, Parry S, Elkousy M et al. A polymorphism in the promoter region of TNF and bacterial vaginosis: preliminary evidence of gene-environment interaction in the etiology of spontaneous preterm birth. Am J Obstet Gynecol 2004; 190: 1504–8.

64. Dizon-Townson DS, Major H, Varner M, Ward K. A promoter mutation that increases transcription of the tumor necrosis factor-alpha gene is not associated with preterm delivery. Am J Obstet Gynecol 1997; 177: 810–13.

65. Simhan HN, Krohn MA, Roberts JM, Zeevi A, Caritis SN. Interleukin-6 promoter-174 polymorphism and spontaneous preterm birth. Am J Obstet Gynecol 2003; 189: 915–18.

66. Lorenz E, Hallman M, Marttila R, Haataha R, Schwartz D. Association between the Asp299Gly polymorphisms in the toll-like receptor 4 and premature births in the Finnish population. Pediatr Res 2002; 52: 373–6.

67. Williams MA, Mittendorf R, Lieberman E, Monson RR. Adverse infant outcomes associated with first-trimester vaginal bleeding. Obstet Gynecol 1991; 78: 14–18.

68. Harger JH, Hsing AW, Tuomala RE et al. Risk factors for preterm premature rupture of fetal membranes: a multicenter case-control study. Am J Obstet Gynecol 1990; 163: 130–7.

69. Salafia CM, Lopez-Zeno JA, Sherer DM et al. Histologic evidence of old intrauterine bleeding is more frequent in prematurity. Am J Obstet Gynecol 1995; 173: 1065–70.

70. Winer N, Hamidou M, El Kouri D, Philippe HJ. Maternal and obstetrical risk factors of placental vascular pathology. Ann Med Interne (Paris) 2003; 154: 316–24.

71. Hladky K, Yankowitz J, Hansen WF. Placental abruption. Obstet Gynecol Surv 2002; 57: 299–305.

72. Roque H, Paidas MJ, Funai EF, Kuczynski E, Lockwood CJ. Maternal thrombophilias are not associated with early pregnancy loss. Thromb Haemost 2004; 91: 290–5.

73. Naeye RL. Maternal age, obstetric complications, and the outcome of pregnancy. Obstet Gynecol 1983; 61: 210–16.

74. Strobino B, Pantel-Silverman J. Gestational vaginal bleeding and pregnancy outcome. Am J Epidemiol 1989; 129: 806–15.

75. Nagase H. Stromelysins 1 and 2. In: Parks WC, Mecham R, eds. Matrix Metalloproteinases. San Diego: Academic Press, 1998: 43–84.

76. Mackenzie AP, Schatz F, Krikun G et al. Mechanisms of abruption-induced premature rupture of the fetal membranes: Thrombin enhanced decidual matrix metalloproteinase-3 (stromelysin-1) expression. Am J Obstet Gynecol 2004; 191: 1996–2001.

77. Rosen T, Schatz F, Kuczynski E et al. Thrombin-enhanced matrix metalloproteinase-1 expression: a mechanism linking placental abruption with premature rupture of the membranes. J Matern Fetal Neonatal Med 2002; 11: 11–17.

78. Lockwood CJ, Toti P, Arcuri F et al. Mechanisms of abruption-induced premature rupture of the fetal membranes: Thrombin-enhanced interleukin-8 expression in term decidua. Am J Pathol 2005; 167: 1443–9.

79. Lathbury LJ, Salamonsen LA. In-vitro studies of the potential role of neutrophils in the process of menstruation. Mol Hum Reprod 2000; 6: 899–906.

80. Phillippe M, Chien EK. Intracellular signaling and phasic myometrial contractions. J Soc Gynecol Invest 1998; 5: 169–77.

81. Martin JA, Hamilton BE, Menacker F, Sutton PD, Matthews TJ. Preliminary births for 2004: Infant and maternal health. Health E-stats. Hyattsville, MD: National Center for Health Statistics. Released November 15, 2005.

82. Levy R, Kanengiser B, Furman B et al. A randomized trial comparing a 30-mL and an 80-mL Foley catheter balloon for pre-induction cervical ripening. Am J Obstet Gynecol 2004; 191: 1632–6.

83. Yoshida M, Sagawa N, Itoh H et al. Prostaglandin F(2alpha), cytokines and cyclic mechanical stretch augment matrix metalloproteinase-1 secretion from cultured human uterine cervical fibroblast cells. Mol Hum Reprod 2002; 8: 681–7.

84. Leguizamon G, Smith J, Younis H, Nelson DM, Sadovsky Y. Enhancement of amniotic cyclooxygenase type 2 activity in women with preterm delivery associated with twins or polyhydramnios. Am J Obstet Gynecol 2001; 184: 117–22.

85. Terakawa K, Itoh H, Sagawa N et al. Site-specific augmentation of amnion cyclooxygenase-2 and decidua vera phospholipase-A2 expression in labor: possible contribution of mechanical stretch and interleukin-1 to amnion prostaglandin synthesis. J Soc Gynecol Invest 2002; 9: 68–74.

86. Terzidou V, Sooranna SR, Kim LU et al. Mechanical stretch up-regulates the human oxytocin receptor in primary human uterine myocytes. J Clin Endocrinol Metab 2005; 90: 237–46.

87. Sooranna SR, Engineer N, Loudon JA et al. The mitogen-activated protein kinase dependent expression of prostaglandin H synthase-2 and interleukin-8 messenger ribonucleic acid by myometrial cells: the differential effect of stretch and interleukin-1{beta}. J Clin Endocrinol Metab 2005; 90: 3517–27.

88. Loudon JA, Sooranna SR, Bennett PR, Johnson MR. Mechanical stretch of human uterine smooth muscle cells increases IL-8 mRNA expression and peptide synthesis. Mol Hum Reprod 2004; 10: 895–9.

89. Lockwood CJ, Radunovic N, Nastic D et al. Corticotropin-releasing hormone and related pituitary-adrenal axis hormones in fetal and maternal blood during the second half of pregnancy. J Perinatol Med 1996; 24: 243.

90. Wadhwa PD, Porto M, Garite TJ, Chicz-DeMet A, Sandman CA. Maternal corticotropin-releasing hormone levels in the early third trimester predict length of gestation in human pregnancy. Am J Obstet Gynecol 1998; 179: 1079–85.

91. Wadhwa PD, Garite TJ, Porto M et al. Placental corticotropin-releasing hormone (CRH), spontaneous preterm birth, and fetal growth restriction: a prospective investigation. Am J Obstet Gynecol 2004; 191: 1063–9.

92. Goland RS, Jozak S, Warren WB et al. Elevated levels of umbilical cord plasma corticotropin-releasing hormone in growth-retarded fetuses. J Clin Endocrinol Metab 1993; 77: 1174–9.

93. Coleman MA, France JT, Schellenberg JC et al. Corticotropin-releasing hormone, corticotropin-releasing hormone-binding protein, and activin A in maternal serum: prediction of preterm delivery and response to glucocorticoids in women with symptoms of preterm labor. Am J Obstet Gynecol 2000; 183: 643–8.

94. Berkowitz GS, Lapinski RH, Lockwood CJ et al. Corticotropin-releasing factor and its binding protein: maternal serum levels in term and preterm deliveries. Am J Obstet Gynecol 1996; 174: 1477–83.

95. Inder WJ, Prickett TC, Ellis MJ et al. The utility of plasma CRH as a predictor of preterm delivery. J Clin Endocrinol Metab 2001; 86: 5706–10.

96. Holzman C, Jetton J, Siler-Khodr T, Fisher R, Rip T. Second trimester corticotropin-releasing hormone levels in relation to preterm delivery and ethnicity. Obstet Gynecol 2001; 97: 657–63.

97. McLean M, Bisits A, Davies J et al. Predicting risk of preterm delivery by second-trimester measurement of maternal plasma corticotropin-releasing hormone and alpha-fetoprotein concentrations. Am J Obstet Gynecol 1999; 181: 207–15.

98. Leung TN, Chung TK, Madsen G et al. Elevated mid-trimester maternal corticotrophin-releasing hormone levels in pregnancies that delivered before 34 weeks. Br J Obstet Gynaecol 1999; 106: 1041–6.

99. Mazor M, Hershkovitz R, Chaim W et al. Human preterm birth is associated with systemic and local changes in progesterone/17 beta-estradiol ratios. Am J Obstet Gynecol 1994; 171: 231–6.

100. Heine RP, McGregor JA, Goodwin TM et al. Serial salivary estriol to detect an increased risk of preterm birth. Obstet Gynecol 2000; 96: 490–7.

101. McGregor JA, Jackson GM, Lachelin GC et al. Salivary estriol as risk assessment for preterm labor: a prospective trial. Am J Obstet Gynecol 1995; 173: 1337–42.

102. Chandra S, Scott H, Dodds L et al. Unexplained elevated maternal serum alpha-fetoprotein and/or human chorionic gonadotropin and the risk of adverse outcomes. Am J Obstet Gynecol 2003; 189: 775–81.

103. Hurley TJ, Miller C, O'Brien TJ, Blacklaw M, Quirk JG Jr. Maternal serum human chorionic gonadotropin as a marker for the delivery of low-birth-weight infants in women with unexplained elevations in maternal serum alpha-fetoprotein. J Matern Fetal Med 1996; 5: 340–4.

104. Morssink LP, Kornman LH, Beekhuis JR, De Wolf BT, Mantingh A. Abnormal levels of maternal serum human chorionic gonadotropin and alpha-fetoprotein in the second trimester: relation to fetal weight and preterm delivery. Prenat Diagn 1995; 15: 1041–6.

105. Gonen R, Perez R, David M et al. The association between unexplained second-trimester maternal serum hCG elevation and pregnancy complications. Obstet Gynecol 1992; 80: 83–6.

106. Lieppman RE, Williams MA, Cheng EY et al. An association between elevated levels of human chorionic gonadotropin in the midtrimester and adverse pregnancy outcome. Am J Obstet Gynecol 1993; 168: 1852–6.

107. Wenstrom KD, Owen J, Boots LR, DuBard MB. Elevated second-trimester human chorionic gonadotropin levels in association with poor pregnancy outcome. Am J Obstet Gynecol 1994; 171: 1038–41.

108. Brajenovic-Milic B, Tislaric D, Zuvic-Butorac M et al. Elevated second-trimester free beta-hCG as an isolated finding and pregnancy outcomes. Fetal Diagn Ther 2004; 19: 483–7.

109. Guvenal T, Kantas E, Erselcan T, Culhaoglu Y, Cetin A. Beta-human chorionic gonadotropin and prolactin assays in cervicovaginal secretions as a predictor of preterm delivery. Int J Gynaecol Obstet 2001; 75: 229–34.

110. Garshasbi A, Ghazanfari T, Faghih Zadeh S. Beta-human chorionic gonadotropin in cervicovaginal secretions and preterm delivery. Int J Gynaecol Obstet 2004; 86: 358–64.

111. Leitich H, Bodner-Adler B, Brunbauer M et al. Bacterial vaginosis as a risk factor for preterm delivery: a meta-analysis. Am J Obstet Gynecol 2003; 189: 139–47.

112. Meis PJ, Goldenberg RL, Mercer B et al. The preterm prediction study: significance of vaginal infections. National Institute of Child Health and Human Development Maternal–Fetal Medicine Units Network. Am J Obstet Gynecol 1995; 173: 1231–5.

113. Hillier SL, Nugent RP, Eschenbach DA et al. Association between bacterial vaginosis and preterm delivery of a low-birth-weight infant. The Vaginal Infections and Prematurity Study Group. N Engl J Med 1995; 333: 1737–42.

114. Leitich H, Brunbauer M, Bodner-Adler B et al. Antibiotic treatment of bacterial vaginosis in pregnancy: a meta-analysis. Am J Obstet Gynecol 2003; 188: 752–8.

115. Romero R, Oyarzun E, Mazor M et al. Meta-analysis of the relationship between asymptomatic bacteriuria and preterm delivery/low birth weight. Obstet Gynecol 1989; 73: 576–8.

116. Villar J, Gulmezoglu AM, de Onis M. Nutritional and antimicrobial interventions to prevent preterm birth: an overview of randomized controlled trials. Obstet Gynecol Surv 1998; 53: 575–85.

117. Krohn MA, Thwin SS, Rabe LK, Brown Z, Hillier SL. Vaginal colonization by Escherichia coli as a risk factor for very low birth weight delivery and other perinatal complications. J Infect Dis 1997; 175: 606–10.

118. El-Bastawissi AY, Williams MA, Riley DE, Hitti J, Krieger JN. Amniotic fluid interleukin-6 and preterm delivery: a review. Obstet Gynecol 2000; 95: 1056–64.

119. Lockwood CJ, Ghidini A, Wein R et al. Increased interleukin-6 concentrations in cervical secretions are associated with preterm delivery. Am J Obstet Gynecol 1994; 171: 1097–102.

120. Kurkinen-Raty M, Ruokonen A, Vuopala S et al. Combination of cervical interleukin-6 and -8, phosphorylated insulin-like growth factor-binding protein-1 and transvaginal cervical ultrasonography in assessment of the risk of preterm birth. Br J Obstet Gynaecol 2001; 108: 875–81.

121. Lange M, Chen FK, Wessel J, Buscher U, Dudenhausen JW. Elevation of interleukin-6 levels in cervical secretions as a predictor of preterm delivery. Acta Obstet Gynaecol Scand 2003; 82: 326–9.

122. Coleman MA, Keelan JA, McCowan LM, Townend KM, Mitchell MD. Predicting preterm delivery: comparison of cervicovaginal interleukin (IL)-1beta, IL-6 and IL-8 with fetal fibronectin and cervical dilatation. Eur J Obstet Gynecol Reprod Biol 2001; 95: 154–8.

123. Holst RM, Mattsby-Baltzer I, Wennerholm UB, Hagberg H, Jacobsson B. Interleukin-6 and interleukin-8 in cervical fluid in

a population of Swedish women in preterm labor: relationship to microbial invasion of the amniotic fluid, intra-amniotic inflammation, and preterm delivery. Acta Obstet Gynecol Scand 2005; 84: 551–7.

124. Trebeden H, Goffinet F, Kayem G et al. Strip test for bedside detection of interleukin-6 in cervical secretions is predictive for impending preterm delivery. Eur Cytokine Netw 2001; 12: 359–60.

125. Rizzo G, Capponi A, Vlachopoulou A et al. The diagnostic value of interleukin-8 and fetal fibronectin concentrations in cervical secretions in patients with preterm labor and intact membranes. J Perinat Med 1997; 25: 461–8.

126. Goldenberg RL, Andrews WW, Mercer BM et al. The preterm prediction study: granulocyte colony-stimulating factor and spontaneous preterm birth. National Institute of Child Health and Human Development Maternal-Fetal Medicine Units Network. Am J Obstet Gynecol 2000; 182: 625–30.

127. Goldenberg RL, Andrews WW, Guerrant RL et al. The preterm prediction study: cervical lactoferrin concentration, other markers of lower genital tract infection, and preterm birth. National Institute of Child Health and Human Development Maternal–Fetal Medicine Units Network. Am J Obstet Gynecol 2000; 182: 631–5.

128. Ramsey PS, Tamura T, Goldenberg RL et al. National Institute of Child Health and Human Development, Maternal–Fetal Medicine Units Network. The preterm prediction study: elevated cervical ferritin levels at 22 to 24 weeks of gestation are associated with spontaneous preterm delivery in asymptomatic women. Am J Obstet Gynecol 2002; 186: 458–63.

129. Vogel I, Grove J, Thorsen P et al. Preterm delivery predicted by soluble CD163 and CRP in women with symptoms of preterm delivery. Br J Obstet Gynaecol 2005; 112: 737–42.

130. Andrews WW, Tsao J, Goldenberg RL et al. The preterm prediction study: failure of midtrimester cervical sialidase level elevation to predict subsequent spontaneous preterm birth. Am J Obstet Gynecol 1999; 180: 1151–4.

131. Wang EY, Woodruff TK, Moawad A. Follistatin-free activin A is not associated with preterm birth. Am J Obstet Gynecol 2002; 186: 464–9.

132. Moawad AH, Goldenberg RL, Mercer B et al. The Preterm Prediction Study: the value of serum alkaline phosphatase, alpha-fetoprotein, plasma corticotropin-releasing hormone, and other serum markers for the prediction of spontaneous preterm birth. Am J Obstet Gynecol 2002; 186: 990–6.

133. Simhan HN, Caritis SN, Krohn MA, Hillier SL. Elevated vaginal pH and neutrophils are associated strongly with early spontaneous preterm birth. Am J Obstet Gynecol 2003; 189: 1150–4.

134. Simhan HN, Caritis SN, Krohn MA, Hillier SL. The vaginal inflammatory milieu and the risk of early premature preterm rupture of membranes. Am J Obstet Gynecol 2005; 192: 213–18.

135. Rosen T, Kuczynski E, O'Neill LM, Funai EF, Lockwood CJ. Plasma levels of thrombin-antithrombin complexes predict preterm premature rupture of the fetal membranes. J Matern Fetal Med 2001; 10: 297–300.

136. Elovitz MA, Baron J, Phillippe M. The role of thrombin in preterm parturition. Am J Obstet Gynecol 2001; 185: 1059–63.

137. Chaiworapongsa T, Espinoza J, Yoshimatsu J et al. Activation of coagulation system in preterm labor and preterm premature rupture of membranes. J Matern Fetal Neonatal Med 2002; 11: 368–73.

138. Lockwood CJ, Senyei AE, Dische MR et al. Fetal fibronectin in cervical and vaginal secretions as a predictor of preterm delivery. N Engl J Med 1991; 325: 669–74.

139. Feinberg RF, Kliman HJ, Lockwood CJ. Is oncofetal fibronectin a trophoblast glue for implantation? Am J Pathol 1991; 138: 537.

140. Zhu BC, Laine RA. Developmental study of human fetal placental fibronectin: alterations in carbohydrates of tissue fibronectin during gestation. Arch Biochem Biophys 1987; 252: 1–6.

141. Peaceman AM, Andrews WW, Thorp JM et al. Fetal fibronectin as a predictor of preterm birth in patients with symptoms: a multicenter trial. Am J Obstet Gynecol 1997; 177: 13–18.

142. Lockwood CJ, Wein R, Lapinski R et al. The presence of cervical and vaginal fetal fibronectin predicts preterm delivery in an inner-city obstetric population. Am J Obstet Gynecol 1993; 169: 798–804.

143. Goldenberg RL, Mercer BM, Meis PJ et al. The preterm prediction study: fetal fibronectin testing and spontaneous preterm birth. NICHD Maternal Fetal Medicine Units Network. Obstet Gynecol 1996; 87: 643–8.

144. Honest H, Bachmann LM, Gupta JK, Kleijnen J, Khan KS. Accuracy of cervicovaginal fetal fibronectin test in predicting risk of spontaneous preterm birth: systematic review. BMJ 2002; 325(7359): 301–4.

145. Roman AS, Koklanaris N, Paidas MJ et al. 'Blind' vaginal fetal fibronectin as a predictor of spontaneous preterm delivery. Obstet Gynecol 2005; 105: 285–9.

146. Roman AS, Rebarber A, Lipkind H et al. Vaginal fetal fibronectin as a predictor of spontaneous preterm delivery after multifetal pregnancy reduction. Am J Obstet Gynecol 2004; 190: 142–6.

147. Roman AS, Rebarber A, Sfakianaki AK et al. Vaginal fetal fibronectin as a predictor of spontaneous preterm delivery in the patient with cervical cerclage. Am J Obstet Gynecol 2003; 189: 1368–73.

148. Goldenberg RL, Iams JD, Miodovnik M et al. The preterm prediction study: risk factors in twin gestations. National Institute of Child Health and Human Development Maternal–Fetal Medicine Units Network. Am J Obstet Gynecol 1996; 175: 1047–53.

149. Lockwood CJ, Nemerson Y, Guller S et al. Progestational regulation of human endometrial stromal cell tissue factor expression during decidualization. J Clin Endocrinol Metab 1993; 76: 231–6.

150. Buyukbayrak EE, Turan C, Unal O, Dansuk R, Cengizoglu B. Diagnostic power of the vaginal washing-fluid prolactin assay as an alternative method for the diagnosis of premature rupture of membranes. J Matern Fetal Neonatal Med 2004; 15: 120–5.

151. O'Brien JM, Peeler GH, Pitts DW et al. Cervicovaginal prolactin: a marker for spontaneous preterm delivery. Am J Obstet Gynecol 1994; 171: 1107–11.

152. Jotterand AD, Caubel P, Guillaumin D et al. Predictive value of cervical-vaginal prolactin in the evaluation of premature labor risk. J Gynecol Obstet Biol Reprod (Paris) 1997; 26: 95–9.

153. Leylek OA, Songur S, Erselcan T, Cetin A, Izgic E. Cervicovaginal washing prolactin assay in prediction of preterm delivery. Int J Gynaecol Obstet 1997; 59: 7–12.

154. Guvenal T, Kantas E, Erselcan T, Culhaoglu Y, Cetin A. Beta-human chorionic gonadotropin and prolactin assays in cervico-vaginal secretions as a predictor of preterm delivery. Int J Gynaecol Obstet 2001; 75: 229–34.

155. Lockwood CJ, Wein R, Chien D et al. Fetal membrane rupture is associated with the presence of insulin-like growth factor-binding protein-1 in vaginal secretions. Am J Obstet Gynecol 1994; 171: 146–50.

156. Vogel I, Gronbaek H, Thorsen P, Flyvbjerg A. Insulin-like growth factor binding protein 1 (IGFBP-1) in vaginal fluid in pregnancy. In Vivo 2004; 18: 37–41.

157. Martina NA, Kim E, Chitkara U et al. Gestational age-dependent expression of insulin-like growth factor binding protein (IGFBP-1) phosphoforms in human extraamniotic cavities, maternal serum, and decidua suggests decidua as the primary source of IGFBP-1 in

these fluids during early pregnancy. J Clin Endocrinol Metab 1997; 82: 1894–8.

158. Kekki M, Kurki T, Karkkainen T et al. Insulin-like growth factor-binding protein-1 in cervical secretion as a predictor of preterm delivery. Acta Obstet Gynecol Scand 2001; 80: 546–51.

159. Lembet A, Eroglu D, Ergin T et al. New rapid bed-side test to predict preterm delivery: phosphorylated insulin-like growth factor binding protein-1 in cervical secretions. Acta Obstet Gynecol Scand 2002; 81: 706–12.

160. Kwek K, Khi C, Ting HS, Yeo GS. Evaluation of a bedside test for phosphorylated insulin-like growth factor binding

protein-1 in preterm labour. Ann Acad Med Singapore 2004; 33: 780–3.

161. Goldenberg RL, Iams JD, Das A et al. The Preterm Prediction Study: sequential cervical length and fetal fibronectin testing for the prediction of spontaneous preterm birth. National Institute of Child Health and Human Development Maternal–Fetal Medicine Units Network. Am J Obstet Gynecol 2000; 182: 636–43.

162. Goldenberg RL, Iams JD, Mercer BM et al. Maternal–Fetal Medicine Units Network. The Preterm Prediction Study: toward a multiple-marker test for spontaneous preterm birth. Am J Obstet Gynecol 2001; 185: 643–51.

12

Biophysical methods of prediction and prevention of preterm labor: uterine electromyography and cervical light-induced fluorescence – new obstetrical diagnostic techniques

Robert E Garfield and William L Maner

INTRODUCTION

Development of effective means to prevent or reduce the occurrence of preterm delivery depends upon the understanding of the conditions that initiate labor. Successful labor is dependent upon forceful uterine contractions, and softening and dilation of the cervix. It is widely accepted that pharmacological control of uterine contractility, and cervix function would allow better management of patients who are in premature labor, or even in term labor.[1] However, to develop a rational approach to the control of either uterine activity or cervical changes associated with labor, a thorough understanding of the underlying mechanisms which regulate uterine contractility and cervical connective tissue is important. Paramount for the appropriate management of labor is the ability to correctly identify true versus false labor. No clinical methods currently exist to objectively evaluate the state and function of the uterus or cervix during pregnancy.

Preparatory phase to labor

In the past, labor was viewed as the transition from an inactive to an active uterine muscle either by the addition of an uterotonin or withdrawal from tonic progesterone inhibition.[2] Although those models recognized the importance of progesterone in controlling uterine quiescence, they neither defined precisely the uterine stages of labor nor identified the mechanism of action of the hormones involved. Such models of parturition

did not usually consider the changes in the cervix as an important component of parturition. Experimental and clinical studies with progesterone and its antagonists indicate, however, that parturition is composed of two major steps: a relatively long conditioning (preparatory) phase, followed by a short secondary phase (active labor) (Figure 12.1).[3,4] The conditioning step leading to the softening of the cervix takes place in a different time frame from the conditioning step of the myometrium, indicating that the myometrium and cervix are regulated in part by independent mechanisms.

Labor

The processes governing changes in the myometrium and cervix ultimately become irreversible, and lead to active labor and delivery. However, there may be a point at which the cervix and uterus are electrochemically and physically prepared for delivery, but during which time there are not effective contractions, nor perceptible dilation. It is during this critical 'interim' phase that there exists the final opportunity to effectively treat the uterus or cervix with tocolytics (in order to prevent preterm labor) by halting, or at least delaying, the process.

After this interim period, which may be exceedingly short, it could be that the uterus is hormonally stimulated to contract (or alternatively freed from inhibition to contract) and the cervix will dilate as a result. Once true active labor has started, delivery might not be delayed for more than a few days in humans because

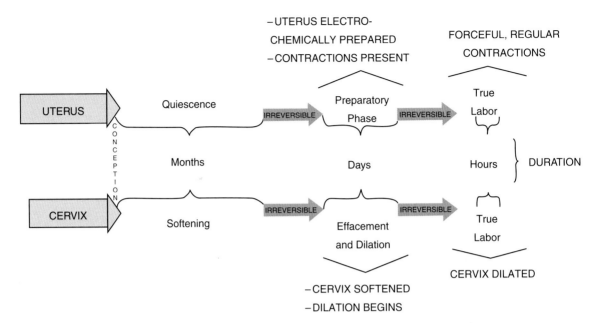

Figure 12.1 A model for the comparison of uterine and cervical evolution through normal parturition (with term delivery). Both organs are regulated by hormonal changes and can be said to exhibit a preparatory phase and a true labor phase. The time period over which the preparatory phase occurs is the primary differing point between the two processes. Note that some phases can be altered with treatments while others presumably cannot. Similarly, some transitions between stages are irreversible.

the changes, which begin in the preparatory phase and culminate with true labor, have by this time become well established and cannot be undone (i.e. irreversible), even with currently available tocolytics. The key to understanding parturition, and to developing suitable treatment methods, is to understand the processes by which the myometrium and the cervix undergo these conditioning, conversion or preparation stages.

Uterus

It has been shown that myometrial cells are coupled together electrically by gap junctions composed of connexin proteins.[5] The grouping of connexins provides channels of low electrical resistance between cells, and so furnishes pathways for the efficient conduction of action potentials. During the greater part of pregnancy, these cell-to-cell channels or contacts are low, causing poor coupling and decreased electrical conductance. This produces quiescence of the muscle for the maintenance of pregnancy. However, at term, cell junctions increase and form an electrical syncytium for producing effective, forceful contractions. The presence of the contacts is controlled by changing estrogen and progesterone levels in the uterus.[5]

As action potentials propagate over the surface of a myometrial cell, the depolarization causes voltage-dependent Ca^{2+} channels (VDCC) to open. Thereafter, Ca^{2+} enters the muscle cell, traveling down its electrochemical gradient to activate the myofilaments, and provokes a contraction. Our research group has demonstrated by reverse transcription polymerase chain reaction (RT-PCR) that the expression of VDCC subunits in the rat myometrium increases during term and preterm labor.[6] The increased expression, which appears to be controlled by progesterone, likely facilitates uterine contractility during labor by increasing portals for Ca^{2+} entry.

Cervix

The composition of the cervix is in the form of smooth muscle (approximately 10%) and a large component of connective tissue (90%), which consists of collagen, elastin and macromolecular components which make up the extracellular matrix.[7] A number of biochemical and functional changes occur in cervical connective tissue at the end of pregnancy.[7–9] Cervical ripening is a process of softening, effacement, and finally dilatation of the cervix, and is required for appropriate progress of labor and delivery of the fetus. It is known that the collagen cross-link, pyridinoline, decreases as the cervix softens. Developing a measure of this system would be useful for monitoring the state and function of the cervix generally.

Physiological cervical ripening is an active biochemical process, which involves connective tissue remodeling,[8] but the mechanism behind this process is not completely understood. Eighty percent of cervical protein is collagen, and 70% of that is in the form of type I collagen and 30% type III collagen.[10] Studies on tissue biopsies have shown that near the end of gestation, and during cervical dilation, the collagen concentration per wet weight is decreasing, the fraction of insoluble collagen shifts towards soluble collagen, and the collagenolytic activity is enhanced in the tissue.[10–13] Electron microscopic investigations show a dissociation and breakdown of collagen fibers.[10,14,15] Little is known about the physiological mediators of cervical ripening. Some investigators suggest the mediators of cervical ripening involve an inflammatory process, and have demonstrated leukocyte infiltration, cytokine activation and prostaglandin (PG) release in the collagen tissue.[10,11,16,17]

Since the exact physiologic mechanism for cervical ripening remains obscure, the action of pharmacologic ripening agents is not entirely clear. PG is widely and successfully used to induce cervical ripening prior to labor induction, but again, the process by which this is accomplished is still unclear. Studies on cervical biopsies from women after PG application demonstrate similar changes in cervical connective tissue as described under physiological ripening, and include an increase in water content, collagenolytic activity, collagen solubility and large proteoglycans.[18–21]

Uterine electromyography (EMG)

Uterine EMG is similar to recording an electrocardiogram (ECG) for heart muscle,[22,23] and amounts to the acquisition of uterine electrical signals taken noninvasively from the abdominal surface (Figure 12.2). Once adopted by physicians, the EMG methodology could benefit obstetrics in much the same way as the ECG benefits cardiology, when utilized as an everyday tool in the perinatal and labor and delivery clinics. Like the function of the ECG for heart-patient monitoring and classification, the capability of the uterine EMG in utilizing electrical recordings for monitoring contractions in normal pregnancies (Figure 12.2) – as well as for diagnosing or even predicting abnormal conditions such as preterm labor, insufficient labor progress and dystocia, and a host of other problems during parturition – would allow for a timely and effective classification of patients.

EMG is based on the actual function of the uterus, and would enable better treatment and management of those patients than with any currently used tool.

This can be accomplished by analyzing several different types of electrical parameters derived from the recorded raw uterine electrical signals, including the power density spectrum (PDS)[24] or wavelet transform,[25,26] either of which will decompose electrical signals into their individual frequency or 'scale' subcomponents. Also, nonlinear signal analysis methods, such as chaoticity or fractal dimension,[26] may be implemented. These types of mathematical functions and transforms allow the uterine electrical signal to be quantified. Receiver-operator-characteristics (ROC) curves can then be used to find the best cut-off values and endpoints to use for patient classification or prediction of labor.

Cervical light-induced fluorescence (LIF)

Examination of LIF is a widely utilized research technique in the biosciences, primarily due to the amount of information that it can reveal in terms of molecular and physical states.[27] Fluorescence spectra offer important details on the structure and dynamics of macromolecules, and their location at microscopic levels. LIF has been used to examine collagen content in a variety of tissues, including changes in collagen content in cancers.[28] This methodology has been used recently to evaluate the cervix (Figure 12.3).

Investigations into the changes in cervical collagen during pregnancy have been noninvasively performed by using the natural fluorescence of collagen. Mature collagen possesses nonreducible hydroxyallysine-based intermolecular cross-links within the primary[29] and secondary structures of collagen fibrils[30] which fluoresce. The greater the amount of collagen in the tissue, the higher the LIF level measured, and therefore the less ripe is the cervix. Near labor and delivery LIF levels are at a minimum, suggesting the possibility of classification of pregnant patients into those who are or are not in true labor, as well as predicting the time of delivery of the fetus. As with the quantified uterine EMG, ROC analysis provides insight into just exactly what are the best cervical LIF cut-off values and measurement-to-delivery time endpoints for consideration. This cervical-assessment methodology, as in the case of uterine EMG, has been shown to be effective in the classification of patients, and in the prediction of labor and delivery.

BENEFITS OF DIAGNOSIS

Diagnosing labor may be the most important (and perhaps the most difficult) task facing obstetricians today.

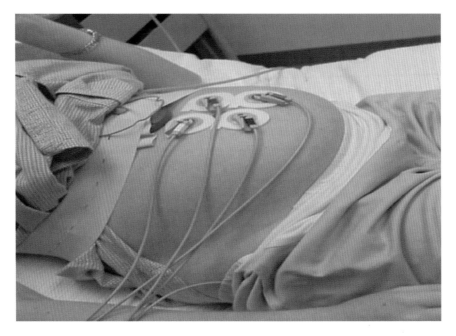

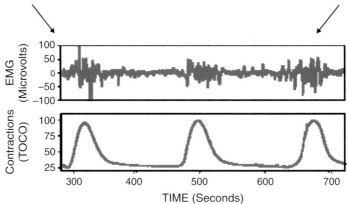

Figure 12.2 The typical uterine electromyography (EMG) setup consists of electrodes placed near the navel close to the midline (which has been determined to yield, generally, the best conduction path from the myometrium to the surface, likely because subcutaneous tissue is thinnest here, especially in late pregnancy). The electrode sites are first prepared by removing excess oils with alcohol, and then by applying a conductive gel. The electrodes are connected to lead wires and cables which pass the uterine EMG signals on to an amplifier/filter. The uterine EMG signals are then displayed on a monitor and stored in a computer for later analysis. Real-time analysis routines are currently being developed to yield a predictive measure while the patient is still being monitored. The tracings at the bottom show the correspondence of uterine EMG burst events to contraction events recorded by tocodynamometer (TOCO) from a laboring patient. The action potentials, as measured by uterine EMG, are actually responsible for the contractions of the uterus, and govern such characteristics as contraction strength, duration, and frequency. The TOCO provides to clinicians only the number of contraction events per unit time and a crude, inaccurate measure of contraction force. Recent studies indicate that the TOCO possesses no objective predictive capability. By contrast, in addition to the number of contraction events per unit time, the uterine EMG signals give critical information about the firing rate and number of action potentials involved during a contraction. As such, the uterine EMG gives a direct measure of the state of myometrial development and preparedness for labor and delivery.

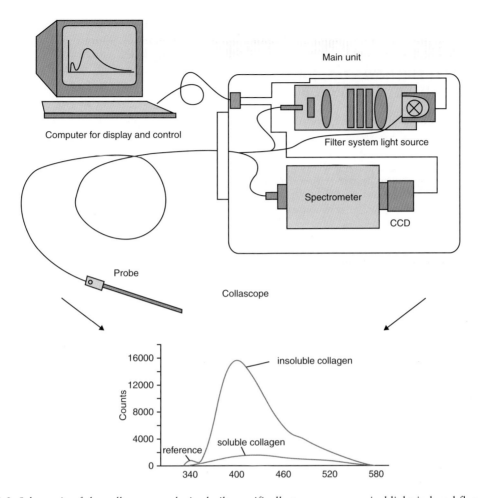

Figure 12.3 Schematic of the collascope, a device built specifically to measure cervical light-induced fluorescence, (LIF). The excitation light source provides light of the proper frequency to elicit fluorescence from cervical collagen pyridinium cross-links, a component which decreases as gestational age increases. The amount of fluorescence produced is proportional to the amount of collagen in the cervix, thereby giving a direct measure of cervical ripeness. The excitation light is applied to the cervix, and fluorescence light is collected from the cervix, via the hand-held probe. The fluorescent light is then separated into frequency components by a spectrometer, and intensity is measured. The results are displayed on a computer screen and stored for later analysis. The trace at the bottom shows the fluorescence spectrum of samples of soluble and insoluble collagen, as measured by the collascope. The LIF ratio value, of the cervix for example, is calculated by taking the peak fluorescent value (which occurs at a wavelength of approximately 390 nm) and dividing by the peak reference value (which occurs at a wavelength of approximately 343 nm). The LIF ratio has been found to be highly predictive of labor in various species, including humans.

Pinpointing exactly when true labor exists – which will lead to delivery – is important for both normal and pathological pregnancies. Predicting labor in normal pregnancies is important for minimizing unnecessary hospitalizations, interventions, and expenses; while accurate prediction and diagnosis of preterm labor will allow practitioners to start treatment earlier in those patients who need it, and avert unnecessary treatment and hospitalization in patients who are having preterm contractions but who are not in true labor. Unfortunately, currently available methods, including those that are based solely on monitoring contractions or on cervical examination, cannot conclusively detect whether a patient has entered the preparatory, or conditioning, phase of parturition, because changes in these variables may be independent of the preparatory stage, or may not become detectable by these methods until a relatively late and inalterable stage has been reached.

WHAT'S OUT THERE NOW – THE CURRENT STATUS OF PARTURITION MONITORING

While several techniques have been adopted to monitor labor, they are either subjective, or do not provide a sufficiently accurate diagnosis or prediction, or both.[31–41] To date, the most important factor for preventing preterm labor has been constant contact and care from health care practitioners.[42]

The applied state-of-the-art in labor monitoring is as follows:

- Present uterine monitors are uncomfortable, inaccurate and/or subjective
- Intrauterine pressure catheters (IUPC) are limited by invasiveness, potential for infection, and the need for ruptured membranes
- No currently used method has consistently/reliably predicted preterm labor
- No currently used method has led to effective treatment of preterm labor
- No currently used method makes a direct measurement of both the function and state of either the uterus or the cervix during pregnancy

Multiple preterm labor symptoms are one currently adopted method for monitoring the state of pregnancy in an effort to predict preterm labor (Table 12.1). Such symptoms include cervical dilation and effacement, vaginal bleeding, and ruptured membranes. These signs are determined by a clinician.

Maximal uterine contractions represent the highest observed number of contraction events seen in any 10 min period. This is assessed by a clinician using a tocodynamometer (TOCO). Most physicians agree that these bulky force-transducer devices provide limited information on labor. Contractions measured with the TOCO can be large or small, and can occur with a similar number of contractions per unit time, regardless of whether the patient is in labor or not. The instruments are largely dependent upon the skill of the clinician, but have not changed treatments or improved outcomes following preterm labor.

The Bishop scoring method was introduced as a means of evaluating the cervix in relationship to successful induction. This scoring system attempts to predict the success of induction by assessing five factors: position of the cervix in relation to the vagina, cervical consistency, dilation, effacement, and station of the presenting part. The higher the score, the higher is the rate of success of the induction. A score less than five indicates an unfavorable cervix for induction.

Measuring the length of the cervix via endovaginal ultrasonography has been used to detect premature labor with some degree of success. However, even in combination with other factors, especially with respect to positive predictive capabilities, there is quite a range of possible predictive values (50–71%), and these are obtained only after the onset of preterm labor symptoms, so the application is limited, as is the potential for treatment upon diagnosis using this method. Furthermore, the measurement of the cervical length is made unreliable by varying amounts of urine in the bladder. This throws considerable doubt on the entire procedure.

Table 12.1 Methods to monitor the state of pregnancy used to try to predict preterm birth

Tests	Sensitivity	Specificity	Positive predictive value (PPV)	Negative predictive value (NPV)
Multiple preterm labor symptoms	86.4	50.0	63.5	21.4
Maximal uterine contractions (TOCO)	84.7	6.7	92.3	25.0
Bishop score	32.0	91.4	42.1	87.4
Cervical length (ultrasound)	88.8	40.8	89.5	42.6
Fetal fibronectin (fFN)	18.0	95.3	42.9	85.6
Salivary estriol	71.0	77.0	66.0	84.0
Uterine electromyography (EMG)	75.0	93.3	81.8	90.3
Cervical light-induced fluorescence (LIF)	59.0	100.0	78.9	80.0

For the first six columns, please see refs 31–41; for uterine EMG and cervical LIF, please see refs 51 and 56, respectively.

In the fetal fibronectin (fFN) test for preterm labor, the practitioner places a speculum in the vagina and takes a sample of cervical secretions with a cotton swab. When analyzing the sample, technicians look for fFN, a protein produced by the fetal membranes that serves as the 'glue' that attaches the fetal sac to the uterine lining. This protein is normally found in the vagina during the first half of pregnancy, but if it leaks out of the uterus and shows up there after 22 weeks, that means the 'glue' may be disintegrating ahead of schedule (due to contractions, an injury to the membranes, or normal softening of the membranes).

Estriol level is a very recently proposed test for preterm labor. Estriol starts to appear in the ninth week of pregnancy, and its plasma concentration continues to increase throughout parturition. Estrogens directly affect myometrial contractility, modulate the excitability of myometrial cells, and increase uterine sensitivity to oxytocin. Plasma and salivary estriol levels both peak 3–5 weeks prior to labor in term deliveries as well as in preterm births. Estriol concentration in saliva very closely measures the free estriol concentration in plasma.

Of the currently used methods, IUPC perhaps provides the best information concerning the state of the pregnancy, but the invasive nature of this procedure can increase the risk of infection or cause more serious complications. Such infections could be a risk factor for preterm labor. At any rate, no real predictive capability exists for IUPC devices, since they are mostly applied only in the cases where labor has already been diagnosed clinically, which is why they do not appear in the Table 12.1.

Although a few of these methods can identify some of the indirect signs of oncoming labor, none of the current methods offer objective data that accurately predict labor over a broad range of patients. Again, this is probably because none of the currently used methods provide direct information about the function and state of the cervix or uterus. In contrast, the uterine EMG and cervical LIF technologies provide both, and the comparative results are demonstrated in Table 12.1.

UTERINE ELECTROMYOGRAPHY (EMG) AND CERVICAL LIGHT-INDUCED FLUORESCENCE (LIF) STUDIES – AN OVERVIEW

Uterine EMG

There are two commonly used methods to acquire uterine EMG signals abdominally: directly from the uterus via needle electrodes through the abdomen and noninvasively through the use of abdominal-surface electrodes. The earliest uterine EMG studies established that the electrical activity of the myometrium is responsible for its contractions.[43,44] Extensive studies have been done over the past 60 years to monitor uterine contractility using the electrical activity measured from needle electrodes placed on the uterus.[45–47] This method, of course, has the advantage of providing electrical data directly from the uterus, but has the disadvantage of being invasive and, hence, less desirable. However, more recent studies indicate that uterine EMG activity can be monitored accurately from the abdominal surface.[48–50]

It has also been established that the uterine electrical signals can be quantified sufficiently with mathematical functions and transforms such as power spectral analysis, so that it is possible to evaluate the state of the uterus for predicting delivery.[51] Experiments have been done to determine whether delivery can be predicted using transabdominal uterine EMG. In one case, a total of 99 patients were grouped as either term delivering (≥ 37 weeks, n = 57) or preterm delivering (< 37 weeks, n = 42), and uterine EMG was recorded for 30 min in the clinic. Uterine EMG 'bursts' were evaluated to determine the PDS. Measurement-to-delivery time was compared with the average PDS peak frequency. ROC curve analysis was performed for 48, 24, 12, and 8 h from measurement to term delivery, and 6, 4, 2, and 1 day(s) from measurement to preterm delivery.

From the analysis, the PDS peak frequency is observed to increase as the measurement-to-delivery interval decreases in both the term (Figure 12.4a) and preterm (Figure 12.4b) groups. ROC curve analysis gives high positive and negative predictive values (PPV and NPV, respectively) for both term and preterm delivery. For term-delivering patients, the maximum overall predictive capability (PPV+NPV) seems to occur at around 24 h from measurement to delivery, with PPV = 85.4% and NPV = 88.9%, and $P < 0.01$. On the other hand, for preterm-delivering patients, the maximum overall predictive capability (PPV+NPV) apparently occurs at around 4 days (96 h) from measurement to delivery, with PPV = 85.7% and NPV = 88.6%, and $P < 0.001$. For term-delivering patients, the average PDS peak frequency is significantly higher for the ≤ 24 h-to-delivery group than for the >24 h-to-delivery group. For preterm-delivering patients, the average PDS peak frequency is significantly higher in the ≤ 4 days-to-delivery group than in the >4 days-to-delivery group ($P < 0.05$).

The purpose of another study was to compare uterine EMG of antepartum patients delivering >24 h from measurement with that of laboring patients delivering <24 h from measurement.[52] Fifty patients (group 1, labor, n = 24; group 2, antepartum, n = 26) were monitored using transabdominal electrodes. Group 2 was recorded at several gestations. Uterine electrical 'bursts' were analyzed by

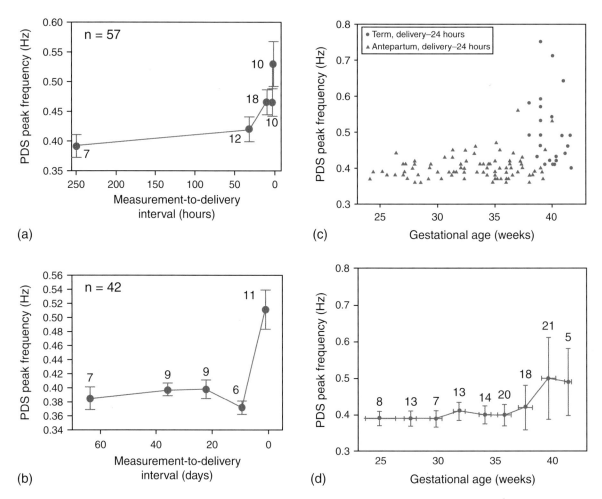

Figure 12.4 (a) and (b) A rapid increase in uterine electromyography (EMG) action potential frequency was seen in both term- and preterm-delivering patients. For patients delivering spontaneously, this increase occurs about 1 day prior to delivery in term-delivering patients (n = 57), and about 4–6 days prior to delivery in preterm-delivering patients (n = 42). Such a change in uterine EMG characteristics can be used to predict the time of delivery with a high degree of success. Note that in these two plots, the number of patients at each time-point is indicated. (c) and (d) An increase in uterine EMG occurs at term (for patients delivering spontaneously at term), especially for patients considered to be in labor. This transition from generally low to high uterine EMG action potential frequencies can be used to discern between those patients who are in true labor and those who are not.

power spectrum from 0.34 to 1.00 Hz. The average PDS peak frequency for each patient was plotted against gestational age, and compared between group 1 and group 2. Frequency was partitioned into 6 bins, and associated burst histograms compared.

These experiments reveal a general increase in uterine electrical frequency content as gestational age increased (Figure 12.4c and d), especially at term and near delivery, and that group 1 is significantly higher than group 2 for gestational age (39.87 ± 1.08 versus

32.96 ± 4.26 weeks) and average PDS peak frequency (0.51 ± 0.10 versus 0.40 ± 0.03 Hz). Histograms are also significantly different between the groups, with a tendency to see a greater number of high-frequency events in the labor group. For PDS versus gestation, a correlation coefficient of 0.41, with significance, is seen.

A further investigation was conducted to determine whether the strength of uterine contractions monitored invasively by IUPC could be acquired noninvasively using transabdominal EMG, and to estimate whether

EMG is a better predictor of true labor compared to TOCO.[53] Uterine EMG was recorded from the abdominal surface in laboring patients simultaneously monitored with an IUPC (n = 13) or TOCO (n = 24). Multiple IUPC-measured contraction events per patient, and their corresponding uterine electrical bursts, were randomly selected and analyzed (integral of the pressure curve for intrauterine pressure; integral, frequency, and amplitude of contraction curve for TOCO; and burst energy for EMG). The Mann–Whitney test, Spearman correlation, and ROC analysis were used as appropriate (significance was assumed at a value of P < 0.05).

From that study, it is seen that uterine EMG energy correlates strongly with intrauterine pressure (r = 0.764; P < 0.005). Uterine EMG burst energy levels are significantly higher in patients who deliver within 48 h compared to those who deliver later [median (25%/75%), 96 640 (26 520–322 240) versus 2960 (1560–10 240), P < 0.001], whereas none of the TOCO parameters are significantly different. In addition, burst energy levels are highly predictive of delivery within 48 h (area under the ROC curve: AUC = 0.9531, P < 0.0001) as assessed by ROC analysis.

Cervical LIF

Previous studies demonstrate that the cross-link molecules, hydroxylysyl-pyridinoline and lysyl-pyridinoline, both of which are found in the cervix, have a natural LIF[29,30] at 390 nm when excited with a 339 nm wavelength light source.[54] Figure 12.3, in addition to showing a schematic of the collascope instrument, also depicts the spectrum from pure insoluble and soluble collagen type I. Soluble collagen has fewer cross-links and therefore smaller LIF values than insoluble collagen. In rats and guinea pigs, it was previously shown that cervical ripening could be monitored by measuring the changes in the LIF value of cervical collagen.[54,55]

It has recently been determined that LIF can also be used to observe cervical ripening in pregnant women approaching delivery, and for prediction of the measurement-to-delivery interval.[56] The purpose of that study was to investigate gestational changes of cervical LIF, and the relationship between LIF and the measurement-to-delivery interval. Fifty patients were included in one of two groups: group 1, 21 healthy pregnant women without signs of labor underwent repeated cervical LIF measurement during the last trimester; group 2, LIF was measured in 29 patients with signs of labor, and the time from measurement to delivery was noted. Cervical LIF was obtained noninvasively with a prototype instrument that was designed specifically for this purpose (collascope). The Spearman correlation, Student t-test and ROC analysis were performed (P < 0.05).

From this investigation, it is now known that: LIF correlates negatively with gestational age and positively with the measurement-to-delivery interval, is significantly lower in patients who deliver <24 h from measurement compared with those patients who deliver >24 h from measurement (Figure 12.5a); and is predictive of delivery within 24 h (using an LIF cut-off value of 0.57, sensitivity is 59%, specificity is 100%, and PPV and NPV are 100 and 63%, respectively, P < 0.01, and AUC is 0.73).

Other work on LIF has sought to define the changes in cervical LIF, after the use of locally applied PG

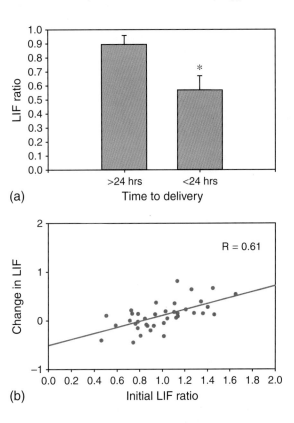

(a)

(b)

Figure 12.5 (a) The light-induced fluorescence (LIF) ratio is significantly lower (P < 0.05) in patients delivering within 24 h of measurement as compared to patients who deliver >24 h from measurement. The lower cervical LIF value indicates the presence of a more ripened cervix. Using receiver-operator-characteristics (ROC) curves with this parameter results in high positive and negative predictive values. (b) A significant correlation (P < 0.05) was found between the initial LIF-ratio value and the change in the LIF ratio value after treatment with prostoglandian (PG). This shows that it may be possible to identify which patients are most likely to benefit from such treatments.

preparations for labor induction at term and the correlation between LIF and the Bishop Score.[57] The characteristic LIF of cervical collagen was measured from the surface of the cervix, again using a specially designed instrument (collascope) in 41 gravidas undergoing labor induction at term by PG. LIF and the Bishop score were obtained directly before (and then again 4 h after) the administration of PG. The paired Student's t-test, Wilcoxon signed rank test, linear regression, Spearman correlation and Fisher exact tests were used as appropriate.

It has been established from this work that the cervical LIF decreases significantly after PG application [0.982 ± 0.04 (before) to 0.885 ± 0.037 (after), P = 0.025]. The decrease in LIF correlates with the initial LIF before PG application (P = 0.61; Figure 12.5b). The Bishop score increased in all 41 patients. However, no correlation is seen between LIF versus the Bishop score.

RECENT PILOT EXPERIMENTS

Uterine EMG

Some of our most recent uterine EMG pilot work includes a test of the hypothesis that uterine EMG activity recorded from the abdominal surface of women with preterm contractions is highest in women with failure of tocolysis. Uterine EMG activity was recorded with bipolar electrodes placed on the abdominal surface in 17 pregnant women with preterm contractions. All measurements were done before the initiation of any treatment. Ten women received either $MgSO_4$, indomethacin, or terbutaline for tocolysis. Three out of the 10 delivered within 7 days (group 1), and seven women delivered >7 days after measurement (group 2). Seven additional women were not treated with tocolytics (group 3). Uterine EMG signals were acquired at 100 Hz and band-pass filtered from 0.05 to 4.00 Hz. Electrical bursts were randomly selected and the frequency of the PDS peak in the 0.34–1.00 Hz region was determined using power spectrum analysis. One-way analysis of variance (ANOVA), Bonferroni post-hoc test, and Pearson's correlation were used for statistical analysis (significance P < 0.05).

In this study, the gestational age at measurement was not significantly different between the groups. Uterine EMG PDS peak frequency within bursts was significantly higher (Figure 12.6) in group 1 (0.55 ± 0.14 Hz) compared to group 2 (0.40 ± 0.03 Hz), (P = 0.011) and group 3 (0.39 ± 0.03 Hz), (P = 0.006). Group 2 and 3 were not significantly different. Gestational age at delivery was lower in group 1 (207 days) compared to group 2 (246 days) and group 3 (262 days), but the difference was statistically significant only between group 1 versus group 3 (P = 0.031).

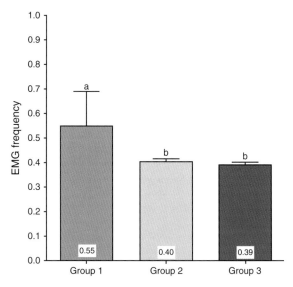

Figure 12.6 For those patients who were treated with tocolytics but who still delivered within 7 days (group 1), the uterine electromyography (EMG) action potential frequency was significantly higher (P < 0.05) than in patients who were treated with tocolytics and did not deliver within 7 days (group 2). The latter value was also comparable to that of patients who had low uterine EMG activity and did not require tocolysis (group 3). This indicates that once the uterus is electrochemically prepared for forceful contractions to deliver, current tocolytics may not be effective. The results of this study also indicate the possibility of using uterine EMG to identify those patients who may benefit from tocolysis and those who likely will not.

In another exploratory study, our objective was to determine whether using two EMG parameters together, in a derived multivariate expression, achieves better results than implementing either one alone. Uterine EMG was recorded with abdominal-surface electrodes for 30 min (at 100 Hz in 0.34–1.00 Hz range) from 22 pregnant 'rule-out' patients (gestation 29–41 weeks; contractions but no definitive clinical evidence of true labor). 'Bursts' of uterine activity were analyzed using power spectrum analysis to determine burst total power (Po) and burst power spectrum peak frequency (F). Measurement-to-delivery time was noted. Patients were divided into two groups: those delivering within 24 h of measurement (G1) and those delivering >24 h from measurement (G2). ROC curves were generated for delivery within 24 h of measurement using Po and F individually, and also when combined (C) in the multivariate parameter $C = Po^{0.25} \times F^4$. Positive and negative predictive values (i.e. PPV and NPV), Z, and AUC were all calculated. The Student t-test was used to compare means of G1 and G2, and True Epistat was used to compare areas under ROC curves (P, Z < 0.05 was considered significant).

The mean value for C was significantly higher for G1 than G2 (Figure 12.7). Po, F, and C were predictive of delivery within 24 h (Po: PPV = 0.58, NPV = 0.90, Z = 2.04, and AUC = 0.72; F: PPV = 0.83, NPV = 0.81, Z = 5.33, and AUC = 0.88; C: PPV = 0.88, NPV = 0.93, Z = 9.21, and AUC = 0.95). Statistical comparison of ROC curves showed that C had significantly higher AUC than Po alone, and C gave higher PPV, NPV, and Z values than either Po or F alone.

Cervical LIF

In one of our recent studies, we used the collascope to examine patients with cervical insufficiency (CI). Significantly lower LIF-measured collagen was found in those patients with CI who required a cerclage. LIF in the cervical insufficiency group at 12–25 weeks of gestation was lower than in groups of patients at later times in gestation.

In another investigation, cervical LIF was measured in 10 patients with CI, in 12 pregnant women (second trimester, 23–26 weeks) without signs of labor, in 27 pregnant women at term without labor, and in 10 women at term with labor. LIF measurements were taken from the anterior lip of the exocervix using the collascope.

LIF values were 0.26 ± 0.23 in women with CI, 0.51 ± 0.26 in the second trimester, 0.77 ± 0.41 in nonlaboring women at term, and 0.52 ± 0.39 in term labor (Figure 12.8). LIF values were lower in patients with CI compared to all groups, and significantly lower (P < 0.001) compared to nonlaboring women at term. Mean gestational age (days) was 111 ± 28 (CI), 176 ± 5 (second trimester), 274 ± 5 (term nonlaboring), and 271 ± 11 (term labor).

Uterine EMG and cervical LIF combined

One of our newest pilot studies characterized differences in uterine EMG and cervical LIF parameters used in conjunction for patients undergoing successful or failed induction. Twelve patients presenting to the labor and delivery area for pitocin induction (for various indications, e.g. postdates, oligo, etc.), had uterine electrical activity and cervical collagen content measured noninvasively using EMG and LIF, respectively, just prior to treatment with pitocin induction agent (standard start dose, 1MU), and then again approximately 4 h later. Patients were divided into two groups: G1, successful induction (n = 8); G2, failed induction (n = 4). Successful induction was deemed to occur for women who ultimately delivered vaginally within 24 h of induction (although future studies will explore different cut-off points). A multivariate expression, namely EMG/LIF,

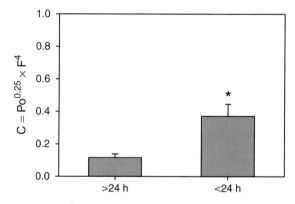

Figure 12.7 Multiple uterine electromyography (EMG) parameters, such as total burst power (Po) and action potential frequency (F), are generally more predictive of labor (in patients delivering spontaneously at term, for example) than are either of the parameters used alone. The values for C in the multivariate expression $C = Po^{0.25} \times F^4$ were significantly higher (P < 0.05) for patients delivering within 24 h of measurement as compared to those patients delivering >24 h from measurement. Note that the exponents in the expression were chosen according to the scale of the two independent variables, and in such a way as to insure that changes in one independent variable were equally weighted (with respect to change in C) as were changes in the other independent variable.

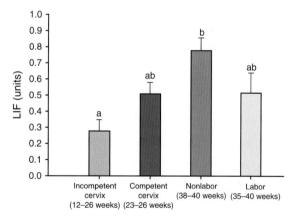

Figure 12.8 Term nonlabor patients have significantly higher (P < 0.05) light-induced fluorescence (LIF) ratio, hence more cervical collagen, than those patients with cervical insufficiency. This result admits the possibility of using the collascope for classifying or identifying patients with cervical insufficiency.

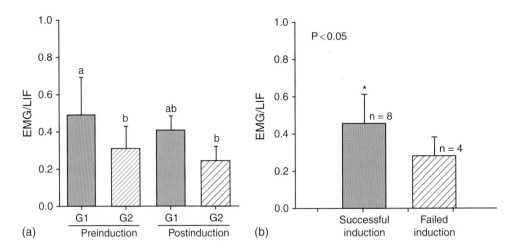

Figure 12.9 (a) Using the electromyography (EMG) and light-induced fluorescence (LIF) ratio, combined in the simple multivariate mathematical expression EMG/LIF, for patients receiving induction agent, showed that the EMG and LIF values, used together in this way, may indicate which patients will benefit from induction and which will not. Both the preinduction and postinduction EMG/LIF values were higher (with the preinduction value having significance, $P < 0.05$) in the group of patients having successful induction (G1) compared to those who had failed induction (G2). (b) Using the composite EMG/LIF value (which is just the average of the pre- and postinduction EMG/LIF values) showed a significantly higher ($P < 0.05$) composite EMG/LIF for G1 compared to G2. The composite score may be useful for determining, after a given period of time, whether such treatment will ultimately succeed, or whether further treatment should be suspended.

was compared for G1 versus G2 between preinduction versus post induction measurements. A composite score, namely the average EMG/LIF activity of each patient, made using the mean of the pre and postinduction values, was also compared between G1 and G2. Initially, one-way ANOVA was used, and post-hoc pair-wise comparisons were then made. The Student t-test was used to compare the composite scores. $P < 0.05$ was considered significant.

For the multivariate expression EMG/LIF, the pre-induction measurement for G1 was significantly higher than either the pre- or postinduction measurements for G2 (0.48 ± 0.20 versus 0.31 ± 0.12 and 0.24 ± 0.08, respectively; Figure 12.9a). The composite score was also significantly higher for G1 compared to G2 (0.45 ± 0.16 versus 0.28 ± 0.10; Figure 12.9b).

CONCLUSIONS

An extensive range of studies using the uterine EMG and cervical LIF diagnostic tools has been performed. From these, a number of conclusions can be reached about the function and state of the uterus and cervix during various conditions of parturition. These observations could not

have been made with any of the other currently available patient assessment and monitoring techniques.

Using a spectral parameter, transabdominal uterine EMG predicts delivery within 24 h at term and within 4 days preterm. With the power spectrum analysis, uterine EMG frequency content in antepartum patients is seen to be significantly lower than in laboring patients delivering <24 h from measurement. This indicates that the uterine muscle tissue is capable of generating more rapid polarizations/depolarizations closer to delivery than those produced far from delivery. Such rapid signal fluctuations are indicative of mature uterine development (extensive gap junctions, plethora of ion channels, etc.) necessary for effective contractions to properly expel the fetus. Furthermore, uterine EMG energy values correlate strongly with the strength of uterine contractions and therefore may be a valuable alternative to invasive measurement of intrauterine pressure.

By contrast, TOCO was seen not to have predictive capability, so unlike TOCO, transabdominal uterine EMG could be used routinely to forecast labor and delivery in an objective manner. For example, transabdominal uterine EMG, specifically the signal frequency within the bursts, is significantly higher in women with consecutive failure of tocolysis. These results suggest that EMG measurements are useful for prediction or monitoring of treatment of preterm contractions. This also indicates that once labor is established, it likely cannot be reversed with present tocolytics.

Uterine EMG parameters can also be combined mathematically for more robust predictive variables. Individually, total burst power and burst spectral frequency content do characterize uterine activity and labor in pregnant humans noninvasively, but together they predict delivery better than each parameter does alone. This predictive nature of combining EMG parameters is born out by the fact that the average value calculated as a result of the mathematical combination of the total power and spectral frequency is higher for patients within 24 h of delivery than those >24 h from delivery. Other multivariate uterine EMG parameters should also be investigated.

Cervical LIF decreases significantly as gestational age increases, and so cervical LIF may be a useful tool to identify patients in whom delivery is imminent. Cervical application of PG decreases the amount of cross-linked collagen as measured by LIF. However, this effect is observed only in patients with a prior high cross-linked collagen level, indicating that once a certain level of cervical ripening is reached, further application of induction agents to the cervix may be futile. Cervical LIF can also be used to identify women with cervical insufficiency so as to aid clinicians in determining the best candidates for cerclage.

Uterine EMG and cervical LIF, in the multivariate expression EMG/LIF, are indicative of successful induction. Specifically, since the pre-pitocin EMG/LIF value was high in those who ultimately had effective treatment, the pretreatment EMG/LIF measurement may determine which patients are most likely to benefit from pitocin induction and which are not. Similarly, in treated patients, the composite score may indicate imminent success or failure of the induction treatment when calculated through 4 h of dosing, and could aid clinicians in deciding on whether or not to continue the treatment.

These methodologies – i.e. uterine EMG and cervical LIF – offer many advantages and benefits not available with present patient monitoring and assessment systems, such as high predictive capability, ease of use and application, and noninvasiveness of measurement. It would likely be of great benefit to obstetrics that these technologies be implemented on a routine basis in the clinic.

REFERENCES

1. US Preventive Services Task Force. Guide to Clinical Preventive Services: An Assessment of the Effectiveness of 169 Interventions. Baltimore, MD: Williams & Wilkins; 1989.

2. Csapo AI. Force of labour. In: Iffy L, Kamientzky HA, eds. Principles and Practice of Obstetrics and Perinatology. New York: John Wiley and Sons; 1981: 761–99.

3. Garfield RE, Yallampalli C. Control of myometrial contractility and labor. In: Chwalisz K, Garfield RE, eds. New York: Springer-Verlag; 1993: 1–28.

4. Chwalisz K, Garfield, RE. Regulation of the uterus and cervix during pregnancy and labor: role of progesterone and nitric oxide. Ann NY Acad Sci 1997; 828: 238–53.

5. Garfield RE, Yallampalli C. Structure and function of uterine muscle. In: Chard T, Grudzinskas JG, eds. The Uterus. Cambridge Reviews in Human Reproduction. 1994: 54–93; Boca Raton: CRC Press: 1994; 40–81.

6. Tezuka N, Ali M, Chwalisz K, Garfield RE. Changes in transcripts encoding calcium channel subunits of rat myometrium during pregnancy. Am J Physiol 1995; 269: C1008–17.

7. Danforth DN. The morphology of the human cervix. Clin Obstet Gynecol 1983; 26: 7–13.

8. Leppert PC. Anatomy and physiology of cervical ripening. Clin Obstet Gynecol 1995; 38: 267–79.

9. Leppert PC. The biochemistry and physiology of the uterine cervix during gestation and parturition. Prenat Neonatal Med 1998; 3: 103–5.

10. Danforth DN. In: Naftolin F, Stubblefield PG, eds. Early Studies of the Anatomy and Physiology of the Human Cervix – and Implication for the Future. New York: Raven Press; 1980: 3–15.

11. Osmers R, Rath W, Adelmann-Grill BC et al. Origin of cervical collagenase during parturition. Am J Obstet Gynecol 1992; 166: 1455–60.

12. Uldbjerg N, Ekman G, Malmstrom A, Olsson K, Ulmsten U. Ripening of the human uterine cervix related to changes in collagen, glycosaminoglycans, and collagenolytic activity. Am J Obstet Gynecol 1983; 147: 662–6.

13. von Maillot K, Zimmermann BK. The solubility of collagen of the uterine cervix during pregnancy and labour. Arch Gynakol 1976; 220: 275–80.

14. Hegele-Hartung C, Chwalisz K, Beier HM, Elger W. Ripening of the uterine cervix of the guinea-pig after treatment with the progesterone antagonist onapristone (ZK 98.299): an electron microscopic study. Hum Reprod 1989; 4: 369–77.

15. Rajabi M, Solomon S, Poole AR. Hormonal regulation of interstitial collagenase in the uterine cervix of the pregnant guinea pig. Endocrinology 1991; 128: 863–71.

16. Junqueira LC, Zugaib M, Montes GS et al . Morphologic and histochemical evidence for the occurrence of collagenolysis and for the role of neutrophilic polymorphonuclear leukocytes during cervical dilation. Am J Obstet Gynecol 1980; 138: 273–81.

17. Winkler M, Fischer DC, Ruck P et al. Parturition at term: parallel increases in interleukin-8 and proteinase concentrations and neutrophil count in the lower uterine segment. Hum Reprod 1999; 14: 1096–100.

18. Ekman G, Uldbjerg N, Malmstrom A, Ulmsten U. Increased postpartum collagenolytic activity in cervical connective tissue from women treated with prostaglandin E2. Gynecol Obstet Invest 1983; 16: 292–8.

19. Osmers R, Rath W, Adelmann-Grill BC et al. Collagenase activity in the human cervix uteri after prostaglandin E2 application during the first trimester. Eur J Obstet Gynecol Reprod Biol 1991; 42: 29–32.

20. Norman M, Ekman G, Malmstrom A. Prostaglandin E2-induced ripening of the human cervix involves changes in proteoglycan metabolism. Obstet Gynecol 1993; 82: 1013–20.

21. Uldbjerg N, Ekman G, Malmstrom A, Ulmsten U, Wingerup L. Biochemical changes in human cervical connective tissue after local application of prostaglandin E2. Gynecol Obstet Invest 1983; 15: 291–9.

22. Olson CW, Wagner G, Albano A, Selvester RH. An interactive instructional program to promote the understanding of normal and abnormal cardiac activation and its resultant electrocardiograph. J Electrocardiol 2003; 36 (Suppl): 170.

23. de Micheli A, Medrano GA, Iturralde P. On the clinical value of electrocardiogram. Arch Cardiol Mex 2003; 73(1): 38–45.

24. Stoica P, Moses RL. Spectral Analysis of Signals. Prentice Hall. 2005.

25. Strang G, Nguyen T. Wavelets and Filter Banks. Cambridge Press. Wellesley, 1996.

26. Maner WL, MacKay LB, Saade GR, Garfield RE. Characterization of abdominally acquired uterine electrical signals in humans, using a non-linear analytic method. Med Biol Eng Comput 2006: 44 (1–2): 117–23.

27. Undenfriend S. Fluorescence Assay in Biology and Medicine (Volume I). New York: Academic Press; 1962.

28. Ramanujam N, Mitchell MF, Mahadevan A et al. Fluorescence spectroscopy: a diagnostic tool for cervical intrepithelial neoplasia (CIN). Gynecol Oncol 1994; 52: 31–8.

29. Fujimoto D, Moriguchi T. Pyridinoline, a non-reducible crosslink of collagen. Quantitative determination, distribution, and isolation of a crosslinked peptide. J Biochem (Tokyo) 1978; 83: 863–7.

30. Eyre DR, Paz MA, Gallop PM. Cross-linking in collagen and elastin. Annu Rev Biochem 1984; 53: 717–48.

31. Iams JD. Prediction and early detection of preterm labor. Obstet Gynecol 2003; 101(2): 402–12.

32. Romero R, Chaiworapongsa T, Espinoza J. Micronutrients and intrauterine infection, preterm birth and the fetal inflammatory response syndrome. J Nutr 2003; 133(5, Suppl 2): 1668S–1673S.

33. Wapner RJ, Cotton DB, Artal R, Librizzi RJ, Ross MG. A randomized multicenter trial assessing a home uterine activity monitoring device used in the absence of daily nursing contact. Am J Obstet Gynecol 1995; 172(3): 1026–34.

34. Dyson DC, Dange KH, Bamber JA et al. Monitoring women at risk for preterm labor. N Engl J Med 1998; 338: 15–19.

35. Colombo D, Iams JD. Cervical length and preterm labor. Clin Obstet Gynecol 2000; 43(4): 735–45.

36. Romero R. Routine obstetric ultrasound. Ultrasound Obstet Gynecol 1993; 3(5): 303–7.

37. Iams JD, Casal D, McGregor JA et al. Fetal fibronectin improves the accuracy of diagnosis of preterm labor (see comments). Am J Obstet Gynecol 1995; 173: 141–5.

38. Lockwood CJ. Predicting premature delivery – no easy task. N Engl J Med 2002; 346(4): 282–4.

39. Hellemans P, Gerris J, Verdonk P. Fetal fibronectin detection for prediction of preterm birth in low risk women (see comments). Br J Obstet Gynecol 1995; 102: 207–12.

40. McGregor JA, Jackson M, Lachelin GCL et al. Salivary estriol as risk assessment for preterm labor: a prospective trial. Am J Obstet Gynecol 1995; 173(4): 1337–42.

41. Goffinet F. Primary predictors of preterm labour. Br J Obstet Gynaecol 2005; 112 (Suppl): 38–47.

42. Goldenberg RL, Cliver SP, Bronstein J et al. Bed rest in pregnancy. Obstet Gynecol 1994; 84: 131–6.

43. Marshall JM. Regulation of the activity in uterine muscle. Physiol Rev 1962; 42: 213–27.

44. Kuriyama H, Csapo A. A study of the parturient uterus with the microelectrode technique. Endocrinology 1967; 80: 748–53.

45. Devedeux D, Marque C, Mansour S, Germain G, Duchene J. Uterine electromyography: a critical review. Am J Obstet Gynecol 1993; 169: 1636–53.

46. Wolfs GMJA, van Leeuwen M. Electromyographic observations on the human uterus during labor. Acta Obstet Gynecol Scand 1979; 90(Suppl): 1–61.

47. Figueroa JP, Honnebier MB, Jenkins S, Nathanielsz PW. Alteration of 24-hour rhythms in the myometrial activity in the chronically catheterized pregnant rhesus monkey after 6-hours shift in the light-dark cycle. Am J Obstet Gynecol 1990; 163: 648–54.

48. Garfield RE, Buhimschi C. Control and assessment of the uterus and cervix during pregnancy and labour. Hum Reprod Update 1998; 4: 673–95.

49. Buhimschi C, Garfield RE. Uterine activity during pregnancy and labor assessed by simultaneous recordings from the myometrium and abdominal surface in the rat. Am J Obstet Gynecol 1998; 178: 811–22.

50. Garfield RE, Chwalisz K, Shi L, Olson G, Saade GR. Instrumentation for the diagnosis of term and preterm labour. J Perinat Med 1998; 26: 413–36.

51. Maner W, Garfield RE, Maul H, Olson G, Saade G. Predicting term and pre-term delivery in humans using transabdominal uterine electromyography. Obstet Gynecol 2003; 101: 1254–60.

52. Garfield RE, Maner WL, MacKay LB, Schlembach D, Saade GR. Comparing uterine electromyography activity of antepartum patients versus term labor patients. Am J Obstet Gynecol 2005; 193: 23–9.

53. Maul H, Maner WL, Olson G, Saade GR, Garfield RE. Non-invasive transabdominal uterine electromyography correlates with the strength of intrauterine pressure and is predictive of labor and delivery. Matern Fetal Neonatal Med 2004; 15: 297–301.

54. Glassman W, Byam-Smith M, Garfield RE. Changes in rat cervical collagen during gestation and after antiprogesterone treatment as measured in vivo with light-induced autofluorescence. Am J Obstet Gynecol 1995; 173: 1550–6.

55. Fittkow CT, Shi SQ, Bytautiene E et al. Changes in light-induced fluorescence of cervical collagen in guinea pigs during gestation and after sodium nitroprusside treatment. J Perinat Med 2001; 29: 535–43.

56. Maul H, Olsen G, Fittkow CT, Saade GR, Garfield RE. Cervical light-induced fluorescence in humans decreases throughout gestation and before delivery. Preliminary observations. Am J Obstet Gynecol 2003; 188(2): 537–41.

57. Fittkow CT, Maul H, Olson G et al. Light-induced fluorescence of the human cervix decreases after prostaglandin application for induction of labor at term. Eur J Obstet Gynecol Reprod Biol 2005; 123: 62–6.

13

Genetics of preterm delivery

Kenneth Ward

INTRODUCTION

Preterm labor is the foremost challenge in obstetrics today. As pointed out by Eastman[1] almost 60 years ago, 'Only when the factors underlying prematurity are completely understood can any progress toward prevention be made.' Unfortunately, the physiological trigger for human labor, both at term and preterm, remains unknown. In many women, pathophysiologic changes occur weeks to months before the clinical diagnosis of preterm labor. These changes include increased inflammatory cytokines in amniotic fluid,[2] elevated fetal fibronectin,[3] decreased cervical length,[4] and increased maternal salivary estriol.[5] These observations suggest that interacting pathways, active long before labor begins, lead to preterm birth. It follows that every ligand, every receptor, every amplification cascade in the programmed responses that orchestrate labor is under the control of either the mother's or the fetus's genes. Uncovering the molecular mechanisms responsible for the onset of preterm labor should lead to improved detection, treatment, and prevention (when appropriate) of preterm birth.

PRETERM LABOR AS A POLYGENIC, MULTIFACTORIAL CONDITION

Preterm birth is said to have a 'multifactorial etiology'.[6] Intrauterine infection, drug abuse, cigarette smoking, low pregnancy weight, uteroplacental insufficiency, and multiple gestation are known causes of preterm delivery (PTD), but together these factors may account for only about 25% of preterm births. The vast majority of PTD have no known cause.[7]

PTD is also familial.[8] Some conditions 'run in families' because of similar diet, habits, or environment, but published reports suggest that PTD is at least in part a genetic disease.[9–11] Analyses of affected families suggest that relatively common alleles act as 'major genes', conferring susceptibility to PTD. It is unlikely that any particular genotype is necessary for PTD to occur; rather 'PTD genes' are susceptibility loci that lower a woman's threshold for delivering prior to term. As is typical for polygenic multifactorial conditions, the number of risk factors and their relative importance will vary for each woman and for each pregnancy. In some women, numerous minor factors will combine to exceed the preterm labor 'threshold', whereas in others one or two major risk factors may predominate.

Mutant genes in any of dozens of pathways could affect a woman's risk of preterm labor.[12] Many women will have 'private' mutations, affecting one woman or only a handful of women. However, analysis of private mutations may give us new insights into the normal mechanism of labor, or lead to a treatment that is applicable to all women. We may also discover mutations with a critical role, and common enough in the population to have epidemiologic importance. A common predisposing mutation might allow predictive testing of obstetric patients or suggest a targeted treatment. Fortunately, linkage analysis and genome-wide association techniques promise discovery of both rare and common alleles which contribute to this serious complication of pregnancy.

The inheritance patterns in preterm birth can be difficult to ascertain given the heterogenous causes of preterm labor (see Table 13.1) and since other obstetric pathologies frequently overlap with PTD. As Iams et al[4] pointed out, 'Risk factors previously considered distinct "causes" of preterm birth (genital infection, abnormal cervical function, physical exertion, sexual activity, uterine volume and contractility, and even vaginal bleeding) should be viewed instead as continuous variables.' Most likely each of the underlying pathologies that predispose women to premature labor vary in the degree to which genes and environment affect their onset. It is unknown which specific causes of PTD

Table 13.1 Heterogenous causes of preterm birth	
Cervix	Iatrogenic/Indicated
Incompetence	
Cervicitis	Uterine
PROM	Malformation
	Overdistention
Idiopathic/Intrinsic	Myomata
	Deciduitis
Maternal	
Systemic illness	Placenta
Abdominal pathology	Abruptio, previa
Illicit drug abuse	Chorioangioma
Trauma	Amnionitis
	Ischemia

Table 13.2 Potential preterm labor subtypes
Hormonal
Increased myometrial activity
Uterine overdistention
Placental
Chorioamnionitis
Membranes
Cervix
Iatrogenic

are familial. Certain etiologic factors may be familial because families also share behaviors and home environments as well as genes.

In order to study PTD using genetic methodologies, a 'phenotype' or clinical picture must be defined.[11] The diagnostic signs of preterm labor are nonspecific. Even if specific diagnostic criteria for PTD existed, there would be a great deal of debate about the proper phenotype to study. Therefore, conditions other than early delivery (such as cervical elasticity or length, cervicitis susceptibility, or placental viability) could prove highly informative for genetic and other etiologic investigations. Table 13.2 lists several clinical subtypes of preterm labor that may need to be distinguished to maximize the chances for success.

Studying the genetics of PTD is complicated by a number of factors.[13] Few convincing animal models of human labor exist, and there are numerous difficulties in identifying and collecting human families. The length of gestation and the rate of fetal maturation are continuous variables, and the line between preterm and term is somewhat arbitrary. Furthermore, gestational age determinations are inherently inaccurate. Record-keeping in obstetrics was extremely limited prior to the last few generations in which there has been a shift to hospitalized birth in many developed countries. Until recently, PTD was a fatal condition for the neonate, making familial cases rarer (and suggesting that a large percentage of cases must be due to new mutations). Medical or obstetric disorders, as well as patient/ physician decision-making factors, often influence time of delivery. Expression of a preterm labor gene could be affected by appropriate medical care. Pregnancy is a gender-limited trait, and expression of any PTD allele is further limited to women in their reproductive years who become pregnant. The gene(s) involved could be extremely common, and therefore males frequently bring PTD genes into pedigrees in a silent manner. Finally, either the genotype of the mother, or the fetus, or an interaction between the two, might be important.

Environmental risk factors clearly contribute to the PTD phenotype. For example, premature rupture of the membranes (PROM), which may occur due to genetic weakness of the membranes, has also been linked to maternal cigarette smoking.[14,15] Infectious agents may produce inflammation at the maternal–fetal interface indistinguishable from that caused by a vascular insult. The mother's response to an infection will be further affected by one or more host factors – such as gestational age, cervical length, or uterine endocrine milieu – each operating as a continuous variable. We have hypothesized that the best opportunity to discover predisposition genes will come from studying an environmentally and culturally homogeneous population with a low prevalence of environmental triggers of preterm labor.[11]

GENETIC ANALYSES

To discover whether a disease is 'genetic', geneticists look for a higher concordance of disease among monozygotic compared with dizygotic twins or a higher risk among relatives (e.g. siblings) of patients with disease than among relatives of controls. Treloar et al[16] published the only formal twin study of preterm labor; they found that heritability was 17% for PTD in first pregnancy, and 27% for PTD in any pregnancy. Unfortunately, their data did not allow for differentiation of the varying etiologies of premature parturition. Few studies have examined the rate of PTD in extended families, possibly due to the inability to obtain accurate information on the length of gestation in family studies.[8,17,18] Most of the published evidence considers: (i) recurrence of PTD in the proband;

(ii) ethnic and racial differences; and (iii) relative risk for close relatives of proband. More recently, molecular genetic studies have added to the evidence for genetic effects.

RECURRENT PRETERM DELIVERY (PTD)

A prior premature birth is one of the best predictors of a premature delivery. Women who experienced an early preterm birth (<32 completed weeks) in their first pregnancy have the highest rate of recurrent preterm birth in subsequent pregnancies. Spontaneous preterm labour and preterm birth in subsequent pregnancies tend to recur at equivalent gestational ages. If a woman herself was born preterm, she is also at an increased risk of spontaneous preterm labour and preterm birth, with the risks being highest for those women who themselves were born most preterm. This predisposition does not apply to men who were born preterm. The risk increases with two or more prior PTD. Of course, nongenetic causes often recur in subsequent pregnancies as well, so recurrence alone does not prove that genes are involved.

The risk of preterm birth was tripled after one previous preterm birth with or without a preceding abortion in a study by Carr-Hill et al[19] of 6572 women, and increased six-fold after two previous preterm births. However, the attributable risk was low, and most multiparous women with preterm births did not have a previous history. Ekwo et al[14] looked at previous pregnancy outcomes and subsequent risk of PROM at two university hospitals. They found that previous preterm birth, abortion and prematurity, and fetal loss/abortion and prematurity all increase risk for subsequent preterm birth with or without PROM.

A series of Danish studies found that women with idiopathic preterm birth in their first or second pregnancies give birth to infants with lower birthweight in previous or subsequent pregnancies. This large cohort (n = 13 967) consisted of all women living in Denmark with a first singleton birth in 1982 and a second in the period of 1982–1987.[20] They also showed that the risk of a second preterm birth was not significantly different between women who had an idiopathic or an indicated first preterm birth (15.2 and 12.8%, respectively), and that women with idiopathic preterm birth in their first or second pregnancies gave birth to infants with lower birthweight in previous or subsequent pregnancies.[21]

The recurrence of spontaneous preterm birth in 1282 parous women was studied by Iams et al.[4] They found that among fetal fibronectin positive women with a prior preterm birth, the estimated recurrence risk of birth <35 weeks of gestation was approximately 65%

when the cervix was ≤25 mm, 45% when the cervix was 26–35 mm, and 25% when the cervix was >35 mm at 24 weeks of gestation. For fetal fibronectin negative women with a prior preterm birth, the recurrence risk was 25% when the cervix was ≤25 mm long, 14% when the cervix was 26–35 mm long, and 7% when the cervix was >35 mm in length. Although the risk of preterm birth was increased in women with a history of preterm birth, the risk was not influenced by the gestational age at delivery of the most recent preterm birth.

More recently, Mercer et al[22] studied 7970 pregnancies delivering at >20 weeks of gestation; periviable birth in the first pregnancy was associated with preterm birth, and periviable birth in the second pregnancy (35.6 and 6.9%, respectively; relative risk, 3.3 and 8.6, respectively; P < 0.0001).[22] Periviable birth and preterm birth in the first pregnancy were insensitive for periviable birth in the second pregnancy (8.8 and 36.8%, respectively).

Various treatment trials confirm the recurrence rate. In a study on the effect of 17 alpha-hydroxyprogesterone caproate on preterm birth in the United States (US), Petrini et al[23] estimated that in 2002, approximately 30 000 women had recurrent preterm births (a recurrent preterm birth rate of 22.5%). A trial in The Netherlands used prophylactic administration of clindamycin vaginal cream to try to reduce the incidence of preterm birth in a high-risk population. Cases and controls showed no difference in the overall preterm birth between clindamycin (23%) and placebo (18%) in the intention-to-treat analysis.[24]

Ghidini and Salafia[25] evaluated whether particular placental histopathology lesions are associated with recurrent preterm birth. Several specific lesions were correlated with the number of prior preterm births by using regression analysis. Only chronic marginating choriodeciduitis (correlation coefficient = 0.13; P = 0.01) and acute choriodeciduitis (correlation coefficient = 0.14; P = 0.008) were correlated. Their data suggest that a prepregnancy endometrial infection, rather than an ascending intrapregnancy pathway, may be responsible for some recurrences of preterm birth.[25]

Maternal medical disorders can contribute to recurrent preterm birth. Rasmussen et al[26] examined the risk of preterm birth subsequent to a birth complicated by placental abruption (PA). They found that the odds ratios (OR) of spontaneous preterm birth in a birth subsequent to a PA was 7.0 (36.3%).[26] In a population-based study in Norway, the recurrence risk of adverse outcomes in women with rheumatic disease was considered. Skomsvoll et al[27] found that women with rheumatic disease and an adverse pregnancy outcome in the first pregnancy had a statistically significant higher recurrence risk of the same event in the second pregnancy than women without rheumatic disease [pre-eclampsia: OR 2.22, 95% confidence interval (CI) 1.18–4.19; preterm birth: OR 1.86, 95% CI 1.12–3.11]. Koike et al[28] found that women who had a history of pre-eclampsia-related preterm birth had a greater risk of pre-eclampsia-related preterm birth in a subsequent pregnancy as compared with women with a previous term birth.

Bloom et al[29] looked at the recurrence of preterm birth in singleton and twin pregnancies (n = 15 945). Women who delivered a singleton before 35 weeks were at a significant increased risk for recurrence (OR 5.6, 95% CI 4.5–7.0), whereas those who delivered twins were not (OR 1.9, 95% CI 0.46–8.14). Of those women with a recurrent preterm birth, 49% delivered within 1 week of the gestational age of their first delivery, and 70% delivered within 2 weeks. Among 15 863 nulliparous women with singleton births at their first delivery, a history of preterm birth in that pregnancy could predict only 10% of the preterm births that ultimately occurred in the entire obstetric population.[29]

A tendency of the occurrence of repeated preterm birth at the same gestational age has been observed.[30] The influence of previous preterm births on future deliveries was shown to be highest when the gestational age of the previous preterm birth was between 23 and 27 weeks.[31]

A preterm prediction study by Mercer et al[32] studied the effect of gestational age and cause of preterm birth on subsequent obstetric outcome. Prospectively evaluating a total of 1711 multiparous women with singleton gestations at 23–24 weeks of gestation, prior pregnancies were coded for the presence or absence of a prior spontaneous preterm birth. If a prior spontaneous preterm birth had occurred, the gestation of the earliest prior birth (13–22, 23–27, 28–34, and 35–36 weeks of gestation) was recorded. They found that those with a prior spontaneous preterm birth carried a 2.5-fold increase in the risk of spontaneous preterm birth in the current gestation over those with no prior spontaneous preterm birth (21.7 versus 8.8%, P ≤ 0.001). Gravid women with an early prior spontaneous preterm birth (23–27 weeks of gestation) had a higher risk of recurrent spontaneous preterm birth (27.1 versus 8.8%, P ≤ 0.001).[32]

A study conducted in Norway by Melve et al[33] looked at the extent to which preterm birth and perinatal mortality are dependent on the gestational ages of previous births within sibships. The data for this study was collected from the Medical Birth Registry of Norway from 1967 to 1995. Newborns were linked to their mothers through Norway's unique personal identification number, yielding 429 554 pairs of mothers and first and second singleton newborns with gestational ages of 22–46 weeks,

based on menstrual dates. Siblings gestational ages were significantly correlated (r = 0.26). They found that the risk of having a preterm second birth was nearly 10 times higher among mothers whose firstborn child had been delivered before 32 weeks of gestation than among mothers whose first child had been born at 40 weeks.[33]

Another study in Norway looked at the correlations of birthweight and gestational age across generations by studying the data of a group of 11 092 pairs of mother–firstborn in the Norwegian Birth Registry. The correlation for gestational age across generations was low, and correlation between maternal and offspring birthweight was a modest 0.242. However, mothers whose own birthweight was <2500 g had a significantly increased risk (OR 3.03, 95% CI 1.79–5.11) of having a low birthweight child compared with mothers with a birthweight >4000 g.[34]

RACIAL DIFFERENCES

Racial and ethnic differences in disease prevalence can be important clues that genes are involved in a disorder. In 1983, Migone et al used US population data to compare birthweight and gestational duration for babies with different parental racial groups. Mean birthweight and mean gestational duration decreased in order from: both parents White; mother White, father Black; mother Black, father White; both parents Black. Adjustment for sociodemographic variables did not alter these trends appreciably. Although group differences were more strongly related to the mother's race than to the father's, the father's race was significant, suggesting that genetic factors are of some importance. Other studies have confirmed that Black women have a markedly higher risk of PTD. However, caution must be used when interpreting these data as race is not a genetically meaningful construct and many nongenetic traits vary by race.[35,36]

Ekwo and Moawad[37] in their study of preterm birth in African-Americans found that the preterm birth rate among African-Americans for the second pregnancy was 30.6%, significantly higher than the rate of 18.2% for the first pregnancy, and 24.5% for the third and fourth pregnancies.[97]

Another study in the African-American population looked at intergenerational effects of socioeconomic status on low birthweight and preterm birth. Persistent differences in birthweight in this high socioeconomic status cohort (OR 3.16, 95% CI 1.89–5.27) suggest that African-American women have birthweight distributions that are somewhat lighter than White women. It is possible that persistent psychosocial and behavioral factors continue to negatively influence birthweight, even in second-generation high socioeconomic African-American mothers.[38]

Using North Carolina birth certificate data for 1988–1989, another study showed that Blacks had 3.3, 2.5, and 3.5 times the risk of Whites to have preterm PROM. The overall prevalence of preterm birth was 8.0 and 16.7% for Whites and Blacks, respectively. The entire gestational age distribution of Blacks was shifted to earlier ages relative to Whites. More highly educated Blacks still had higher risks of moderately and very PTD than less educated Whites. Multivariate analysis, controlling for other factors, showed that Blacks had 3.3, 2.5, and 3.5 times the risk of Whites to have preterm PROM, complication-related, and idiopathic delivery, respectively, among very preterm births, and 1.6, 1.9, and 2.0 times the risk of Whites for moderately preterm births of the same three types.[39]

McGrady et al[40] looked at preterm birth among first-born infants of Black and White college graduates using a mail survey from graduates (1973–1985) of four Atlanta, GA, colleges between February and June 1988. The results of this survey found that compared with White graduates, Black graduates had 1.67 times the risk of preterm delivery.

A study conducted by Reagan and Salsberry[41] looked at race and ethnic differences in determinants of preterm birth in the US. They found evidence that neighborhood poverty rates and housing vacancy rates increased the rate of very preterm birth and decreased the rate of moderately preterm birth for Blacks. The rate of very preterm birth increased with the fraction of female-headed households for Hispanics and decreased with the fraction of people employed in professional occupations for Whites.[41] Another study looked at the epidemiology of PTD in two birth cohorts with an interval of 20 years.[42] It was found that the overall incidence (percentage) of PTD fell from 9.1 to 4.8, including a reduction from 8.8 to 3.4 for spontaneous PTD. The increase in the proportion of iatrogenic PTD was accompanied by these being more common at lower than at higher socioeconomic levels in 1985–1986, whereas the social gradient appeared to be reversed in 1966.

Another study examining the racial and ethnic disparities in preterm birth found that Black women and American Indian/Alaska Native women reported the highest number of stressful life events in the 12 months before delivery. Compared with nonHispanic White women, Black women were 24% more likely to report emotional stressors, 35% more likely to report financial stressors, 163% more likely to report partner-related stressors, and 83% more likely to report traumatic stressors. Although they found that there are significant racial/ethnic disparities in the experience of stressful life events before and during pregnancy, they concluded that these stressful life events do not contribute significantly to racial/ethnic disparities in preterm birth.[43]

Black women have an increased risk for all subtypes of preterm birth – 1.9 for preterm PROM, 2.1 for preterm labor, and 1.7 for medically induced births. Hispanic women also have increased risk – 1.7 for preterm PROM, 1.9 for preterm labor, and 1.6 for medically induced births. For those who had had a previous preterm birth the risks are 3.2 for preterm PROM, 4.5 for preterm labor, and 3.3 for medically induced births. For those who began prenatal care after the first trimester the risks are 1.4 for preterm PROM, 1.3 for preterm labor, and 1.3 for medically induced births.[44]

Heaman et al[45] studied the risk of preterm birth in Aboriginal and non-Aboriginal women in Manitoba, Canada, using a multivariable logistic regression model. They found that although the rate of preterm birth had been increasing among Aboriginal women, a significant risk factor for all women in the study included previous preterm birth.

CANDIDATE GENES

The candidate gene approach looks for epidemiologic associations with variations in the genes coding for proteins known to be involved in some aspect of pregnancy or labor. Dozens of genes have been considered as candidates already (see Table 13.3). The molecular genetics of preterm labor have been recently reviewed by Crider et al[46] and Varner and Esplin:[10] some of this work is considered in other chapters of this book so only selected examples will be considered here. Unfortunately, most of these association studies included relatively small numbers of subjects, and they don't adequately address heterogeneity. Few have been replicated to date, and replication is critical to be certain that hidden biases in the control populations are not causing false associations.

Hartel et al[47] considered hemostasis genes polymorphisms as risk factors for PTD using a multivariate regression analysis. They found that previous preterm delivery (OR 3.8, 95% CI 1.7–8.4), the maternal carrier status of the factor VII-121del/ins polymorphism (OR 1.7, 95% CI 1.12–2.5, P = 0.007), and the lower frequency of the infant's factor XIII-Val34Leu polymorphism (OR 0.53, 95% CI 0.29–0.96, P = 0.038) were independently associated with preterm birth. Gene–environment interactions were considered in a study of the common dihydrofolate reductase (DHFR) 19-base pair deletion allele. Women with a DHFR deletion allele and low folate intake (<400 μg/day from diet

Table 13.3 Examples of candidate genes for preterm labor

Gene name	Symbol	Location
Alcohol dehydrogenase 1C	ADH1C	4q21-q23
Aldehyde dehydrogenase 2	ALDH2	12q24.2
3eta 2 Adrenergic Receptor	ADRB2	5q32-q34
Coagulation factor V	F5	1q23
Colony stimulating factor 3	CSF3	17q11.2-q12
Corticotropin releasing hormone	CRH	8q13
Corticotropin-releasing hormone binding protein	CRHBP	5q11.2-q13.3
Cytochrome P450IA1	CYP1A1	15q22-q24
Cytochrome P450IIE1	CYP2E1	10q24.3-qter
Cytochrome P450IID6	CYP2D6	22q13.1
Dopamine receptor D2	DRD2	11q23
Epidermal growth factor	EGF	4q25
Epoxide hydrolase	EPHX	1p11-qter
Fibronectin	FN1	2q34
Glutathione S-transferase theta 1	GSTT1	22q11.2
Glutathone S-transferase mu 1	GSTM1	1p13.3
Inteferon gamma receptor 1	IFNFG1	6q23-q24
Interleukin 1 receptor antagonist	IL-1RN	2q14.2
Interleukin 1 receptor, type II	IL-1R2	2q12-q22
Interleukin 1, alpha	IL-1A	2q14
Interleukin 1, beta	IL-1B	2q13-q21
Interleukin 4	IL-4	5q31.1
Interleukin 6	IL-6	7p21-p25
Interleukin 8	IL-8	4q13-q21
Interleukin 10	IL-10	1q31-32
Interleukin 10 receptor, alpha	IL-10RA	11q23
Interleukin 11	IL-11	19q13.3.-q13.4
Interleukin 12A	IL-12A	3p12-q13.2
Interleukin 18	IL-18	11q22.2-q22.3
Lymphotoxin alpha	LTA	6p21.3
Matrix metalloproteinase 1	MMP-1	11q22-q23
Methylenetretra-hydrofolate reductase	MTHFR	1p36.3
N-acetyltransferase 2	NAT2	8p23.1-p21.3
NAD(P)H quinone oxidoreductase 1	NQO1	16q22.1
Nitric oxide synthase 2A	NOS2A	17q11.2-q12
Nitric oxide synthase 3	NOS3	7q36
Opioid receptor, mu 1	OPRM1	6q24-q25
Oxytocin receptor	OXTR	3p26.2
Paraoxonase-2	PON2	7q21.3
Progesterone receptor	PGR	11q22-q23
Prostaglandin E receptor 2	PTGER2	14q22
Prostaglandin E synthase	PTGES	9q34.3
Prostaglandin F receptor	PTGFR	1p31.1
Protein C	PROC	2q13-q14
Toll-like receptor 4	TLR-4	9q32-q33
Tumour necrosis factor α	TNF-α	6p21.3

plus supplements) had a significantly greater risk of preterm birth (OR 5.5, 95% CI 1.5–20.4, P = 0.01).[48]

An A>G polymorphism at position -670 in the Fas gene promoter was examined for its relationship to preterm PROM in multifetal pregnancies. Buccal swabs from 119 mother–infant sets were analyzed for the single nucleotide substitution in the TNFRSF6 promoter. Maternal homozygosity for the G allele (TNFRSF6*G) was observed in 42.4% of 33 preterm PROM pregnancies as opposed to 19.5% of 77 term births (P = 0.01). Similarly, homozygosity for the G allele was present in 37.5% of 32 first-born neonates from preterm PROM pregnancies as opposed to 18.7% of 75 uncomplicated pregnancies (P = 0.04). Preterm PROM occurred in 8/14 (57.1%) pregnancies in which mother and all neonates were TNFRSF6*G homozygotes, as opposed to 25/105 (23.8%) cases in which uniform TNFRSF6*G homozygosity was not observed (P = 0.02).[49]

It is well established that upper genital tract infection and/or inflammation is seen in association with spontaneous preterm labor and preterm birth. Previous investigations have focused primarily on an infectious etiology for this finding. This association may represent an exaggerated inflammatory response.[50] The frequent association of spontaneous preterm labor and preterm birth with histological infection/inflammation and elevated body fluid concentrations of inflammatory cytokines has focused investigations on single gene polymorphisms of these cytokines in both mother and fetus. The polymorphisms tumor necrosis factor (TNF) α-308 interleukin (IL) 1β +3953/3954 and IL-6-174 have been most consistently associated with spontaneous preterm labor and preterm birth. Toll-like receptors (TLR) are important components of the innate immune systems, which have also been linked to spontaneous preterm labour and preterm birth. Both maternal and fetal polymorphisms of the TLR-4 gene have been associated with spontaneous preterm labour and preterm birth in certain populations, but in others no apparent link has been observed.

An Australian study considered the relationship between preterm birth and 22 single nucleotide polymorphisms in genes that encode cytokines, and mediators of apoptosis and host defense.[51] Using multivariate analyses, they found that clinical risk factors such as alcohol exposure, substance use, and smoking are significant. The authors found that polymorphisms in immunoregulatory genes also influence susceptibility to preterm birth or PROM. For instance, one haplotype for the TNF gene (+488A/-238G/-308G) had an OR of 2.4 (P = 0.04). Homozygosity for IL-10-1082G/-819C/-592C haplotype was twice as common in women with preterm PROM.

An investigation into the association among preterm birth, cytokine gene polymorphisms and periodontal disease by Moore et al[52] found that a higher proportion of women who delivered preterm carried the polymorphic TNF-α-308 gene. In this study, there did not appear to be any interaction between either of the genotypes and periodontal disease with preterm birth as has been reported for bacterial vaginosis and the TNF-α-308 polymorphic gene.

A large number of candidate gene studies can be completed in parallel using high-throughput genotyping technologies. Hao et al[12] performed case-control studies exploring the associations of 426 single-nucleotide polymorphisms in 300 mothers with preterm birth and 458 mothers with term deliveries at the Boston Medical Center. A significant association of a factor V gene haplotype with preterm birth was revealed, and remained significant after Bonferroni correction for multiple testing (P = 0.025). Other candidate genes showed associations only within particular ethnic cohorts [IL-1R2 (P = 0.002 in Blacks), NOS2A (P < 0.001 in Whites) and OPRM1 (P = 0.004 in Hispanics)].

Ethnic differences of polymorphisms in cytokine and innate immune system genes in pregnant women were also uncovered by Nguyen et al.[53] They found that allele 2 of the IL-1ra gene (IL-1RN*2) and IL-4 -590C homozygosity was four-fold less common in Blacks than in Whites or Hispanics (P < 0.001). The IL-4 -590T allele was almost two-fold more common in Hispanics than in Whites (P < 0.001). The frequency of the 70 kDa heat-shock protein 1267G allele was at least 1.4 times greater in Blacks compared with Whites (P < 0.001) or Hispanics (P = 0.002), whereas the homozygous mannose-binding lectin codon 54G allele was observed at least 4.5 times more often in Hispanics compared with Whites (P = 0.007) or Blacks (P = 0.02).[53]

POPULATION STUDIES

At first, difficulties in studying humans forced scientists to use animal models. Studies from the 1950s on calves attribute 5–8% of the variance in gestation length in calves to maternal genotype, and 42–45% of the variance to the genotype of the calves.[17] A genetic effect from the father is seen in some mammals. Human population studies have been hampered by the inability to obtain accurate information on the length of gestation in past generations and the heterogeneous nature of this disorder.[17]

Wang et al[54] reported familial clustering of low birthweight infants born to both Whites and Blacks in the US. Porter et al[18] used the Utah Genealogy database to suggest a genetic component for PTD. He found that the risk for premature delivery of offspring became significantly greater in mothers who were born before 34 weeks of gestation, and that this was inversely correlated with the maternal gestation age at birth. As mentioned above, a recent twin study in Australia estimated that the heritability was 17% for delivery before 38 weeks in the first pregnancy and 27% for premature delivery in any pregnancy.[16] An earlier study of the Old Order Amish suggested that prematurity is related to the maternal genotype.[55]

My group recently asked women who delivered a singleton infant at <36 weeks of gestation at the University of Utah about their family history.[11] Twenty-eight families were identified in which the proband had at least five first- or second-degree relatives with PTD. We used a unique genealogy database that documents the relationships between over 21 million ancestors of people living in Utah. This database was searched for the names, birth dates, and birthplaces of the four grandparents for each of the 28 familial PTD probands. Pairwise coefficients of kinship were determined for the 93 PTD grandparents identified in GenDB and for 1000 randomly selected sets of 100 individuals born in the 1920s.[56] The coefficient of kinship quantifies the degree of relatedness between two individuals. This coefficient is defined as the probability that randomly selected homologous genes from two individuals are identical by descent from a common ancestor. Siblings have a coefficient of kinship of 0.25; first cousins have a coefficient of kinship of 0.0625; and nth degree relatives have a coefficient of kinship equal to $(0.5)^n$. In this study, the mean coefficient of kinship for the familial PTD probands was calculated by considering all possible unique pairings of the grandparents of the familial PTD probands from the 28 families.[57]

The coefficient of kinship for familial PTD grandparents [3.4×10^{-5} (P < 0.0001)] was over 50 standard deviations (SD) higher than the kinship coefficient in controls [1.5×10^{-6} (SD = 0.6×10^{-6})]. On average, gravidae randomly selected from our population are 23rd-degree relatives, while these PTD probands are 8th-degree relatives. Obviously, the calculated mean coefficient of kinship will vary depending upon how cases are selected. We focused on familial clusters since our long-term aim is to discover the genes involved. Many of the families currently living in Utah, and most of the subjects in this study, are genetically representative of a Northern European population.[58] Due to a continued influx of immigrant workers and converts to the Mormon religion from around the world, the Utah population does not have unusual levels of inbreeding.[59] Due to the Mormon Church proscriptions against consumption of tobacco and alcohol, and relatively low rates of sexually transmitted diseases and substance abuse, this population may have a lower rate of environmental triggers for premature labor. Relatively complete and accurate knowledge of the

---

Table 13.4 Insights available from the GenDB database[*]

How genetic is the disorder?
Likely inheritance patterns?
Penetrance, expression, variability?
Is there a 'founder effect'?
Does sample size assure statistical power?
Is there locus heterogeneity?
How many loci are involved?

[*]GenDB also lessens false-positive results during data analysis.

---

ancestral histories of many of our research subjects should help us to sort out the genetic heterogeneity and map genes through 'identity-by-descent'.[60] A genome-wide search for preterm labor genes is underway in this population. Table 13.4 lists some of the other genetic insights that can be derived from analyzing the families in GenDB prior to actually mapping the genes involved.

GENE MAPPING

We and other investigators are using family studies and genome-wide association studies to map the genetic defects which predispose to preterm labor to their location on particular chromosomes. No knowledge of the biochemistry of the condition, or even the location or timing of gene expression, is required for these gene-mapping efforts. The identified chromosomal region is narrowed down until the correct gene can be identified, and then the function of normal and diseased associated forms of the gene can be studied.

Linkage analyses involve large families in which several women delivered preterm. We use genetic markers evenly spaced in the human genome to identify a chromosomal region (locus) segregating with the disease in families. Markers and genes located close to each other on the same chromosome are inherited together more often than expected by chance. Genes that are far apart will not inherit together because recombination disrupts the association of the marker and the disease locus. Whenever, marker alleles are segregating with the disease in a family, those markers are assumed to be located near a disease-associated gene. Using maximal likelihood analyses, a 'lod score' is calculated. The lod score is the logarithm OR (the odds that the loci are linked divided by the odds that the loci are independent given the observed data). A lod score of ≥3 is used as an indication of statistically significant linkage.

Once disease genes are mapped, the relatively small number of genes in the region can be sequenced in cases and controls.

Linkage analysis is best suited for Mendelian disorders or common diseases in which the correlation between the genotype and the phenotype is very high.[61] Linkage analysis works best when genetic parameters such as mode of inheritance, penetrance, age of onset, etc. are known. Errors in phenotypic classification will cause false conclusions. Unfortunately, locus heterogeneity (more than one causal gene) and clinical heterogeneity (multiple forms of the same disease with different etiology) are likely in preterm labor, and these will make linkage analysis more difficult.

In contrast to linkage analysis, genetic-association studies are generally model free, or nonparametric.[62] As with the candidate gene studies presented above, genetic-association analysis examines whether affected individuals share the common allele more often than controls. Variant alleles are often identical-by-descent; affected patients share a common ancestor from whom the shared allele originated. The number of subjects required for genetic-association studies can be large, particularly if the heritability of the disorder is low. Hundreds of thousands of loci need to be tested to test genome-wide for associations, creating significant statistical and computational challenges. Despite stringent approaches, selected controls may have differences in their genetic background which introduce variables unrelated to the disease. Spurious associations due to confounding population stratification and hidden bias are common in the genetic-association literature. The frequency of false-positive results requires replication in an independent study or computer simulation.[63,64]

IMPLICATIONS

Morbidity from premature delivery may extend well into adulthood. Epidemiologic studies in Britain suggest that low birthweight may also be associated with an increased risk of hypertension and death due to cardiovascular disease. The first cohorts of extremely premature children who have survived since the introduction of neonatal intensive care are only now entering adulthood. It appears that this cohort is also having a high rate of preterm labor.

Preterm labor is difficult to predict and treat, and erroneous diagnoses are common. More than 50% of PTD occur in women who have been identified as 'low risk' during their pregnancy. The factor most likely to accurately predict the likelihood of premature delivery is a history of PTD in a prior pregnancy, but at least 50% of women who deliver prematurely are pregnant for the first time. Despite widespread use, the available technologies (home uterine activity monitoring, tocolytic drugs, bed rest, and cervical cerclage) appear to have had little impact on reducing the incidence of preterm birth. With the possible exception of antibiotics to treat vaginal and cervical infections, no current treatment has any effect on the causes of preterm birth. When proposed treatments are evaluated against placebos, it is found that the diagnosis of preterm labor is erroneous up to 80% of the time.

Once PTD is understood at a molecular level, and genetic determinants can be examined directly, the clinical classification, as well as the diagnosis and treatment, of PTD are likely to be redefined.[65] Proceeding from molecular pathways to clinical manifestations or 'phenotypes' constitutes a radical alternative in the logic of scientific inference. Since genetic risk factors are stable through the mother's and child's lifespan, they are easier to observe than other transient factors such as cervical shortening or fetal inflammation, which can only be observed proximate to the delivery. Ultimately, genetic and environmental factors operate on the same critical molecular pathways, genetic approaches to preterm birth may uncover these pathways more efficiently than the approaches that have been tried to date.

ACKNOWLEDGMENTS

This work was supported by grants from the National Institutes of Health (5 K24 HD01315-02), and from the Research Centers in Minority Institutions program in the National Center for Research Resources (2 U 54 RR014607-06 and P20).

REFERENCES

1. Eastman NJ. Prematurity from the viewpoint of the obstetrician. Am Pract 1947; 1: 343–52.
2. Dudley DJ, Trautman MS, Araneo BA, Edwin SS, Mitchell MD. Decidual cell biosynthesis of interleukin-6: regulation by inflammatory cytokines. J Clin Endocrinol Metab 1992; 74: 884–9.
3. Goldenberg RL, Mercer BM, Meis PJ et al. The preterm prediction study: fetal fibronectin testing and spontaneous preterm birth. NICHD Maternal Fetal Medicine Units Network. Obstet Gynecol 1996; 87: 643–8.
4. Iams JD, Goldenberg RL, Mercer BM et al. The Preterm Prediction Study: recurrence risk of spontaneous preterm birth. National Institute of Child Health and Human Development Maternal–Fetal Medicine Units Network. Am J Obstet Gynecol 1998; 178: 1035–40.
5. McGregor JA, Jackson GM, Lachelin GC et al. Salivary estriol as risk assessment for preterm labor: a prospective trial. Am J Obstet Gynecol 1995; 173: 1337–42.
6. Lumley J. Recent work on the epidemiology of preterm birth. Acta Obstet Gynecol Scand 2005; 84: 541–2.

7. Adams MM, Sarno AP, Harlass FE, Rawlings JS, Read JA. Risk factors for preterm delivery in a healthy cohort. Epidemiology 1995; 6: 525–32.

8. Hennessy E, Alberman E. Intergenerational influences affecting birth outcome. II. Preterm delivery and gestational age in the children of the 1958 British birth cohort. Paediatr Perinat Epidemiol 1998; 12 (Suppl) 1: 61–75.

9. Adams KM, Eschenbach DA. The genetic contribution towards preterm delivery. Semin Fetal Neonatal Med 2004; 9: 445–52.

10. Varner MW, Esplin MS. Current understanding of genetic factors in preterm birth. Br J Obstet Gynaecol 2005; 112 (Suppl 1): 28–31.

11. Ward K, Argyle V, Meade M, Nelson L. The heritability of preterm delivery. Obstet Gynecol 2005; 106: 1235–9.

12. Hao K, Wang X, Niu T et al. A candidate gene association study on preterm delivery: application of high-throughput genotyping technology and advanced statistical methods. Hum Mol Genet 2004; 13: 683–91.

13. Wang X, Zuckerman B, Kaufman G et al. Molecular epidemiology of preterm delivery: methodology and challenges. Paediatr Perinat Epidemiol 2001; 15 (Suppl 2): 63–77.

14. Ekwo EE, Gosselink CA, Moawad A. Previous pregnancy outcomes and subsequent risk of preterm rupture of amniotic sac membranes. Br J Obstet Gynaecol 1993; 100: 536–41.

15. Wang X, Zuckerman B, Pearson C et al. Maternal cigarette smoking, metabolic gene polymorphism, and infant birth weight. JAMA 2002; 287: 195–202.

16. Treloar SA, Macones GA, Mitchell LE, Martin NG. Genetic influences on premature parturition in an Australian twin sample. Twin Res 2000; 3: 80–2.

17. Wildschut HI, Lumey LH, Lunt PW. Is preterm delivery genetically determined? Paediatr Perinat Epidemiol 1991; 5: 363–72.

18. Porter TF, Fraser AM, Hunter CY, Ward RH, Varner MW. The risk of preterm birth across generations. Obstet Gynecol 1997; 90: 63–7.

19. Carr-Hill RA, Hall MH. The repetition of spontaneous preterm labour. Br J Obstet Gynaecol 1985; 92: 921–8.

20. Kristensen J, Langhoff-Roos J, Kristensen FB. [Significance of idiopathic preterm birth in relation to previous and future pregnancies]. Ugeskr Laeger 1998; 160: 3732–5.

21. Kristensen J, Langhoff-Roos J, Kristensen FB. Implications of idiopathic preterm delivery for previous and subsequent pregnancies. Obstet Gynecol 1995; 86: 800–4.

22. Mercer B, Milluzzi C, Collin M. Periviable birth at 20 to 26 weeks of gestation: proximate causes, previous obstetric history and recurrence risk. Am J Obstet Gynecol 2005; 193: 1175–80.

23. Petrini JR, Callaghan WM, Klebanoff M et al. Estimated effect of 17 alpha-hydroxyprogesterone caproate on preterm birth in the United States. Obstet Gynecol 2005; 105: 267–72.

24. Vermeulen GM, Bruinse HW. Prophylactic administration of clindamycin 2% vaginal cream to reduce the incidence of spontaneous preterm birth in women with an increased recurrence risk: a randomised placebo-controlled double-blind trial. Br J Obstet Gynaecol 1999; 106: 652–7.

25. Ghidini A, Salafia CM. Histologic placental lesions in women with recurrent preterm delivery. Acta Obstet Gynecol Scand 2005; 84: 547–50.

26. Rasmussen S, Irgens LM, Dalaker K. Outcome of pregnancies subsequent to placental abruption: a risk assessment. Acta Obstet Gynecol Scand 2000; 79: 496–501.

27. Skomsvoll JF, Baste V, Irgens LM, Ostensen M. The recurrence risk of adverse outcome in the second pregnancy in women with rheumatic disease 1. Obstet Gynecol 2002; 100: 1196–202.

28. Koike T, Minakami H, Izumi A et al. Recurrence risk of preterm birth due to preeclampsia. Gynecol Obstet Invest 2002; 53: 22–7.

29. Bloom SL, Yost NP, McIntire DD, Leveno KJ. Recurrence of preterm birth in singleton and twin pregnancies. Obstet Gynecol 2001; 98: 379–85.

30. Bakketeig LS, Hoffman HJ, Harley EE. The tendency to repeat gestational age and birth weight in successive births. Am J Obstet Gynecol 1979; 135: 1086–103.

31. Ward K. Genetic factors in preterm birth. Br J Obstet Gynaecol 2003; 110 (Suppl 20): 117.

32. Mercer BM, Goldenberg RL, Moawad AH et al. The preterm prediction study: effect of gestational age and cause of preterm birth on subsequent obstetric outcome. National Institute of Child Health and Human Development Maternal–Fetal Medicine Units Network. Am J Obstet Gynecol 1999; 181: 1216–21.

33. Melve KK, Skjaerven R, Gjessing HK, Oyen N. Recurrence of gestational age in sibships: implications for perinatal mortality. Am J Epidemiol 1999; 150: 756–62.

34. Magnus P, Bakketeig LS, Skjaerven R. Correlations of birth weight and gestational age across generations. Ann Hum Biol 1993; 20: 231–8.

35. Bamshad M. Genetic influences on health: does race matter? JAMA 2005; 294: 937–46.

36. Fiscella K. Race, genes and preterm delivery. J Natl Med Assoc 2005; 97: 1516–26.

37. Ekwo E, Moawad A. The risk for recurrence of premature births to African-American and white women. J Assoc Acad Minor Phys 1998; 9: 16–21.

38. Foster HW, Wu L, Bracken MB, Semenya K, Thomas J. Intergenerational effects of high socioeconomic status on low birthweight and preterm birth in African Americans. J Natl Med Assoc 2000; 92: 213–21.

39. Zhang J, Savitz DA. Preterm birth subtypes among blacks and whites. Epidemiology 1992; 3: 428–33.

40. McGrady GA, Sung JF, Rowley DL, Hogue CJ. Preterm delivery and low birth weight among first-born infants of black and white college graduates. Am J Epidemiol 1992; 136: 266–76.

41. Reagan PB, Salsberry PJ. Race and ethnic differences in determinants of preterm birth in the USA: broadening the social context. Soc Sci Med 2005; 60: 2217–28.

42. Olsen P, Laara E, Rantakallio P et al. Epidemiology of preterm delivery in two birth cohorts with an interval of 20 years. Am J Epidemiol 1995; 142: 1184–93.

43. Lu MC, Chen B. Racial and ethnic disparities in preterm birth: the role of stressful life events. Am J Obstet Gynecol 2004; 191: 691–9.

44. Berkowitz GS, Blackmore-Prince C, Lapinski RH, Savitz DA. Risk factors for preterm birth subtypes. Epidemiology 1998; 9: 279–85.

45. Heaman MI, Blanchard JF, Gupton AL, Moffatt ME, Currie RF. Risk factors for spontaneous preterm birth among Aboriginal and non-Aboriginal women in Manitoba. Paediatr Perinat Epidemiol 2005; 19: 181–93.

46. Crider KS, Whitehead N, Buus RM. Genetic variation associated with preterm birth: a HuGE review. Genet Med 2005; 7: 593–604.

47. Hartel C, von Otte S, Koch J et al. Polymorphisms of haemostasis genes as risk factors for preterm delivery. Thromb Haemost 2005; 94: 88–92.

48. Johnson WG, Scholl TO, Spychala JR et al. Common dihydrofolate reductase 19-base pair deletion allele: a novel risk factor for preterm delivery. Am J Clin Nutr 2005; 81: 664–8.

49. Kalish RB, Nguyen DP, Vardhana S et al. A single nucleotide A>G polymorphism at position -670 in the Fas gene promoter: relationship to preterm premature rupture of fetal membranes in multifetal pregnancies. Am J Obstet Gynecol 2005; 192: 208–12.

50. Romero R, Chaiworapongsa T, Kuivaniemi H, Tromp G. Bacterial vaginosis, the inflammatory response and the risk of preterm birth: a role for genetic epidemiology in the prevention of preterm birth. Am J Obstet Gynecol 2004; 190: 1509–19.

51. Annells MF, Hart PH, Mulligan CG et al. Interleukins-1, -4, -6, -10, tumor necrosis factor, transforming growth factor-beta,

FAS, and mannose-binding protein C gene polymorphisms in Australian women: Risk of preterm birth. Am J Obstet Gynecol 2004; 191: 2056–67.

52. Moore S, Ide M, Randhawa M et al. An investigation into the association among preterm birth, cytokine gene polymorphisms and periodontal disease. Br J Obstet Gynaecol 2004; 111: 125–32.

53. Nguyen DP, Genc M, Vardhana S et al. Ethnic differences of polymorphisms in cytokine and innate immune system genes in pregnant women. Obstet Gynecol 2004; 104: 293–300.

54. Wang X, Zuckerman B, Coffman GA, Corwin MJ. Familial aggregation of low birth weight among whites and blacks in the United States. N Engl J Med 1995; 333: 1744–9.

55. Khoury MJ, Cohen BH. Genetic heterogeneity of prematurity and intrauterine growth retardation: clues from the Old Order Amish. Am J Obstet Gynecol 1987; 157: 400–10.

56. Malecot-G. Les Mathematiques de l'Heredite. Paris: Masson et Cie, 1948.

57. Gholami K, Thomas A. A linear time algorithm for calculation of multiple pairwise kinship coefficients and the genetic index of familiarity. Comput Biomed Res 1994; 27: 342–50.

58. McLellan T, Jorde LB, Skolnick MH. Genetic distances between the Utah Mormons and related populations. Am J Hum Genet 1984; 36: 836–57.

59. Jorde LB. Consanguinity and prereproductive mortality in the Utah Mormon population. Hum Hered 2001; 52: 61–5.

60. Marchini J, Donnelly P, Cardon LR. Genome-wide strategies for detecting multiple loci that influence complex diseases. Nat Genet 2005; 37: 413–17.

61. Terwilliger JD, Goring HH. Gene mapping in the 20th and 21st centuries: statistical methods, data analysis, and experimental design. Hum Biol 2000; 72: 63–132.

62. Hirschhorn JN, Daly MJ. Genome-wide association studies for common diseases and complex traits. Nat Rev Genet 2005; 6: 95–108.

63. Neale BM, Sham PC. The future of association studies: gene-based analysis and replication. Am J Hum Genet 2004; 75: 353–62.

64. Gordon D, Finch SJ. Factors affecting statistical power in the detection of genetic association. J Clin Invest 2005; 115: 1408–18.

65. Esplin MS, Varner MW. Genetic factors in preterm birth – the future. Br J Obstet Gynaecol 2005; 112 (Suppl 1): 97–102.

SECTION IV

CURRENT STATUS OF INTERVENTIONS

14

Calcium-channel blockers and betamimetics

John J Morrison and Sharon M Cooley

INTRODUCTION

While fetal and neonatal outcome rely on a variety of diverse factors, the main factor of importance is the gestation at which the baby is born. Preterm delivery, or delivery at less than <37 completed weeks of gestation, accounts for 6–15% of all births,[1,2] depending on the socioeconomic variables of the population studied. This proportion of births results in 75% of perinatal deaths, and is responsible for the majority of neonatal morbidity in current practice.[3] Because neonatal survival is close to 100% by 32 weeks of gestation, and morbidity is much reduced after this time, prenatal therapeutic interventions are targeted predominantly at the 2–3% of births that occur prior to this gestation.[4,5] While the etiology of preterm birth is multifactorial[6,7] there is a consensus from published reports that approximately 25–50% of all preterm births arise from causes that are unexplained in nature (i.e. idiopathic) or related to mechanisms for which there is no evident benefit from delivery (i.e. cervical incompetence, congenital uterine malformation, multiple pregnancy), and hence are suitable for appropriate pharmacological intervention to inhibit uterine contractions, i.e. tocolysis.[8,9] Attempts to develop an ideal tocolytic drug have been ongoing for 50 years now, and scrutiny of the literature has revealed the progression from case reports,[10] to small observational series,[11] to randomized controlled trials,[12] and ultimately combinations of the latter in the form of meta-analyses.[13] However, this major expansion in information on management of preterm labor has not resulted in a definitive answer to the central questions of whether tocolytic treatments have a role, if so which tocolytic drug is the most effective, and, finally, which compound is the safest for use from a maternal and fetal point of view. For this reason, clinical practice in relation to tocolytic drugs varies from one hospital and country to the next, and controversy remains in relation to indications, choice of agent, dosage regimens and duration of therapy for tocolytic drugs. The aim of this chapter is to examine the evidence, clinically and scientifically, for the use of calcium-channel blockers (CCB) and betamimetic agents, as tocolytic compounds, in the light of the current literature, and in comparison to no treatment (or placebo) and other compounds.

TOCOLYSIS

Since the 1960s a host of different drug compounds, all of which exert the end result of relaxing myometrial smooth muscle, have been used in an attempt to stop or inhibit preterm labor.[14–23] These agents include betamimetic compounds, CCB, cyclooxygenase (COX) inhibitors, nitric oxide donor compounds, indomethacin, magnesium sulfate, and oxytocin antagonists. These agents have all been subjected to randomized controlled trials of varying size and quality, for many of them in comparison with the use of placebo compounds, and for nearly all of them in comparison to another tocolytic agent. There are difficulties in performing such trials, and these difficulties have been addressed in some studies and largely ignored in others. The 'placebo effect' has a major influence on studies carried out to test the efficacy of potential tocolytic compounds, whereby a large proportion of women who present with uterine contractions are not in true preterm labor, and a placebo will be as effective as a putative drug compound. The concept that the overall time period or duration of preterm labor, i.e. 23–37 weeks of gestation, provides for vastly different outcomes in terms of neonatal wellbeing, is poorly addressed in the design of some studies. In order to evaluate fully the subtle differences in terms of neonatal morbidity, large international studies are required which involve significant recruitment. In addition, while it is possible to document objective evidence of infection in only approximately 15% of women who go into preterm labor,[24] it is frequently believed that delivery may be advantageous for the fetus in preterm labor, from an infection point of view, because of the so-called 'chorio-decidual inflammatory syndrome'. Finally, many studies have focused on the period of delay achieved by drug compounds evaluated, from onset of preterm labor to final delivery, but fail to recognize or address the issue of the perinatal benefit derived from the use of these drugs.

For tocolytics as a group in general, it is apparent that their use will delay delivery after the onset of preterm labor for >24 h and up to 1 week compared with placebo, or no treatment.[16,19–23] However, scrutiny of the data pertaining to outcome in terms of neonatal wellbeing, i.e. perinatal death, respiratory distress syndrome, birthweight, necrotizing enterocolitis, intraventricular hemorrhage, seizures, hypoglycemia, patent ductus arteriosus or neonatal sepsis, reveals that there is no difference between the treatment and control (no treatment or placebo) groups. In other words, the delay in timing of delivery achieved by this group of drugs cannot be translated into objectively defined perinatal benefit.

The question therefore arises whether or not tocolytic drugs should be used in current obstetric practice. The recommendation of the Royal College of Obstetricians and Gynaecologists, London, UK, states that it is reasonable not to use tocolytic drugs as there is no clear evidence that outcome is improved by such practice, but that their use should be considered if a few days gained could be put to good use for corticosteroids or in utero transfer.[25] This summarizes the current state of the literature. Interpreted another way, there is no clear evidence that clinical obstetric practice involving the use of these drugs is superior to their omission from such practice, but there remains the possibility, as yet unproven, that the delay achieved could result in some benefit.

CALCIUM-CHANNEL BLOCKERS (CCB)

CCB act on the voltage-dependent L-type calcium channels in the cell membrane, and result in blocking the influx of calcium into the intracellular compartment. This leads to a reduction in the amplitude and frequency of myometrial activity, by inhibiting the calcium-dependent myosin light-chain kinase phosphorylation.[26] Relaxation of uterine smooth muscle, and a decrease in the basal tone, follows.[27] The potent effects of nifedipine on isometric recordings of in vitro spontaneous uterine contractility (Figure 14.1), and uterine contractility elicited by oxytocin (Figure 14.2), are demonstrated. Nifedipine, the most frequently used drug of this group, exerts a negative inotropic and chronotropic effect on the heart.

However, the cardiac effects of nifedipine are less marked than the systemic effects. Sympathetic vasodilation occurs in response to the inotropic and chronotropic effects of nifedipine. This precipitates a drop in maternal blood pressure and pulse.[28]

Nifedipine has the advantage that it is cheap, readily available with a variety of release formulations, and easy to administer. It is not licensed for use as a tocolytic in any country, to the authors' knowledge. Transplacental transfer of CCB occurs with slightly lower fetal/umbilical serum levels reported than those noted in the maternal serum (ratio of 0.9).[29,30] While the implications of this are not entirely clear, it must be taken into consideration when prescribing CCB in pregnancy.

There are two common dosage regimes for nifedipine usage as a tocolytic.[31] The first is to administer an initial loading dose of 30 mg orally, followed by an additional 20 mg orally in 90 min. An alternative regimen is to administer 10 mg orally every 20 min, up to four doses, followed by 20 mg orally every 4–8 h. The half-life of nifedipine is approximately 2–3 h, and the duration of action of a single orally administered dose is up to 6 h. Plasma concentrations peak in 30–60 min. Nifedipine is almost completely metabolized in the liver and excreted by the kidney.

Nifedipine is a peripheral vasodilator, and thus may cause symptoms such as nausea, dizziness, headache, dizziness, facial flushing and palpitations. Serious complications include marked hypotension, congestive cardiac failure (CCF), and myocardial infarction.[32,33] Nifedipine relaxes arteriolar smooth muscle, precipitating a decrease in mean arterial pressure and a reflex increase in heart rate. However, these changes are usually mild and less severe than those seen after beta-adrenergic agonist (β-AR) treatment.[34,35] CCB are contraindicated in women with known hypersensitivity to the drug, and should be used with caution in women with cardiac disease, in particular congestive cardiac failure or left ventricular dysfunction. The concomitant use of a CCB with magnesium sulfate may exacerbate muscular contractility inhibition and result in respiratory paralysis.[36]

The majority of trial data refers to oral nifedipine but intravenous nicardipine usage has also been reported.[37] The data relating to the use of intravenous nicardipine was based on a single clinical trial however, and acute pulmonary edema has been a reported association, even with the limited numbers in the trial.[38] Further evaluation is therefore required, and the remainder of the discussion in relation to CCB in this review pertains to nifedipine.

There are approximately 40 studies, 12 randomized trials and seven meta-analyses available, which have been undertaken to assess the efficacy and impact of nifedipine as a tocolytic compound, and its effects in relation to

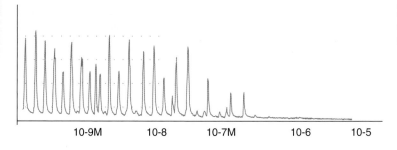

Figure 14.1 The effect of nifedipine on spontaneous myometrial contractions.

10-9M   10-8   10-7M   10-6   10-5

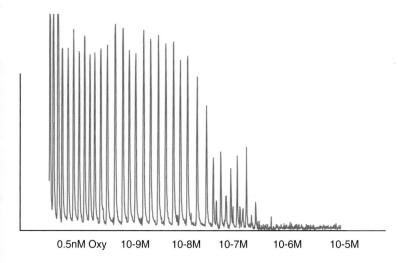

Figure 14.2 The effect of nifedipine on oxytocin-induced contractions.

0.5nM Oxy   10-9M   10-8M   10-7M   10-6M   10-5M

maternal and neonatal wellbeing.[13,14,23,26–35,37–39] Most of these trials have compared nifedipine with other tocolytic agents, in particular betamimetics. A small number of reports have addressed the efficacy of nifedipine in comparison to no treatment or placebo, but the numbers recruited are small and the studies are of poor methodology, and hence there are no reliable data on this topic.

In recent years, a renewed enthusiasm for nifedipine as a tocolytic compound has emerged, secondary to reports that have outlined the possibility that it may actually confer perinatal benefit, unlike other compounds studied, in addition to delaying onset of labor, and that its safety profile is satisfactory, or even more satisfactory than other compounds.[13,23,39,40] Essentially, these reports have demonstrated that CCB used for inhibiting preterm labor reduce the number of preterm deliveries within 7 days of receiving treatment [relative risk (RR) 0.76, 95% confidence interval (CI) 0.6–0.97]. They also reduced the number of deliveries at <34 weeks of gestation (RR 0.83, 95% CI 0.69–0.99), and the number of women having to stop treatment secondary to adverse side effects (RR 0.1, 95% CI 0.05–0.36). In relation to neonatal morbidity, a reduction was noted in intra-ventricular hemorrhage (RR 0.59, 95% CI 0.36–0.98),

neonatal respiratory distress syndrome (RR 0.63, 95% CI 0.46–0.88), neonatal jaundice (RR 0.73, 95% CI 0.57–0.93), and necrotizing enterocolitis (RR 0.21, 95% CI 0.05–0.96).[39] These data are derived from a meta-analysis including 12 RCT involving 1029 women, and all studies have compared the use of CCB versus any other tocolytic agent. The exciting aspect of these results is the actual benefit in neonatal terms arising from the use of nifedipine, and the fact that it was well tolerated by patients. This combined with the attractive cost, and the ease of administration, led the authors to suggest that, when tocolysis is indicated, CCB are preferable to other agents.

However, there many issues which give rise to caution in interpreting these results for clinical use. There are no reliable placebo-controlled/no-treatment trials. The overall results are heavily weighted by the two trials carried out by Papatsonis and his team of researchers.[37,41] These studies used rather high dosage regimes and prolonged maintenance therapy. The safety aspect of nifedipine, and particularly in relation to higher dosage regimes, needs further investigation. From a clinical governance point of view it must be borne in mind that nifedipine is not licensed for this indication. It is reasonable to infer that further trials, carried out to address some of these issues, and involving large numbers, are required to reassure clinicians that nifedipine is preferable to other tocolytic agents.[42]

BETAMIMETICS

Betamimetics, also known as β-AR agonists, were the first drugs used from a research perspective to prevent preterm delivery. In 1980, the US Drug and Food administration approved the use of ritodrine for inhibition of preterm labor. Other betamimetics used, but not licensed, for this purpose include salbutamol and terbutaline. The β-AR agonists, on binding with $β_2$-AR, activate adenylate cyclase, resulting in increased intracellular concentrations of cyclic adenosine monophosfate (cAMP). This in turn activates protein kinase and phosphorylation of intracellular proteins, including membrane proteins in the sarcoplasmic reticulum, leading ultimately to decreased availability of free intracellular calcium to actin and myosin.[43] Myosin light-chain kinase is also phosphorylated, which decreases its affinity for calmodulin.[43,44] The cumulative result of these actions is that uterine smooth muscle is relaxed. Unfortunately, in terms of clinical effectiveness, the inhibition of contractions by betamimetics is often short-lived. Escape from their tocolytic effect is well described in vitro and in vivo.[45–49]

Historically, there were initially two major reports outlining the efficacy of betamimetics as tocolytic agents, in the 1980s[39] and early 1990s.[16] In their meta-analyses, King et al[39] reviewed 16 controlled trials in which tocolytic agents, chiefly ritodrine, were evaluated. Betamimetics were found to be effective in reducing the proportion of women who delivered within 24 h and within 48 h of treatment [odds ratio (OR) 0.5, 95% CI 0.42–0.83]. However, this treatment did not decrease the likelihood of preterm delivery, and had no effect on perinatal mortality or neonatal morbidity.[39]

A later randomized, controlled, multicenter study – the Canadian Preterm Labor Trial – which involved 708 women receiving either ritodrine or placebo, concluded that the use of ritodrine in the treatment of preterm labor had no significant beneficial effect on perinatal mortality, the frequency of prolongation of pregnancy to term, or birthweight.[16] The accumulated evidence at that time therefore showed that treatment with a betamimetic reduced the rate of delivery within 48 h, but that this effect did not lead to clinically significant reductions in the rates of preterm birth, or low birthweight, and, most importantly, did not result in improvement in outcome in terms of severe neonatal respiratory distress syndrome or perinatal death. Little has changed since then, with the more recent meta-analysis by Mary Hannah's group,[14] demonstrating effectively the same findings.

Gyetvai et al, with a sample size >1000 patients, found that the use of β-AR agonists, in comparison to placebo or no treatment, was associated with similar infant death rates (9 versus 8%, OR 1.08, 95% CI 0.72–1.62). There was a trend towards a reduction in respiratory distress syndrome (18 versus 25%, OR 0.76, 95% CI 0.57–1.01), and in infants born with a birthweight <2500 g (50 versus 63%, OR 0.79, 95% CI 0.61–1.01). However, these observations were not statistically significant.

β-AR agonists impact significantly on maternal health, having serious side effects such as palpitations, pulmonary edema, nausea, hyperglycemia, and hypokalemia, all of which limit their clinical applicability.[14,50] Many of the maternal side effects of the β-AR agonists are the result of stimulation of both $β_1$- and $β_2$-AR. The resulting increase in maternal heart rate, combined with peripheral vasodilation and diastolic hypotension, give rise to maternal tachycardia and palpitations. The incidence of serious complications, such as pulmonary edema is rare, and can be limited by strict fluid management and regular pulmonary system examination of women receiving β-AR agonists for prevention of preterm labor.[51,52] However, there are clear documented reports of maternal mortality associated with the use of ritodrine, largely due to pulmonary edema and cardiac dysrhythmmias, and it is important for clinicians to be aware of this.

Metabolic complications are more common, and necessitate regular serum assessment of glucose and potassium levels during tocolytic therapy with β-AR.[53] Strict control of maternal systemic and metabolic complications during therapy will subsequently reduce the incidence of fetal tachycardia and neonatal hypoglycemia resulting from β-AR agonist therapy.[54] Tachyphylaxis, a process of desensitization of the β-AR, occurs with prolonged use of β-AR agonists, decreasing their effectiveness.[55] The use of β-AR agonists is contraindicated in women with cardiac disease. They are also relatively contraindicated among women with poorly controlled hyperthyroidism or diabetes, because of potential exacerbation of the chronotropic and glycemic side effects, respectively.

Terbutaline is the most commonly used β-AR agonist for tocolysis in the United States (US). It may be administered intravenously, subcutaneously or via intermittent injections. The most common route of administration is intravenously as part of a continuous intravenous infusion, with an initial rate of 2.5–5 μg/min, which is increased slowly to a maximum of 25 μg/min. The infusion rate may also be reduced gradually once uterine myometrial activity has ceased. As β-AR agonists are relatively inexpensive they are still the mainstay of treatment in underdeveloped countries.[56] However, the variety of adverse effects seen with their use has understandably limited their applicability and universal uptake. In addition, the availability of newer, potentially safer, tocolytic agents has made the use of the more controversial β-AR agonists, such as ritodrine, obsolete.

β₃-ADRENOCEPTOR (β₃-AR) AGONISTS

In the last 10 years knowledge concerning the role of the β₃-AR in smooth muscle tissues has expanded significantly. For uterine smooth muscle, two separate research groups – that led by Marc Bardou in Dijon, France, and our group in Galway, Ireland – have reported in relation to the expression and modulation of β₃-AR in human myometrium. The first reports outlined that the β₃-AR was expressed in human myometrium,[57] and that BRL37344, a β₃-AR, was of equal potency to the β₂-AR agonist ritodrine for inhibiting uterine contractions in vitro.[58] This raised the question of whether or not specific β₃-AR agonist activity might be mediated solely through the β₃-AR, or whether it may have non specific effects on the β₁- or β₂-AR. In parallel with this concept was the fact that there was substantial in vitro and other evidence suggesting that the potency of β₃-AR agonists was less in vascular tissue then that of their β₂-AR agonist counterparts.[59,60] If this were truly the case, then the possibility that β₃-AR agonists may exert the same uterorelaxant affect, but without the adverse systemic cardiovascular effects of β₂-AR agonists, was an attractive concept for development of novel tocolytic compounds.

To this end Dennedy et al[58] evaluated the effects of the β₃-AR agonist BRL37344, and those of the β₂-AR agonist ritodrine, in the presence and absence of various β-AR antagonists, to filter out the specificity of each of the above agents in human myometrial tissue. In addition, the effects of both compounds were investigated on umbilical artery rings, as a model of human vascular tissue, albeit a model with limitations. The net result of these investigations was that BRL37344 appeared to be mediated solely through the β₃-AR, while ritodrine exerted its effects on β₁-, β₂-, and β₃-AR. The dose–response curve outlining the effects of BRL37344 is demonstrated in Figure 14.3, outlining the antagonism of its uterorelaxant activity by bupranolol. In addition, it was observed that BRL37344 had a much reduced effect in vascular tissue in comparison to ritodrine. Taken together, these findings indicated that β₃-AR modulation may provide a novel scientific approach to tocolysis with fewer unwanted vascular effects.

The above pharmacological data are very encouraging in terms of a scientific outline or basis for β₃-AR modulation as a tocolytic possibility. More recently, Marc Bardou and his group,[61] have investigated the physiological functionality and expression of the β-AR in human myometrium. They have demonstrated that inhibition of spontaneous contractions by a specific β₃-AR agonist was significantly greater in pregnant, compared with nonpregnant, myometrium. The opposite was observed with the use of salbutamol, i.e. the use of salbutamol as a β₂-AR agonist was significantly less efficient or potent in pregnant myometrium as compared to nonpregnant myometrium. Using binding studies, they have demonstrated that there is a clear predominance of the β₃-AR subtype in myometrium with a two-fold upregulation at the end of pregnancy. In addition, expression of the β₃-AR transcripts and immunoreactive proteins was increased in pregnant compared with nonpregnant myometrium. These findings taken together all clearly indicate a predominant role for the β₃-AR in the regulation of human myometrial contractility over that of the β₂-AR, and particularly in the third trimester of pregnancy. These objective scientific findings point to the possibility that modulation of the β₃-AR provides much

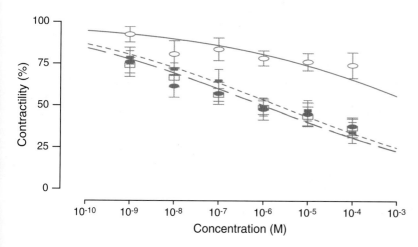

Figure 14.3 Dose–response curves show the uterorelaxant effect of the β₃-adrenoreceptor (β₃-AR) agonist BRL373449 (closed squares), and after-bath pre-exposure to one of the β₃-AR antagonists, bupranolol (open circles), propanolol (open squares), or butoxamine (closed circles). The points represent the mean and the error bars represent the SEM. (Reproduced with permission from Dennedy et al, Br J Obstet Gynaecol 2001; 108: 605–9.)

more exciting potential than the previous approach via the β_2-AR. There are, however, no clinical data currently available pertaining to β_3-AR use in human preterm labor.

The mechanism of relaxation elicited by the β_3-AR agonist is as yet unknown, but one might speculate that it is also linked to increased production of cAMP. We hypothesized that it may also have other mechanisms of action, and in particular be linked to the large conductance, calcium-activated, potassium channel (BK_{Ca} or Maxi K). To this end, the effects of BRL37344 on single-channel and whole-cell recordings from human myometrial cells were carried out to evaluate the potential

electrophysiological effects of BRL37344.[62] Alongside these experiments, the effects of BRL37344 on contractile activity in vitro, in the presence and absence of iberiotoxin as a BK_{Ca} blocking agent, and in the presence and absence of bupranolol and SR59230a, both of which are β_3-AR blocking compounds, were evaluated. These experiments identified clearly that the BK_{Ca} channel is a target of BRL37344, with this latter compound significantly increasing the open-state probability of the channel in a concentration-dependent manner. This effect was completely blocked with both of the β_3-AR blocking compounds used, bupranolol as a nonselective blocker and SR59230a as a selective blocker. While BRL37344

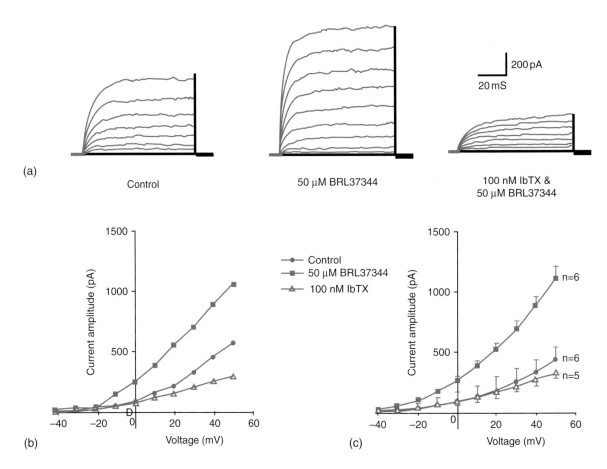

Figure 14.4 BRL37344 increases whole-cell currents in human uterine smooth muscle myocytes. (a) Perforated patch recordings from the same myocyte before and 15 min after exposure to 50 μM BRL37344, and then 5–10 min after cumulative addition of 100 nM iberiotoxin (IbTX). (b) The complete current versus voltage relationship for the steady-state outward current from the same cell as in (a). Treatment conditions are the same as described for control, 50 μM BRL37344 and BRL37344, and 100 nM IbTX. (c) Average current versus voltage relationship for uterine myocytes before and after 50 μM BRL37344, and then cumulative addition of 100 nM IbTX. Each point represents the mean number of cells ±SEM. (Reproduced with permission from Doheny et al, J Clin Endocrinol Metab 2005; 90: 5786–96.)

increased whole-cell currents from human myometrial cells over a range of membrane potentials, this effect was reversed by iberiotoxin. Iberiotoxin also attenuated the functional relaxant effect of BRL37344 on spontaneous and oxytocin-induced contractions in isometric recordings from human myometrial tissue. These findings therefore clearly outline that activation of the BK_{Ca} channel may partially explain the potent uterorelaxant effect of the β_3-AR agonist BRL37344. The effects of BRL37344 on myometrial whole-cell current recordings, in the presence and absence of iberiotoxin, are shown in Figure 14.4.

In conclusion, the above data are novel and point to the exciting finding that β_3-AR may have greater potential as a potent uterorelaxant compounds than their β_2-AR counterparts. There is now clear evidence that the β_3-AR has clear predominance in the myometrium over the β_2-AR, and that this is upregulated in pregnancy. β_3-AR agonists appear to have greater potency in pregnant myometrial tissue than nonpregnant tissue, unlike their β_2-AR counterparts. Finally, the potential mechanisms of relaxation elicited by β_3-AR compounds include modulation of the large conductance, calcium-activated channel, which is a very potent and central mechanism of myometrial relaxation. As there are no clinical studies on the β_3-AR agonists in human preterm labor, the scientific ground is well prepared to outline their importance for the future.

CONCLUSION

In summary, there are very clear scientific data in relation to the role of CCB and betamimetics as uterorelaxant compounds. In terms of clinical use, the recent renewed enthusiasm for CCB, concomitant with a much reduced enthusiasm for β_2-AR agonist, has to be interpreted in the light of the potential limitations of CCB. It would be most reassuring to have further trials from different groups in relation to their effectiveness, and the issue of safety, particularly for higher dosage regimens, remains unanswered. In many parts of the world the use of β_2-AR agonists has now been largely discontinued, particularly outside of the US. While there are very exciting scientific data about β_3-AR agonists, there are no clinical data as yet, but they offer promising potential for the future.

ACKNOWLEDGMENTS

The authors would like to acknowledge the members of the research group whose published work has contributed to this review, namely Drs Michael Dennedy and Helen Doheny.

REFERENCES

1. Martin JA, Hamilton BE, Ventura SJ et al. Births: final data for 2001. Natl Vital Stat Rep 2002; 51: 1.
2. Kiely JL. What is the population-based risk of preterm birth among twins and other multiples? Clin Obstet Gynecol 1998; 41: 3.
3. Arias E, MacDorman MF, Strobino DM et al. Annual summary of vital statistics – 2002. Pediatrics 2003; 112: 1215.
4. Morrison JJ, Rennie JM. Clinical, scientific and ethical aspects of fetal and neonatal care at extreme preterm periods of gestation. Br J Obstet Gynaecol 1997; 104: 1341–50.
5. Demissie K, Rhoads GG, Anath CV et al. Trends in preterm birth and neonatal mortality among blacks and whites in the United States from 1989 to 1997. Am J Epidemiol 2001; 154: 307–15.
6. To MS, Alfirevic Z, Heath VC et al. Cervical cerclage for prevention of preterm delivery in women with short cervix: randomised controlled trial. Lancet 2004; 363: 1849.
7. Mercer BM, Goldenberg RL, Moawad AH et al. The preterm prediction study: effect of gestational age and cause of preterm birth on subsequent obstetric outcome. National Institute of Child Health and Human Development Maternal–Fetal Medicine Units Network. Am J Obstet Gynecol 1999; 181: 1216.
8. Joseph KS, Kramer MS, Marcoux S et al. Determinants of preterm birth rates in Canada from 1981 through 1983 and from 1992 through 1994. N Engl J Med 1998; 339: 1434.
9. Kiely JL, Kiely M. Epidemiological trends in multiple births in the United States, 1971–1998. Twin Res 2001; 4(3): 131–3.
10. Van Kets H, Thiery M, Derom R et al. Perinatal hazards of chronic antenatal tocolysis with indomethacin. Prostaglandins 1979; 18(6): 893–907.
11. Creasy RK, Golbus MS, Laros Jr RK et al. Oral ritodrine maintenance in the treatment of preterm labor. Am J Obstet Gynecol 1980; 137(2): 212–19.
12. Hollander DI, Nagey DA, Pupkin MJ. Magnesium sulfate and ritodrine hydrochloride: a randomized comparison. Am J Obstet Gynecol 1987; 156(3): 631–7.
13. Sanchez-Ramos L, Kaunitz AM, Gaudier FL et al. Efficacy of maintenance therapy after acute tocolysis: a meta-analysis. Am J Obstet Gynecol 1999; 181(2): 484–90.
14. Gyetvai K, Hannah ME, Hodnett ED et al. Tocolytics for preterm labour: a systematic review. Obstet Gynecol 1999; 94(5 Pt 2): 869–77.
15. Slattery M, Morrison JJ. Preterm delivery. Lancet 2002; 360: 1489–97.
16. The Canadian Preterm Labor Investigators Group. Treatment of preterm labor with the beta-adrenergic agonist ritodrine. N Engl J Med 1992; 327: 308–12.
17. Morrison JJ, Ashford ML, Khan RN et al. The effects of the potassium channel openers on isolated pregnant human myometrium before and after the onset of labor: potential for tocolysis. Am J Obstet Gynecol 1993; 169: 1277–85.
18. Terrone DA, Rinehart BK, Kimmel ES et al. A prospective randomized, controlled trial of high and low maintenance doses of magnesium sulphate for acute tocolysis. Am J Obstet Gynecol 2000; 182: 1477–82.
19. Hannah M, Amankwah K, Barret J et al. The Canadian consensus on the use of tocolytics for preterm labour. J SOGC 1995; 17: 1089–115.
20. Lees CC, Lojacono A, Thompon C et al. Glyceryl trinitrate and ritodrine in tocolysis: an international multicenter randomised study. Obstet Gynecol 1999; 94: 403–8.
21. Romero R, Sibai BM, Sanchoz-Ramos L et al. An oxytocin receptor antagonist (atosiban) in the treatment of preterm labor: a randomized, double-blind, placebo-controlled trial with tocolytic rescue. Am J Obstet Gynecol 2000; 182: 1173–83.

22. The Worldwide Atosiban versus Beta-agonists Study Group. Effectiveness and safety of the oxytocin antagonist atosiban versus beta-adrenergic agonists in the treatment of preterm labour. Br J Obstet Gynaecol 2001; 108: 133–42.

23. Tsatsaris V, Papatsonis D, Goffnet F et al. Tocolysis with nifedipine or beta-adrenergic agonists: a meta-analysis. Obstet Gynaecol 2001; 97: 840–7.

24. Romero R, Avila C, Breuke CA et al. The role of systemic and intrauterine infection in preterm parturition. Ann NY Acad Sci 1991; 622: 355–75.

25. Royal College of Obstetricians and Gynaecologists. Clinical Green Top Guidelines Tocolytic Drugs for Women in Preterm Labour (1B) – Oct 2002.

26. Andersson KE, Ingemarsson I, Ulmsten U et al. Inhibition of prostaglandin induced uterine activity by nifedipine. Br J Obstet Gynaecol 1979; 86: 175–9.

27. Ulmsten U, Anderson KE, Forman A. Relaxing effects of nifedipine on the pregnant uterus in vitro and vivo. Obstet Gynecol 1978; 52: 536–41.

28. Scholz H. Pharmacological aspects of calcium channel blockers. Cardiovasc Drugs Ther 1997; 10 (Suppl 3): 869–72.

29. Ferguson JE, Schutz T, Pershe R et al. Nifedipine pharmacokinetics during preterm labour tocolysis. Am J Obstet Gynecol 1989; 161: 145–9.

30. Prevost PR, Pharm D, Sherif A et al. Oral nifedipine: pharmacokinetics in pregnancy induced hypertension. Pharmacotherapy 1992; 12: 174–7.

31. van Geijn HP, Lenglet JE, Bolte AC. Nifedipine trials: effectiveness and safety aspects. Br J Obstet Gynaecol 2005; 112 (Suppl 1): 79–83.

32. Impey L. Severe hypotension and fetal distress following sublingual administration of nifedipine to a patient with severe pregnancy induced hypertension at 33 weeks. Br J Obstet Gynaecol 1993; 100: 959.

33. van Veen AJ, Pelinck MJ, van Pampus MG et al. Severe hypotension and fetal death due to tocolysis with nifedipine. Br J Obstet Gynaecol 2005; 112: 509.

34. Ferguson 2nd JE, Dyson DC, Schutz T et al. A comparison of tocolysis with nifedipine or ritodrine: analysis of efficacy and maternal, fetal, and neonatal outcome. Am J Obstet Gynecol 1990; 163: 105.

35. Bracero LA, Leikin E, Kirshenbaum N et al. Comparison of nifedipine and ritodrine for the treatment of preterm labor. Am J Perinatol 1991; 8: 365.

36. Feldman, S, Karalliedde, L. Drug interactions with neuromuscular blockers. Drug Saf 1996; 15: 261.

37. Vaast P, Dubreucq-Fossaert S, Houfflin-Debarge V et al. Acute pulmonary oedema during nicardipine therapy for premature labour. Report of five cases. Eur J Obstet Gynecol Reprod Biol 2004; 113: 98–9.

38. Jannet D, Abankwa B, Guyard B et al. Nicardipine versus salbutamol in the treatment of preterm labour. Eur J Obstet Gynecol Reprod Biol 1997; 73: 11–16.

39. King JF, Flenady VJ, Papatsonis D et al. Calcium channel blockers for inhibiting preterm labour. Cochrane Database Syst Rev 2003; (1): CD002255.

40. Papatsonis D, Flenady V, Cole S et al. Oxytocin receptor antagonists for preventing preterm labour. Cochrane Database Syst Rev 2005; (3): CD004452.

41. Papatsonis DN, Van Geijn HP, Ader HJ et al. Nifedipine and ritodrine in the management of preterm labor: a randomized multicenter trial. Obstet Gynecol 1997; 90(2): 230–4.

42. Beattie RB, Helmer H, Khan KS et al. Emerging issues over the choice of nifedipine, beta-agonists and atosiban for tocolysis in spontaneous preterm labour – a proposed systematic review by the International Preterm Labour Council. J Obstet Gynaecol 2004; 24(3): 213–15.

43. Roberts JM. Current understanding of pharmacological mechanisms in the prevention of preterm birth. Clin Obstet Gynecol 1984; 27: 592–605.

44. Schneid CR, Honeyman TW, Fay FS. Mechanism of β-adrenergic relaxation of smooth muscle. Nature 1979; 277: 32–6.

45. Caritis SN, Chiao JP, Kridgen P. Comparison of the pulsatile and continuous ritodrine administration. Effects on uterine contractility and β-adrenergic cascade. Am J Obstet Gynecol 1991; 164: 1005–12.

46. Casper RF, Lye SJ. Myometrial desensitization to continuous but not to intermittent β-adrenergic agonist infusion in sheep. Am J Obstet Gynecol 1986; 154: 301–5.

47. Ke R, Vohra M, Casper R. Prolonged inhibition of human myometrial contractility by intermittent isoproterenol. Am J Obstet Gynecol 1984; 149: 841–3.

48. Lam F, Gill P, Smith M et al. Use of the subcutaneous terbutaline pump for long-term tocolysis. Obstet Gynecol 1988; 72: 810–13.

49. Ryden G, Andersson RGG, Berg G. Is the relaxing effect of β-adrenergic agonists on the human myometrium only transitory? Acta Obstet Gynecol Scand (Suppl) 1982; 108: 47–51.

50. Guid Oei S, Koen Oei S, Brolmann HA. Myocardial infarction during nifedipine therapy for preterm labour. N Engl J Med 1999; 340: 154: 1–3.

51. Perry KG Jr, Morrison JC, Rust OA et al. Incidence of adverse cardiopulmonary effects with low-dose continuous terbutaline infusion. Am J Obstet Gynecol 1995; 173: 1273.

52. Lamont RF. The pathophysiology of pulmonary oedema with the use of beta-agonists. Br J Obstet Gynaecol 2000; 107: 439.

53. Main DM, Main EK. Preterm birth. In: Gabbe SG, Niebyl JR, Simpson JL, eds. Obstetrics: Normal and Problem Pregnancies, 2nd ed. New York: Churchill Livingstone, 1991: 829.

54. Golichowski AM, Hathaway DR, Fineberg N et al. Tocolytic and hemodynamic effects of nifedipine in the ewe. Am J Obstet Gynecol 1985; 151: 1134.

55. Caritis SN, Chiao JP, Moore JJ, Ward SM. Myometrial desensitization after ritodrine infusion. Am J Physiol 1987; 253: E410.

56. Anotayananth S, Subhedar NV, Garner P et al. Betamimetics for inhibiting preterm labour. Cochrane Database Syst Rev 2004 Oct 18; (4): CD004352.

57. Bardou M, Loustalot C, Cortijo J et al. Functional, biochemical and molecular biological evidence for a possible beta(3)-adrenoceptor in human near-term myometrium. Br J Pharmacol 2000; 130(8): 1960–6.

58. Dennedy MC, Friel AM, Gardeil F et al. Beta-3 versus beta-2 adrenergic agonists and preterm labour: in vitro uterine relaxation effects. Br J Obstet Gynaecol 2001; 108(6): 605–9.

59. Gauthier C, Langin D, Balligand JL. β₃-adrenoreceptors in the cardiovascular system. Trends Pharmacol Sci 2000; 21: 426–31.

60. Trochu JN, Leblais V, Rautureau Y et al. Beta 3-adrenoceptor stimulation induces vasorelaxation mediated essentially by endothelium-derived nitric oxide in rat thoracic aorta. Br J Pharmacol 1990; 101: 569–74.

61. Rouget C, Bardou M, Breuiller-Fouche M et al. Beta3-adrenoceptor is the predominant beta-adrenoceptor subtype in human myometrium and its expression is up-regulated in pregnancy. J Clin Endocrinol Metab 2005; 90(3): 1644–50.

62. Doheny HC, Lynch CM, Smith TJ et al. Functional coupling of beta3-adrenoceptors and large conductance calcium-activated potassium channels in human uterine myocytes. J Clin Endocrinol Metab 2005; 90(10): 5786–96.

15

Prostaglandins, oxytocin, and antagonists

A López Bernal

INTRODUCTION

The mechanism for parturition in women remains a mystery, but in most cases delivery occurs following the spontaneous onset of labor at around 39–41 weeks of gestation. It is not known whether women who go into labor and deliver preterm do so as a consequence of a different physiopathological mechanism, or as a result of the mis-timing or acceleration of the same process that operates at term. From a practical point of view, it is useful to subdivide preterm deliveries (deliveries at <37 weeks of gestation) into very early preterm birth (<32 weeks of gestation) and extremely preterm birth (<28 weeks of gestation) because the rates of perinatal mortality or disability in the newborns are considerably different in each subgroup.[1,2] The prevention of all preterm births is an unattainable goal because this would mean resolving every medical and obstetric complication of pregnancy (e.g. pregnancy-induced hypertension; pre-eclampsia, antepartum hemorrhage, premature rupture of the membranes). These complications contribute to iatrogenic preterm deliveries. However, by focusing our efforts on spontaneous preterm labor we have the potential to improve neonatal mortality and morbidity rates quite substantially. Our ignorance of the mechanism of parturition at term, let alone preterm labor, has made this very difficult; and the prevention of preterm labor remains the most important challenge in obstetrics in the 21st century. In this chapter the role of prostaglandins (PG) and oxytocin (OT) in human labor, and the rationale behind the use of PG and OT antagonists in an attempt to stop preterm labor, are reviewed.

EICOSANOID HORMONES

von Euler[3] discovered in 1935 bioactive lipid compounds in extracts of prostate gland and seminal vesicles which he called 'prostaglandins'. However, interest in the possible role of these lipid mediators in parturition started with the observations of Karim and Devlin,[4] and others,[5,6] that the primary prostaglandins PGE_2 and $PGF_{2\alpha}$ accumulated in the amniotic fluid of women in labor. PG are products of arachidonic acid, a polyunsaturated fatty acid derived from linoleate; the availability of linoleate/arachidonate is dependent on the diet because linoleate cannot be synthesized by mammals (i.e. it is an essential fatty acid). Arachidonate is stored in phospholipids and diacylglycerols, and it is liberated by phospholipase A_2 from the former and by diacylglycerol lipase from the latter. These enzymes provide important points of regulatory control. The systematic name of arachidonate is all-cis-$\Delta^5,\Delta^8,\Delta^{11},\Delta^{14}$-eicosatetraenoate (a 20 carbon chain with four double bonds; 20:4). Hence the term 'eicosanoid hormones', which is used to describe several classes of signaling molecules derived from arachidonate. Eicosanoids include the leukotrienes, prostacyclin, thromboxanes and PG (Figure 15.1).[7] The formation of leukotrienes is catalysed by lipoxygenases. The rest of eicosanoid hormones are formed via an intermediary compound called PGH_2, which is formed from arachidonic acid in two steps: a cyclooxygenase (COX) reaction yielding PGG_2, followed by a peroxidase exchange that converts PGG_2 to PGH_2. These steps are catalysed by a membrane-associated protein called prostaglandin H_2 synthase (PGHS), also referred to simply as COX. The attachment of COX to the cell membrane is essential for its action, because arachidonic acid is lypophilic and once liberated from membrane phospholipids it enters the active site of the enzyme through a hydrophobic channel without contact with the aqueous cytosolic environment.[7]

The synthesis of PG from PGH_2 is catalysed by terminal PG synthases; in many cells PGH_2 is also a substrate for prostacyclin synthase or thromboxane synthases. The major classes of PG are designated with a letter (A–I, depending on the chemical structure of the

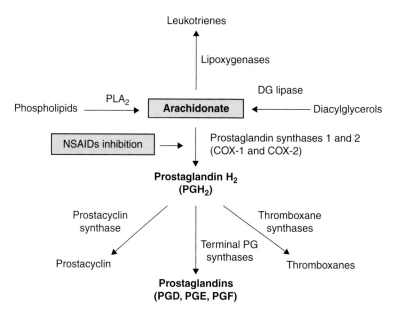

Figure 15.1 Synthesis of eicosanoid hormones from arachidonic acid. Nonsteroidal anti-inflammatory drugs (NSAID) block prostaglandin (PG) synthesis by interfering with the cyclooxygenase (COX) reaction. (Modified from Berg et al, Biochemistry, New York: WH Freeman & Co, 2002.)

cyclopentane ring in the eicosanoid molecule), and a subscript denoting the number of carbon–carbon double bonds. PGD_2, PGE_2, and $PGF_{2\alpha}$ are all readily produced by intrauterine tissues such as the placenta, fetal membranes and decidua. Each tissue or cell type has different PG production profile depending on the relative activities of PGD, PGE or PGF synthases.

PROSTAGLANDINS (PG) AND PARTURITION

The role of PG in human parturition is still a subject of considerable investigation. Factors in favor of an involvement of PG in labor include: (i) PG release increases in association with labor;[5,6,8] (ii) PG analogs have useful pharmacological effects on uterine contractility and cervical ripening;[9] (iii) COX inhibitors delay labor and delivery by inhibiting uterine activity.[10] However, little is known about the factors that promote PG release at the onset of labor. Surfactant in amniotic fluid, derived from the maturing fetal lung, is an important intrauterine source of arachidonic acid, and increases the rate of PG synthesis in the fetal membranes.[11] This effect is due to the release of fatty acids, including arachidonate, from the lipids of fetal surfactant by the sequential action of phospholipase C and diglyceride lipase activities in amniotic fluid,[12] and by the transfer of arachidonate from surfactant phosphatidylcholine to phosphatidylethanolamine and phosphatidylinositol in amnion cells.[13] There is also evidence that platelet-activating factor, a phosphoacylglycerol component of fetal lung surfactant, may activate myometrial contractility at term through interaction with Toll-like receptor (TLR) 4.[14] It is likely that these pathways are involved in the mechanism of parturition, for they provide a link between the process of maturation of the fetus in preparation for birth and the potentially labor-initiating activation of PG release.

USE OF PROSTAGLANDIN (PG) SYNTHESIS INHIBITORS

The COX activity of PGHS has been the target of drug design for decades and continues to be so.[15] Felix Hoffman made the acetylated form of salicylic acid (aspirin) in 1897, creating the most widely used medical drug of all time. Unknowingly he designed the first COX inhibitor.[16] Aspirin works by transferring an acetyl group to a serine residue in PGHS, thus blocking the path of arachidonate through the hydrophobic channel to the active COX site. The synthesis of ibuprofen in 1961 started a new generation of 'nonsteroidal anti-inflammatory drugs' (NSAID). Ibuprofen also inhibits PG release[17] by blocking the hydrophobic channels of PGHS. The anti-PG effect of NSAID, and their ease of administration, made them attractive as a way of inhibiting contractions in preterm labor. Indometacin – 1-(4-chlorobenzoyl)-5-methoxy-2-methyl-1-H-indole-3-acetic acid – was discovered in 1963, and shown to be an anti-inflammatory drug by inhibiting PG release.[18] Indometacin became one of the most popular NSAID drugs in obstetrics and has been utilized to inhibit uterine contractions for over 30 years.[19,20] Indometacin is an effective tocolytic agent and delays delivery for at least 48 h. However, its use has been associated with risks to the fetus and neonate, including pulmonary hypertension, necrotizing enterocolitis, intraventricular hemorrhage, toxicity on fetal kidney, persistent patent ductus arteriosus, and bronchopulmonary dysplasia. Unfortunately, the effects of indometacin on neonatal mortality and morbidity are difficult to assess, due to the limited power of published randomized trials.[21]

Indometacin and other NSAID inhibit PGHS at pharmacological concentrations, but they have COX-independent effects as well, leading to various functional alterations. For instance, indometacin inhibits members of the aldo-keto reductase family, including the human enzyme AKR1C3, also known as 3α-hydroxysteroid dehydrogenase type 2; 17β-hydroxysteroid dehydrogenase type 5; and PGD_2 11-ketoreductase. Thus, administration of NSAID may disrupt local steroid and PG interconversion in many tissues.[22] Indometacin and ibuprofen also disrupt the transport of PG, cyclic nucleotides and other molecules across the plasma membrane.[23] A common side effect of indometacin is the reduction in fetal urinary output, and recent research has demonstrated direct effects of the drug on aquaporin water channels in the kidney.[24]

COX-2 inhibitors

In 1990 a report appeared of a COX activity that was modulated by steroids,[25] and the gene responsible, which is homologous to PGHS, was quickly identified.[26,27] The known enzyme was renamed PGHS-1 (COX-1), and the newly discovered isozyme was named PGHS-2 (COX-2). In most tissues COX-1 is constitutively expressed, whereas COX-2 can be induced or repressed by a variety of hormones and inflammatory mediators. Aspirin and indometacin inhibit both the constitutively expressed COX-1 and the inducible COX-2, and therefore have effects on many organs, notably the gastrointestinal tract. This opened the race to design new drugs selective against COX-2 but sparing COX-1, thus offering better protection against the undesired effects of NSAID. Celocoxib and rofecoxib were introduced in the mid-90s as specific COX-2 inhibitors, primarily to reduce pain and inflammation with no gastric side effects.

In pregnant women, the expression of COX-2 in the fetal membranes is relatively high at term,[28,29] and this isozyme is thought to be the one responsible for the increased intrauterine PG release associated with labor. The possibility to use COX-2 inhibitors for the management of preterm labor, reducing potential fetal side effects, soon caught the attention of obstetricians. COX-1 expression remains relatively stable in many tissues during pregnancy, however, COX-2 increases towards term not only in the fetal membranes but also in the fetal lung and kidneys where it has important physiological roles,[30] so the risk of fetal side effects by using COX-2-selective drugs is not completely eliminated. In fact, use of the selective COX-2 inhibitors rofecoxib and nimesulide has been associated with impaired fetal renal function.[31] Moreover, at pharmacological doses, COX-2 inhibitors may have residual COX-1 effects in many organs. Considerable anxiety was generated when rofecoxib was withdrawn in September 2004 for increased risk of myocardial infarction.

The amino acid arrangement and crystal structure of the COX-2 active site is known in detail, which has allowed the design of a new class of potent drugs with extremely high COX-2 selectivity.[32] It may be possible to use these novel drugs at low doses to inhibit uterine and decidual PG production in the mother, minimizing the risk of fetal side effects. At present it is not possible to recommend the use of COX-2 inhibitors over the more traditional drugs such as indometacin. More evidence, both from randomized controlled trials and from laboratory studies on the role of PG in parturition, is needed.

Is the inhibition of PG synthesis the best strategy to stop labor?

This question is difficult to answer in women because the mechanism of parturition is not known, and the role of eicosanoid hormones is not completely elucidated. However, we can make some extrapolations from experiments in mice, a species in which the role of PG has been clearly established. The timely onset of labor in mice involves a decrease in progesterone production from the corpus luteum. Luteolysis is caused by the release of PG from the uterus before the onset of labor. Mice lacking cytosolic phospholipase A_2 produce only small litters and the pups do not survive.[33] This suggests that blocking the release of arachidonic acid from phospholipids disrupts fertility and birth. Mice lacking the PGHS-1 gene have delayed onset of parturition and high neonatal mortality, indicating that arachidonate metabolism via PGHS-1 is important for normal labor.[34]

Decidual expression of PGHS-1 is essential for the onset of labor.[35] On the other hand, mice lacking the $PGF_{2\alpha}$ receptor (FP receptor) maintain elevated serum progesterone levels in late gestation, and have severe disruption of labor with high neonatal loss.[36] These combined observations demonstrate that decidual $PGF_{2\alpha}$ production, and activation of the luteal FP receptor, are necessary and sufficient for the spontaneous onset of labor. Thus, mice provide an excellent model to test the hypothesis that blocking PG synthesis inhibits labor. Yet, it has been shown that inhibition of intrauterine PG release by as much as 90% (using low-dose aspirin or by controlled disruption of the PGHS-1 gene) has no effect on parturition or rate of survival of the pups.[37] Parturition is delayed only when uterine $PGF_{2\alpha}$ levels fall <1% of normal levels at term.[37] In the FP null mice, disruption of the OT gene can restore parturition,[35] demonstrating that alternative luteolytic mechanisms can step in when the $PGF_{2\alpha}$ pathway is absent. The murine model shows that only a profound blockade of PG production is effective to inhibit labor. If the same is true in women, we will have to use COX inhibitors at such high concentrations that maternal or fetal side effects will be difficult to eliminate. Moreover, PG synthesis blockade alone may not always be sufficient to stop preterm labor because alternative mechanisms may come into action.

Other approaches

The use of FP receptor antagonists to block parturition has been proposed following encouraging experiments in sheep.[38] The FP receptor is present in the human uterus and it stimulates calcium entry into myometrial cells through a G protein (Gq) coupled to a phospholipase C pathway.[39] Moreover, $PGF_{2\alpha}$ release is differentially increased in decidual cells obtained from women in labor compared to women not in labor,[40] suggesting that activation of the terminal PGF synthase may be a trigger for spontaneous labor. The idea of blocking one specific PG receptor without interfering with overall eicosanoid synthesis is attractive because this would minimize the risk of side effects. However, the FP receptor is present in many organs outside the pregnant uterus and further evaluation of candidate drugs is needed.

The effect of PGE_2 and $PGF_{2\alpha}$ on isolated myometrial strips from pregnant women is biphasic, with a rapid stimulatory component mediated by calcium entry, and a slow inhibitory component mediated by sodium/potassium adenosine triphosphate (ATP)ase pumps.[41] The precise signaling pathway responsible for each component is not known, but further investigations in this area might lead to the possibility of designing compounds which will enhance the inhibitory effect of PG receptors while blocking the stimulatory component. Myometrial cells contain both stimulatory (FP, EP1) and inhibitory (EP2) prostanoid receptors,[42–44] and the development of drugs selective for each receptor subtype would be a sensible approach. Such compounds might be useful in the management of preterm labor.

In the myometrium of pregnant women there is very good correlation between the increase in intracellular calcium and the development of force. Calcium is bound to calmodulin and this complex activates myosin light-chain kinase (MLCK). Phosphorylated myosin interacts with actin and becomes an enzyme capable of turning the chemical energy of ATP into mechanical energy for contraction. Relaxation occurs when myosin is dephosphorylated by a specific myosin light-chain phosphatase (MLCP). Myometrial cells have calcium-independent pathways which enhance contractility by inhibiting MLCP, so that the cells achieve the same level of myosin phosphorylation at lower rates of MLCK activity. This phenomenon is called 'calcium sensitization' because the more inhibition of MLCP, the more effective MLCK becomes at a given level of intracellular calcium.[45] Activation of RhoA-dependent kinase (ROK) leads to MLCP inhibition by phosphorylation, and this pathway can be stimulated by OT, lysophosphatidic acid and other agonists in human myometrium.[46,47] Interestingly, ROK is induced by thromboxane analogs in human myometrial cells.[48] Thus, inhibition of thromboxane action may facilitate uterine relaxation in pregnancy, especially if inhibitors are designed against thromboxane receptors (TP), such as TP-β which are stimulatory in myometrium, while sparing TP-α receptors which are inhibitory.[49]

INFECTION, INFLAMMATION, AND PRETERM LABOR

There are situations when the production of PG and leukotrienes by decidua, fetal membranes and placenta are exacerbated are a consequence of severe inflammatory reactions, usually triggered by infection. We observed that women who delivered following spontaneous preterm labor could be divided into two subgroups depending on gestational age and rate of eicosanoid production (Figure 15.2): very early preterm births, <32 weeks of gestation, were associated with inflammatory changes in the placenta and other intrauterine tissues (chorioamnionitis, deciduitis, villitis, and/or funisitis), whereas late preterm births (33–37 weeks) usually had normal histology. The production of PGE_2, $PGF_{2\alpha}$ and leukotriene B_4 by the fetal membranes and placenta was orders of magnitude higher in

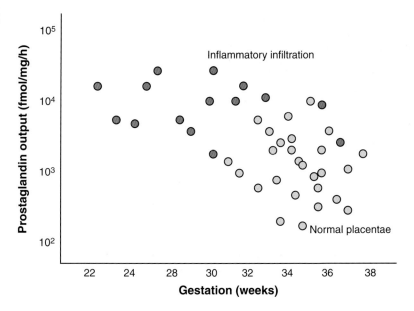

Figure 15.2 Prostaglandin (PG) production by the fetal membranes, following spontaneous preterm labor. Early preterm deliveries were associated with inflammatory infiltration (red) in the placental tissues had much higher PG production rates than preterm deliveries >32 weeks with normal histology (blue). Note the logarithmic scale. (Modified from López Bernal et al, Br J Obstet Gynecol 1989; 96: 113–9.)

the very early preterm group with inflammatory infiltration compared with the late preterm labor group with normal histology.[50,51] The fetal membranes and decidua in late pregnancy are rich in tissue macrophages, which have important immune defence roles,[52] and these cells have a high capacity for $PGF_{2\alpha}$ production in response to inflammatory mediators.[53] A murine model in which fetal surfactant proteins may trigger labor by activating tissue macrophages has been proposed.[54] In some instances, very early preterm labor may be caused by the premature release of PG and other inflammatory mediators by decidual macrophages, triggered by infection. In these situations attempts to block PG production would be contraindicated.

OXYTOCIN (OT) AND RELATED PEPTIDES

OT is a nonapeptide hormone that belongs to a very primitive hormone system, dating back 500 million years in evolution. Components of this system include annetocin (involved in egg-laying behavior in the earthworm), vasotocin (present in nonmammalian vertebrates and cyclostomes), mesotocin (found in marsupials, amphibians, reptiles, and birds) and vasopressin, a hormone typical of mammals. OT has been found in placental mammals, some marsupials and even sharks. The physiological roles of OT include the stimulation of uterine contractility and of lactation, but it is also involved in penile erection and ejaculation, prostate growth, luteal function and cardiovascular function. The uterotonic effect of posterior pituitary extracts was noted more than 100 years ago,[55,56] and they were

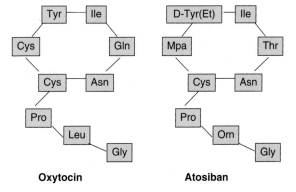

Figure 15.3 Structures of oxytocin[58] and atosiban[69], the first oxytocin antagonist approved for use in preterm labor.

used by Sir William Blair Bell for the treatment of postpartum hemorrhage.[57] However, it took several decades for the active uterotonic principle in the posterior pituitary to be characterized. In 1953, the year that the Society for Gynecologic Investigation was founded, Du Vigneaud et al[58] published the structure of OT: a cyclic hexapeptide ring with a three-residue tail (Figure 15.3). The chemical synthesis of OT made the peptide available in a relatively cheap and pure form. OT was soon incorporated in obstetric practice for the induction and augmentation of labor.[59] The bovine OT-neurophysin gene was cloned in 1983 by Land et al,[60] and in 1992 Tadashi Kimura, a Japanese obstetrician, cloned the human oxytocin receptor (OTR), beating several other investigators to the pole. Kimura attributed his success to the fact that he chose human pregnant myometrium

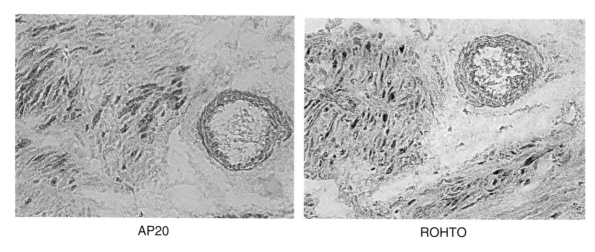

AP20   ROHTO

Figure 15.4 Immunochemical localization of oxytocin receptors in human term myometrial sections using two different antibodies: one raised in-house against the third intracellular loop of the receptor (AP20), and another against the N-terminal end (ROHTO Pharmaceutical Co Ltd., Osaka, Japan). Horse-radish peroxidase/diaminobenzidine/hematoxylin staining at 400× magnification. Note the staining for receptors in the bundles of myometrial smooth muscle cells, and also in the round arteriolar wall.

as a starting material, a tissue with very high level of expression.[61] OTR is present in term uterine tissue, especially in myometrial cells, but also in arteriolar smooth muscle (Figure 15.4).

Is OT involved in human parturition?

The main evidence for a role of OT in parturition in women arises from the fact that OT is a potent uterotonic agent both in vivo and in vitro, and is widely used for the induction and augmentation of labor. The pulsatile release of OT by the maternal pituitary,[62] and baseline maternal plasma OT concentrations, increase in the later stages of labor.[63] There is also local production of OT in uterine tissues.[64,65] Uterine OTR (but not the closely related vasopressin receptors) increase in late pregnancy, making the uterus very sensitive to OT.[66–68] OT antagonists may delay preterm labor[69] but their effect on neonatal outcome is not proven. However, there is also evidence against a role for OT in the onset of spontaneous labor. For instance, women with diabetes insipidus who may produce little pituitary OT have normal labors and deliveries,[70] but this condition is rare and more data on OT pulses and concentrations in these patients are needed. OT-gene-depleted mice have normal deliveries, although the pups tend to die because lactation is defective;[71] moreover, OTR-deficient mice exhibit normal parturition but have defects in lactation and maternal nurturing.[72] Although there is general agreement that spontaneous

uterine contractility and uterine sensitivity to OT increase towards term, there is no clear evidence of a significant increase in OT sensitivity prior to labor.[73–75] Thus, it is difficult to ascribe to OT an essential role in the initiation of labor in women; most likely this ancient peptide has been preserved as a protective hormone against uterine postpartum hemorrhage and to facilitate lactation.

OTR signaling

The OTR belongs to the G-protein coupled receptor (GPCR) family and is a member of the vasopressin receptor group. Activation of myometrial OTR results in phospholipase C (PLC)-mediated hydrolysis of phosphatidylinositol 4,5-bisphosphate and the production of 1,2-diacylglycerol, which activates protein kinase C (PKC), and inositol 1,4,5-trisphosphate, which mobilizes calcium from intracellular stores. These effects of OT are well established, and are mediated by heterotrimeric G proteins of the G_q and G_i families. OTR mediates not only a transient increase in Ca^{2+} in myometrial cells, but it has more sustained effects on other signaling pathways such as the mitogen-activated protein kinase (MAPK) pathway, which is part of a complex mitogenic signaling cascade. OT upregulates the expression of COX-2 and promotes the activation of cytosolic PLA_2, leading to increased PG production in human myometrial and amnion cells. These effects are mediated by a G_i protein and involve the activation of the MAPK ERK2.[76,77] It could be argued that some effects of OT on uterine activation are actually mediated by stimulation of MAPK and consequent release of prostanoids.[78] The concentration of OTR in human myometrial tissue increases during gestation,[79,80] and in some cases spontaneous preterm labor may be due to increased sensitivity to OT.[75] OT induces stress fiber formation in human myometrial cells by a pathway involving ROK.[46] It is likely that activation of ROK-mediated pathways enhances the efficiency of uterine contractions at the time of labor. The possibility that ROK contributes to increased sensitivity of the uterus to OT deserves to be investigated.[47] However, the contribution of the ROK pathway to uterine sensitivity to OT may be relatively minor compared to the PLC/Ca^{2+} pathway.[81] These findings illustrate the complexity of OTR signaling in myometrium, and the need to carry out further research into the regulation of PLC, MAPK and ROK pathways in order to improve the effectiveness and selectivity of potential OT antagonists.

OTR desensitization, internalization and downregulation

Sustained stimulation of GPCR typically causes desensitization (a reduction in receptor response in the face of a constant stimulus), which protects cells from overstimulation and involves numerous adaptive mechanisms in characteristic time frames. Within seconds to minutes of stimulation, most GPCR desensitize as a consequence of receptor phosphorylation by G protein receptor kinases (GRKs) or second-messenger regulated protein kinases (PKA, PKC). We have found that GRK2 and GRK6 are upregulated in pregnant compared to nonpregnant myometrial tissue.[82] Phosphorylation inhibits G-protein activation (i.e. it causes receptor desensitization), but the most important effect of the GRK-mediated phosphorylation is to facilitate the binding of specialized proteins called β-arrestins. This not only prevents G-protein activation but also targets the desensitized receptor for internalization. Internalization and association of the OTR with β-arrestins may actually mediate MAPK activation, as shown for the related vasopressin receptor and other GPCR.[83] The consequent reduction in cell surface receptor number can also underlie desensitization in the intermediate time frame of minutes to hours. Over longer periods (hours to days) numerous adaptive processes serve to either reinforce or reverse the earlier desensitization by changing rates of synthesis and degradation of receptors and downstream effectors. These processes may explain the apparent decrease in OTR binding with advancing labor in women.[66,79,80] The density of OTR increases from 85 fmol/mg in nonpregnant myometrium to 480 fmol/mg in late pregnancy

(>37 weeks), and this is associated with increased responsiveness to OT. It then reduces to 220 fmol/mg during spontaneous labor, probably as a consequence of OTR downregulation.[80] The apparent loss of myometrial OTR binding sites also occurs in vivo in women after OT-induced labor.[80] In vitro, the number of OTR in myometrial cells is reduced by exposure to OT, and this effect is associated with a pronounced reduction in OTR mRNA and a corresponding reduction in OTR-mediated PLC activation and Ca^{2+} mobilization.[84]

Clathrin-mediated pathway

Agonist occupancy of GPCR promotes the association of GRK2 with tubulin and tubulin phosphorylation, which suggests a role for GRK2 in the internalization of receptors by the cytoskeleton. OTR is rich in putative phosphorylation sites for PKA and PKC, casein kinase and calmodulin II kinase, making it a target for regulatory influences through activation of heterologous receptors which operate through these pathways.[84] Moreover, after phosphorylation by GRK receptors may be internalized by several pathways, involving either specialized proteins such as caveolins, or through the classical dynamin- and clathrin-coated pit pathway.[85] We have recently demonstrated the involvement of the clathrin pathway in OTR desensitization and internalization.[86] The functional significance of these associations is under investigation.

DEVELOPMENT OF OXYTOCIN RECEPTOR (OTR) ANTAGONISTS

GPCR are the largest family of signaling proteins and are targets for the majority of current therapeutics. Despite the uncertainty about its physiological role in the onset of labor, OTR are clearly stimulatory and are present in high density in the pregnant uterus in relation to other tissues, so they are an attractive pharmacological target. The discovery of the cyclical structure of OT[58] led to renewed interest in neurohypophyseal hormones, and for several decades extensive laboratory work was carried out on a number of OT and arginine vasopressin (AVP) analogs. None of these compounds was developed into therapeutically useful drugs until the late 1980s. OT and AVP antagonists were of interest in obstetrics and gynecology because of the possible involvement of these hormones in preterm labor[66] and dysmenorrhea.[87] The task of developing OT antagonists was made much easier by the cloning of the OTR,[61] allowing structural modeling of the OT–OTR complex.

Early attempts to develop OT analogs with decreased uterotonic activity were based on structure-activity studies, and it was noted that modifications of the amino acids at positions 1, 2, 4 and 8 led to excellent uterotonic antagonism.[69] One of these compounds – 1-(3mercaptopropanoic acid)-2-(O-ethyl-D-tyrosine)-4-L-threonine-8-L-ornithine-oxytocin – was chosen for its tocolytic effect,[88] and investigated in clinical trials under the approved name atosiban (Figure 15.3).[89] In 2000, atosiban became the first OT antagonists specifically approved for the management of preterm labor. Atosiban is a competitive inhibitor of the OTR and it blocks OT binding: OT-induced PLC activation and Ca^{2+} increase in a dose-dependent manner.[90,91] The relative binding affinity of atosiban for the OTR in pregnant human myometrium is 3.5%, and for the AVP (V_{1a}) receptor 24%; atosiban is actually a better inhibitor of the vasopressin V_{1a} receptor than of the OTR.[91] High doses of atosiban can block OT binding and OTR signaling completely, with no evidence of residual agonist effect. This makes atosiban a useful drug to block OT action in reproductive tissues; however, the fact that it also blocks V_{1a} receptors may result in unwanted effects.

Several approaches have been taken to improve the specificity and potency of OTR antagonists.[69] These include: shortening the carboxy-terminal tail, the synthesis of linear, rather than cyclic, structures,[92] the bicyclization of OT-like structures, and even the use of nonanimal peptides as templates, e.g. cyclic hexapeptides from *Streptomyces*.[93] The use of napthylalanine isomers to replace residues in OT analogs has led to the development of antagonists with very high affinity for both OTR and V_{1a} receptors.[94] Barusiban is a new generation OTR antagonist with increased potency and specificity in the human pregnant uterus compared to atosiban.[95]

A significant drawback of atosiban and other peptide OTR antagonists is their low bioavailability, requiring parenteral administration to achieve therapeutic doses. This problem was addressed in the early 1990s with the development of nonpeptide OTR antagonists of high bioavailability.[96] There are several orally active compounds available[97,98] with very potent and OTR selective effects. Medicinal chemistry has delivered the goods and we now have an excellent range of selective OTR antagonists, with a choice of short- or long-lasting effects. The use of these drugs in obstetrics, in the context of well-designed and well-conducted clinical trials, will decide whether OTR antagonists have a future in the management of preterm labor.

SEARCH FOR THE IDEAL TOCOLYTIC AGENT

PG synthesis inhibitors and OT antagonists may well become established as safe and effective drugs to inhibit uterine contractility in women in preterm labor, but at the present time their efficacy and benefit in terms of infant outcomes remains to be demonstrated. From a conceptual point of view, an ideal tocolytic agent would have to meet a number of criteria:

- Effective at 23–29 weeks of gestation: This is the time in gestation when maximum benefit would be obtained in terms of neonatal survival and rates of disability. It must be emphasized that our knowledge of myometrial physiology and receptor function at this stage of gestation is limited; conclusions derived from studies on myometrial samples taken at term may not be directly applicable to the uterus at <30 weeks of gestation.
- High potency: Requiring small doses to achieve the desired effect.
- Pure antagonist: This is important when targeting a stimulatory receptor (e.g. OTR or FP receptors). The best drugs would be those without any intrinsic stimulatory effect on the myometrium. (The opposite would be true when targeting an inhibitory receptor, e.g. the PG EP2 receptor; in this case a perfect agonist would be desirable).
- Minimal side effects: This is achieved with drugs that are both organ and receptor selective.
- High bioavailability: Allowing oral or other nonparenteral administration.
- Long versus short half-life: Resistance to catabolism may be an advantage because stability to degradation would maintain effective doses for a long time (long-term tocolysis). However, in some instances, it may be better to use drugs with a short half-life for acute obstetric emergencies which might benefit from a brief period of tocolysis.
- Is it indicated? Even the perfect drug can be harmful if the indication for its administration is wrong. For instance, using a tocolytic agent in infection-associated preterm labor or in antepartum hemorrhage may do more harm than good to the fetus and mother.

CONCLUSIONS

- Preterm labor remains a major cause of perinatal mortality and morbidity, and efforts to prevent this problem are hampered by our poor understanding of the mechanism of labor in women. We don't know whether preterm labor is caused by an acceleration of the physiological mechanism that triggers labor at term, or whether it is due to a different physiopathological mechanism. More research is needed into the factors involved in uterine activation and cervical ripening. We also need better biomarkers to predict the onset of labor.

- There is insufficient information on how to base decisions about the role of PG synthesis inhibitors for women in preterm labor. However, our understanding of the mechanism of action of eicosanoid hormones is increasing rapidly. It is worth exploring new myometrial-specific mechanisms to inhibit/modulate PG and thromboxane action.

- Oxytocin remains closely associated with parturition in animals and humans because of its ability to stimulate uterine contractility. OT is released in pulses by the neurohypophysis, and it is thought to be important for the normal progress of labor, although its involvement in the initiation of labor is controversial. The concentration of myometrial OTR increases in pregnancy, making the uterus very responsive to exogenous OT, which is widely used for the induction and augmentation of labor.

- From a clinical point of view, efforts should concentrate on the prevention and management of early preterm births which are associated with the highest rates of mortality and disability; babies born >32 weeks of gestation tend to do very well, although they still require specialized neonatal care. It is likely that only a subset of spontaneous preterm labors not associated with infection, hemorrhage, uterine abnormalities or other maternal or fetal complications will benefit from tocolytic treatment.

- The clinical safety and efficacy of any tocolytics need to be proven by appropriate randomized controlled trials. Many studies have reported a strong placebo effect in delaying delivery, which probably reflects our inability to diagnose preterm labor accurately. More than 50% of women admitted with 'threatened preterm labor' may not be in labor at all.

- It is said that the most beneficial use of tocolytic agents is to delay labor to allow the administration of glucocorticoids to accelerate fetal maturation.[99] However, there is no evidence that the use of tocolytics increases the percentage of women who are able to complete a single course of glucocorticoids therapy when compared with placebo-treated controls.[100] There is also controversy as to whether the use of tocolytic agents to allow the transport of a patient to a medical center with good neonatal facilities does more harm than good.

- Future research in preterm labor should combine efforts to increase the understanding of the mechanism of parturition with the discovery of better biomarkers and tests for the prediction of preterm labor.

ACKNOWLEDGMENTS

I am grateful to Dr Mike Smith for the staining in Figure 15.4; to Dr Tadashi Kimura for making the ROHTO OTR antibody available; and to Dr John Lartey for reading the manuscript.

REFERENCES

1. Morrison JJ, Rennie JM. Clinical, scientific and ethical aspects of fetal and neonatal care at extremely preterm periods of gestation. Br J Obstet Gynaecol 1997; 104: 1341–50.
2. Marlow N, Wolke D, Bracewell MA, Samara M. Neurologic and developmental disability at six years of age after extremely preterm birth. N Engl J Med 2005; 352: 9–19.
3. von Euler US. History and development of prostaglandins. Gen Pharmacol 1983; 14: 3–6.
4. Karim SM, Devlin J. Prostaglandin content of amniotic fluid during pregnancy and labor. J Obstet Gynaecol Br Commonw 1967; 74: 230–4.
5. Keirse MJ, Flint AP, Turnbull AC. F prostaglandins in amniotic fluid during pregnancy and labor. J Obstet Gynaecol Br Commonw 1974; 81: 131–5.
6. Dray F, Frydman R. Primary prostaglandins in amniotic fluid in pregnancy and spontaneous labor. Am J Obstet Gynecol 1976; 126: 13–19.
7. Berg J, Tymoczko J, Stryer L. Fatty acid metabolism. In Berg J, Tymoczko J, Stryer L eds. Biochemistry. New York: WH Freeman & Co, 2002; pp. 601–632.
8. Granstrom E, Kindahl H. Radioimmunoassay for urinary metabolites of prostaglandin F2alpha. Prostaglandins 1976; 12: 759–83.
9. Karim SM, Hillier K. Prostaglandins in the control of animal and human reproduction. Br Med Bull 1979; 35: 173–80.
10. Wiqvist N, Lindblom B, Wikland M, Wilhelmsson L. Prostaglandins and uterine contractility. Acta Obstet Gynecol Scand Suppl 1983; 113: 23–9.
11. López Bernal A, Newman GE, Phizackerley PJ, Turnbull AC. Effect of lipid and protein fractions from fetal pulmonary surfactant on prostaglandin E production by a human amnion cell line. Eicosanoids 1989; 2: 29–32.
12. López Bernal A, Phizackerley PJ. Fetal surfactant as a source of arachidonate in human amniotic fluid. Prostaglandins Other Lipid Mediat 2000; 60: 59–70.
13. Newman GE, Phizackerley PJ, López Bernal A. Utilization by human amniocytes for prostaglandin synthesis of [1-14C]arachidonate derived from 2-[1-14C]arachidonylphosphatidylcholine associated with human fetal pulmonary surfactant. Biochim Biophys Acta 1993; 1176: 106–12.
14. Elovitz MA, Wang Z, Chien EK, Rychlik DF, Phillippe M. A new model for inflammation-induced preterm birth: the role of platelet-activating factor and Toll-like receptor-4. Am J Pathol 2003; 163: 2103–11.
15. Fitzpatrick FA. Cyclooxygenase enzymes: regulation and function. Curr Pharm Des 2004; 10: 577–88.
16. Vane JR, Botting RM. The mechanism of action of aspirin. Thromb Res 2003; 110: 255–8.
17. Vane JR. Inhibition of prostaglandin synthesis as a mechanism of action for aspirin-like drugs. Nat New Biol 1971; 231: 232–5.
18. Ferreira SH, Moncada S, Vane JR. Indomethacin and aspirin abolish prostaglandin release from the spleen. Nat New Biol 1971; 231: 237–9.

19. Wiqvist N, Lundstrom V, Green K. Premature labor and indomethacin. Prostaglandins 1975; 10: 515–26.

20. Niebyl JR, Blake DA, White RD et al. The inhibition of premature labor with indomethacin. Am J Obstet Gynecol 1980; 136, 1014–19.

21. Loe SM, Sanchez-Ramos L, Kaunitz AM. Assessing the neonatal safety of indomethacin tocolysis: a systematic review with meta-analysis. Obstet Gynecol 2005; 106: 173–9.

22. Lovering AL, Ride JP, Bunce CM et al. Crystal structures of prostaglandin D(2) 11-ketoreductase (AKR1C3) in complex with the nonsteroidal anti-inflammatory drugs flufenamic acid and indomethacin. Cancer Res 2004; 64: 1802–10.

23. Reid G, Wielinga P, Zelcer N et al. The human multidrug resistance protein MRP4 functions as a prostaglandin efflux transporter and is inhibited by nonsteroidal antiinflammatory drugs. Proc Natl Acad Sci USA 2003; 100: 9244–9.

24. Kim SW, Kim JW, Choi KC et al. Indomethacin enhances shuttling of aquaporin-2 despite decreased abundance in rat kidney. J Am Soc Nephrol 2004; 15: 2998–3005.

25. Fu JY, Masferrer JL, Seibert K, Raz A, Needleman P. The induction and suppression of prostaglandin H2 synthase (cyclooxygenase) in human monocytes. J Biol Chem 1990; 265: 16 737–40.

26. Xie WL, Chipman JG, Robertson DL, Erikson RL, Simmons DL. Expression of a mitogen-responsive gene encoding prostaglandin synthase is regulated by mRNA splicing. Proc Natl Acad Sci USA 1991; 88: 2692–6.

27. Kujubu DA, Fletcher BS, Varnum BC, Lim RW, Herschman HR. TIS10, a phorbol ester tumor promoter-inducible mRNA from Swiss 3T3 cells, encodes a novel prostaglandin synthase/ cyclooxygenase homologue. J Biol Chem 1991; 266: 12 866–72.

28. Hirst JJ, Teixeira FJ, Zakar T, Olson DM. Prostaglandin endoperoxide-H synthase-1 and -2 messenger ribonucleic acid levels in human amnion with spontaneous labor onset. J Clin Endocrinol Metab 1995; 80: 517–23.

29. Slater D, Dennes W, Sawdy R, Allport V, Bennett P. Expression of cyclo-oxygenase types-1 and -2 in human fetal membranes throughout pregnancy. J Mol Endocrinol 1999; 22: 125–30.

30. Olson DM, Mijovic JE, Zaragoza DB, Cook JL. Prostaglandin endoperoxide H synthase type 1 and type 2 messenger ribonucleic acid in human fetal tissues throughout gestation and in the newborn infant. Am J Obstet Gynecol 2001; 184: 169–74.

31. Loudon JA, Groom KM, Bennett PR. Prostaglandin inhibitors in preterm labour. Best Pract Res Clin Obstet Gynaecol 2003; 17: 731–44.

32. Chen QH, Rao PN, Knaus EE. Design, synthesis, and biological evaluation of linear 1-(4-, 3- or 2-methylsulfonylphenyl)-2-phenylacetylenes: a novel class of cyclooxygenase-2 inhibitors. Bioorg Med Chem 2005; 13: 6425–34.

33. Bonventre JV, Huang Z, Taheri MR et al. Reduced fertility and postischaemic brain injury in mice deficient in cytosolic phospholipase A2. Nature 1997; 390: 622–5.

34. Langenbach R, Morham SG, Tiano HF et al. Prostaglandin synthase 1 gene disruption in mice reduces arachidonic acid-induced inflammation and indomethacin-induced gastric ulceration. Cell 1995; 83: 483–92.

35. Gross GA, Imamura T, Luedke C et al. Opposing actions of prostaglandins and oxytocin determine the onset of murine labor. Proc Natl Acad Sci USA 1998; 95: 11 875–9.

36. Sugimoto Y, Yamasaki A, Segi E et al. Failure of parturition in mice lacking the prostaglandin F receptor. Science 1997; 277. 681–3.

37. Yu Y, Cheng Y, Fan J et al. Differential impact of prostaglandin H synthase 1 knockdown on platelets and parturition. J Clin Invest 2005; 115: 986–95.

38. Hirst JJ, Parkington HC, Young IR et al. Delay of preterm birth in sheep by THG113.31, a prostaglandin F2alpha receptor antagonist. Am J Obstet Gynecol 2005; 193: 256–66.

39. Carrasco MP, Phaneuf S, Asboth G, Lopez Bernal A. Fluprostenol activates phospholipase C and Ca2+ mobilization in human myometrial cells. J Clin Endocrinol Metab 1996; 81: 2104–10.

40. Norwitz ER, Starkey PM, Lopez Bernal A. Prostaglandin D2 production by term human decidua: cellular origins defined using flow cytometry. Obstet Gynecol 1992; 80: 440–5.

41. Parkington HC, Tonta MA, Davies NK, Brennecke SP, Coleman HA. Hyperpolarization and slowing of the rate of contraction in human uterus in pregnancy by prostaglandins E2 and f2alpha: involvement of the Na1 pump. J Physiol 1999; 514(Pt 1), 229–43.

42. Asboth G, Phaneuf S, Lopez Bernal AL. Prostaglandin E receptors in myometrial cells. Acta Physiol Hung 1997; 85: 39–50.

43. Asboth G, Phaneuf S, Europe-Finner GN, Toth M, Bernal AL. Prostaglandin E2 activates phospholipase C and elevates intracellular calcium in cultured myometrial cells: involvement of EP1 and EP3 receptor subtypes. Endocrinology 1996; 137: 2572–9.

44. Myatt L, Lye SJ. Expression, localization and function of prostaglandin receptors in myometrium. Prostaglandins Leukot Essent Fatty Acids 2004; 70: 137–48.

45. Somlyo AP, Somlyo AV. Ca2+ sensitivity of smooth muscle and nonmuscle myosin II: modulated by G proteins, kinases, and myosin phosphatase. Physiol Rev 2003; 83: 1325–58.

46. Gogarten W, Emala CW, Lindeman KS, Hirshman CA. Oxytocin and lysophosphatidic acid induce stress fiber formation in human myometrial cells via a pathway involving Rho-kinase. Biol Reprod 2001; 65: 401–6.

47. Woodcock NA, Taylor CW, Thornton S. Effect of an oxytocin receptor antagonist and rho kinase inhibitor on the [Ca++]i sensitivity of human myometrium. Am J Obstet Gynecol 2004; 190: 222–8.

48. Moore F, Lopez Bernal A. Chronic exposure to TXA2 increases expression of ROCKI in human myometrial cells. Prostaglandins Other Lipid Mediat 2003; 71: 23–32.

49. Moore F, Asboth G, Lopez BA. Thromboxane receptor signaling in human myometrial cells. Prostaglandins Other Lipid Mediat 2002; 67: 31–47.

50. López Bernal A, Hansell DJ, Khong TY, Keeling JW, Turnbull AC. Prostaglandin E production by the fetal membranes in unexplained preterm labor and preterm labor associated with chorioamnionitis. Br J Obstet Gynaecol 1989; 96: 1133–9.

51. López Bernal A, Hansell DJ, Khong TY, Keeling JW, Turnbull AC. Placental leukotriene B4 release in early pregnancy and in term and preterm labor. Early Hum Dev 1990; 23: 93–9.

52. Singh U, Nicholson G, Urban BC et al. Immunological properties of human decidual macrophages – a possible role in intrauterine immunity. Reproduction 2005; 129: 631–7.

53. Norwitz ER, Lopez Bernal A, Starkey PM. Tumor necrosis factor-alpha selectively stimulates prostaglandin F2 alpha production by macrophages in human term decidua. Am J Obstet Gynecol 1992; 167: 815–20.

54. Condon JC, Jeyasuria P, Faust JM, Mendelson CR. Surfactant protein secreted by the maturing mouse fetal lung acts as a hormone that signals the initiation of parturition. Proc Natl Acad Sci USA 2004; 101: 4978–83.

55. Oliver G, Schaefer E. On the physiological action of extracts of pituitary body and and certain other glandular organs. J Physiol 1895; 18: 272–9.

56. Dale H. On some physiological actions of ergots. J Physiol 1906; 34: 163–206.

57. Blair Bell W. The pituitary body and the therapeutic value of the infundibular extract in shock, uterine atony and intestinal paresis. BMJ 1909; 2: 1609–13.

58. Du Vigneaud V, Ressler C, Trippett S. The sequence of amino acids in oxytocin, with a proposal for the structure of oxytocin. J Biol Chem 1953; 205: 949–57.

59. Theobald GW. Active labor. BMJ 1969; 3: 653–4.

60. Land H, Grez M, Ruppert S et al. Deduced amino acid sequence from the bovine oxytocin-neurophysin I precursor cDNA. Nature 1983; 302: 342–4.

61. Kimura T, Tanizawa O, Mori K, Brownstein MJ, Okayama H. Structure and expression of a human oxytocin receptor. Nature 1992; 356: 526–9.

62. Fuchs AR, Romero R, Keefe D, Parra M, Oyarzun E, Behnke E. Oxytocin secretion and human parturition: pulse frequency and duration increase during spontaneous labor in women. Am J Obstet Gynecol 1991; 165: 1515–23.

63. Leake RD, Weitzman RE, Glatz TH, Fisher DA, Plasma oxytocin concentrations in men, nonpregnant women, and pregnant women before and during spontaneous labor. J Clin Endocrinol Metab 1981; 53: 730–3.

64. Chibbar R, Miller FD, Mitchell BF. Synthesis of oxytocin in amnion, chorion, and decidua may influence the timing of human parturition. J Clin Invest 1993; 91: 185–92.

65. Blanks AM, Vatish M, Allen MJ et al. Paracrine oxytocin and estradiol demonstrate a spatial increase in human intrauterine tissues with labor. J Clin Endocrinol Metab 2003; 88: 3392–400.

66. Fuchs AR, Fuchs F, Husslein P, Soloff MS. Oxytocin receptors in the human uterus during pregnancy and parturition. Am J Obstet Gynecol 1984; 150: 734–41.

67. Rivera J, Lopez Bernal A, Varney M, Watson SP. Inositol 1,4,5-trisphosphate and oxytocin binding in human myometrium. Endocrinology 1990; 127: 155–62.

68. Maggi M, Del Carlo P, Fantoni G et al. Human myometrium during pregnancy contains and responds to V1 vasopressin receptors as well as oxytocin receptors. J Clin Endocrinol Metab 1990; 70: 1142–54.

69. Melin P. Oxytocin antagonists in preterm labor and delivery. Baillières Clin Obstet Gynaecol 1993; 7: 577–600.

70. Hime MC, Richardson JA. Diabetes insipidus and pregnancy. Case report, incidence and review of literature. Obstet Gynecol Surv 1978; 33: 375–9.

71. Nishimori K, Young LJ, Guo Q et al. Oxytocin is required for nursing but is not essential for parturition or reproductive behavior. Proc Natl Acad Sci USA 1996; 93: 11 699–704.

72. Takayanagi Y, Yoshida M, Bielsky IF et al. Pervasive social deficits, but normal parturition, in oxytocin receptor-deficient mice. Proc Natl Acad Sci USA 2005; 102: 16 096–101.

73. Caldeyro-Barcia R, Theobald GW. Sensitivity of the pregnant human myometrium to oxytocin. Am J Obstet Gynecol 1968; 102: 1181.

74. Turnbull AC, Anderson AB. Uterine contractility and oxytocin sensitivity during human pregnancy in relation to the onset of labor. J Obstet Gynaecol Br Commonw 1968; 75: 278–88.

75. Takahashi K, Diamond F, Bieniarz J, Yen H, Burd L. Uterine contractility and oxytocin sensitivity in preterm, term, and post-term pregnancy. Am J Obstet Gynecol 1980; 136: 774–9.

76. Molnar M, Rigo Jr J, Romero R, Hertelendy F. Oxytocin activates mitogen-activated protein kinase and up-regulates cyclooxygenase-2 and prostaglandin production in human myometrial cells. Am J Obstet Gynecol 1999; 181: 42–9.

77. Soloff MS, Jeng YJ, Copland JA, Strakova Z, Hoare S. Signal pathways mediating oxytocin stimulation of prostaglandin synthesis in select target cells. Exp Physiol 2000; 85 Spec No, 51S–58S.

78. Ohmichi M, Koike K, Nohara A et al. Oxytocin stimulates mitogen-activated protein kinase activity in cultured human puerperal uterine myometrial cells. Endocrinology 1995; 136: 2082–7.

79. Bossmar T, Akerlund M, Fantoni G et al. Receptors for and myometrial responses to oxytocin and vasopressin in preterm and term human pregnancy: effects of the oxytocin antagonist atosiban. Am J Obstet Gynecol 1994; 171: 1634–42.

80. Phaneuf S, Rodriguez Linares B, TambyRaja RL, MacKenzie IZ, López Bernal A. Loss of myometrial oxytocin receptors during oxytocin-induced and oxytocin-augmented labor. J Reprod Fertil 2000; 120: 91–7.

81. Szal SE, Repke JT, Seely EW et al. [Ca2+]i signaling in pregnant human myometrium. Am J Physiol 1994; 267: E77–87.

82. Brenninkmeijer CB, Price SA, López Bernal A, Phaneuf S. Expression of G-protein-coupled receptor kinases in pregnant term and non-pregnant human myometrium. J Endocrinol 1999; 162: 401–8.

83. Tohgo A, Choy EW, Gesty-Palmer D et al. The stability of the G protein-coupled receptor-beta-arrestin interaction determines the mechanism and functional consequence of ERK activation. J Biol Chem 2003; 278: 6258–67.

84. Phaneuf S, Asboth G, Carrasco MP et al. The desensitization of oxytocin receptors in human myometrial cells is accompanied by down-regulation of oxytocin receptor messenger RNA. J Endocrinol 1997; 154: 7–18.

85. Koenig JA, Edwardson JM. Endocytosis and recycling of G protein-coupled receptors. Trends Pharmacol Sci 1997; 18: 276–87.

86. Smith MP, Ayad VJ, Mundell SJ et al. Internalization and desensitization of the oxytocin receptor is inhibited by dynamin and clathrin mutants in HEK-293 cells. Mol Endocrinol 2006; 20(2): 379–388.

87. Akerlund M, Stromberg P, Forsling ML. Primary dysmenorrhoea and vasopressin. Br J Obstet Gynaecol 1979; 86: 484–7.

88. Akerlund M, Stromberg P, Hauksson A et al. Inhibition of uterine contractions of premature labor with an oxytocin analogue. Results from a pilot study. Br J Obstet Gynaecol 1987; 94: 1040–4.

89. Goodwin TM, Paul R, Silver H et al. The effect of the oxytocin antagonist atosiban on preterm uterine activity in the human. Am J Obstet Gynecol 1994; 170: 474–8.

90. López Bernal A, Phipps SL, Rosevear SK, Turnbull AC. Mechanism of action of the oxytocin antagonist 1-deamino-2-D-Tyr-(OEt)-4-Thr-8-Orn-oxytocin. Br J Obstet Gynaecol 1989; 96: 1108–10.

91. Phaneuf S, Asboth G, MacKenzie IZ, Melin P, Lopez Bernal A. Effect of oxytocin antagonists on the activation of human myometrium in vitro: atosiban prevents oxytocin-induced desensitization. Am J Obstet Gynecol 1994; 171: 1627–34.

92. Manning M, Stoev S, Kolodziejczyk A et al. Design of potent and selective linear antagonists of vasopressor (V1-receptor) responses to vasopressin. J Med Chem 1990; 33: 3079–86.

93. Pettibone DJ, Clineschmidt BV, Anderson PS et al. A structurally unique, potent, and selective oxytocin antagonist derived from *Streptomyces silvensis*. Endocrinology 1989; 125: 217–22.

94. Manning M, Cheng LL, Stoev S et al. Design of peptide oxytocin antagonists with strikingly higher affinities and selectivities for the human oxytocin receptor than atosiban. J Pept Sci 2005; 11: 593–608.

95. Nilsson L, Reinheimer T, Steinwall M, Akerlund, M. FE 200 440: a selective oxytocin antagonist on the term-pregnant human uterus. Br J Obstet Gynaecol 2003; 110: 1025–8.

96. Evans BE, Leighton JL, Rittle KE et al. Orally active, nonpeptide oxytocin antagonists. J Med Chem 1992; 35: 3919–27.

97. Serradeil-Le Gal C, Valette G, Foulon L et al. SSR126768A (4-chloro-3-[(3R)-(1)-5-chloro-1-(2,4-dimethoxybenzyl)-3-methyl-2-oxo-2,3-dihydro-1H-indol-3-yl]-N-ethyl-N-(3-pyridylmethyl)-benzamide, hydrochloride): a new selective and orally active oxytocin receptor antagonist for the prevention of preterm labor. J Pharmacol Exp Ther 2004; 309: 414–24.

98. Quattropani A, Dorbais J, Covini D et al. Discovery and development of a new class of potent, selective, orally active oxytocin receptor antagonists. J Med Chem 2005; 48: 7882–905.

99. Crowley P. Prophylactic corticosteroids for preterm birth. Cochrane Database Syst Rev 2000; CD000065.

100. Mitchell BF, Olson DM. Prostaglandin endoperoxide H synthase inhibitors and other tocolytics in preterm labor. Prostaglandins Leukot Essent Fatty Acids 2004; 70: 167–87.

16

Progestational agents and labor

Paul J Meis

Progesterone, the hormone of the corpus luteum, has been known to be important in maintaining pregnancy since the classic work of Corner and Allen.[1] Soon after progestational agents became commercially available, these drugs were employed to treat pregnancy problems. Most of these early applications of progesterone, and trials of treatment, concerned infertility or threatened early pregnancy loss. However, interest also began in administering progestational drugs to prevent preterm delivery, and the first randomized trial of progesterone for this purpose was by Papiernik in 1970.[2] Several other small trials of progesterone therapy were reported over the next two decades. Recently, interest in this therapy has been re-invigorated, as evidenced by the recent publication of six review articles and an ACOG Committee Opinion.[3–9] The origin of this new enthusiasm and interest in progesterone was sparked by the publication, in 2003, of two randomized trials; one used progesterone vaginal suppositories and the other 17 alpha hydroxyprogesterone capoate (17P) injections to prevent recurrent preterm delivery.[10,11]

The results of the early reported trials of progesterone were evaluated by three different meta-analyses. The first of these, by Goldstein et al[12] published in 1989, gave the results of a meta-analysis of randomized controlled trials involving the use of progesterone or other progestogenic agents for the maintenance of pregnancy. Fifteen trials of variously defined high-risk subjects were felt to be suitable for analysis. The trials employed six different progestational drugs. The pooled odds ratios (OR) for these trials showed no statistically significant effect on rates of miscarriage, stillbirth, neonatal death or preterm birth. The authors concluded that '... progestogens should not be used outside of randomized trials at present'. The second meta-analysis, by Daya,[13] and published at the same time in the same journal, evaluated progesterone efficacy in treating women with a history of recurrent miscarriage, and found that progesterone therapy was effective in

increasing the likelihood of pregnancies reaching at least 20 weeks of gestation [OR 3.09, 95% confidence interval (CI) 1.28–7.42]. In a separate response to Goldstein, Keirse[14] presented, in 1990, the results of an analysis of a more focused selection of trials. This meta-analysis was restricted to trials that employed 17P, the most fully studied progestational agent, and included all placebo-controlled trials which used this drug. Pooled OR found no significant effect on rates of miscarriage, perinatal death or neonatal complications. However, in contrast to Goldstein's review, the OR for preterm birth was significant (OR 95% CI 0.30–0.85), as was the OR for birthweight <2500 g (OR 0.46, 95% CI 0.27–0.80). Keirse remarked that the results demonstrated by these trials contrast markedly with the poor effectiveness of other efforts to reduce the occurrence of preterm birth, but that since no effect was demonstrated to result in lower perinatal mortality or morbidity, '... further well-controlled research would be necessary before it is recommended for clinical practice'.

A large trial of an oral progestational drug was reported in 1994 by Hobel.[15] As part of a larger preterm birth prevention program, 823 patients were identified as being at risk for preterm birth by a high-risk pregnancy scoring system. The drug used was Provera (medroxyprogesterone acetate), and 411 patients were assigned to take 20 mg orally daily. The control group of 412 patients was given placebo tablets. The allocation to drug or placebo was on the basis of the particular prenatal clinic in which the patient attended. The subjects were enrolled prior to 31 weeks of gestation. The outcome of interest was delivery at <37 weeks. The rate of preterm delivery in the treatment group was 11.2%, compared with 7.3% in the placebo group. The rate of compliance for the subjects was low, with only 55% of the patients assigned to the Provera group actually taking the drug. This remains the only large reported trial of an oral progestational agent to prevent preterm birth.

Recently, two large trials have been reported of the use of progestational drugs to prevent preterm birth. In 2003 da Fonseca et al[10] reported the results of a randomized, placebo-controlled trial of vaginal progesterone suppositories in 142 women. The subjects were selected as being at high risk for preterm birth. The risk factor in >90% of the subjects was that of a previous preterm delivery. The patients were randomly assigned to daily insertion of either a 100 mg progesterone suppository or a placebo suppository. The treatment period was 24–34 weeks of gestation. All patients were monitored for uterine contractions once weekly for 1h with an external tocodynamometer. Although 81 progesterone and 76 placebo patients were entered into the study, several patients were excluded from analysis because of premature rupture of the fetal membranes, or were lost to follow-up, leaving 72 progesterone and 70 placebo subjects. The rate of preterm delivery <37 weeks in the progesterone patients was 13.8%, significantly less than the rate in the placebo patients of 28.5%. The rate of preterm delivery <34 weeks in the treatment group was 2.8% compared with 18.6% in the placebo group. These differences were statistically significant. The rate of uterine contractions measured by the weekly 1h recording was significantly less between 28 and 34 weeks in the progesterone patients compared with the placebo patients. Analysis of the results by 'intent-to-treat' showed smaller differences between the groups, but these differences remained statistically significant.[16]

Meis et al[11] reported the results of a large multicenter trial of 17P conducted by the Maternal Fetal Medicine Units Network of the National Institute of Child Health and Human Development. The study enrolled women with a documented history of a previous spontaneous preterm delivery, which occurred as a consequence of either spontaneous preterm labor or preterm premature rupture of the fetal membranes. After receiving an ultrasound examination to rule out major fetal anomalies, and to determine gestational age, the subjects were offered the study and given a test dose of the placebo injection to assess compliance. If they chose to continue, they were randomly assigned, using a 2:1, weekly injections of 250 mg 17P or a placebo injection. Treatment was begun between 16 and 20 weeks of gestation, and was continued until delivery or 37 weeks of gestation, which ever came first. The study planned to enroll 500 subjects, a sample size estimated to be sufficient to detect a 37% reduction in the rate of preterm birth. However, enrollment was halted at 463 subjects – 310 in the treatment group and 153 in the placebo group – following a scheduled evaluation by the Data Safety and Monitoring Committee, which found that the evidence of efficacy for the primary outcome was such that further entry of patients was unnecessary. In this study, delivery at less than 37 weeks was reduced from 54.9% in the placebo group to 36.3% in the treatment group. Similar reductions were seen in delivery at <35 weeks, from 30.7 to 20.6%, and in delivery <32 weeks from 19.6 to 11.4%. All of these differences were statistically significant. Rates of birthweight <2500 g were significantly reduced, as were rates of intraventricular hemorrhage, necrotizing enterocolitis, and need for supplemental oxygen and ventilatory support. Rates of neonatal death were reduced from 5.9% in the placebo group to 2.6% in the treatment group, though this difference did not reach statistical significance. The women enrolled in this study had unusually high rates of preterm birth. This could be explained in part by the fact that the mean gestational age of their previous preterm delivery was quite early, at 31 weeks. In addition, one third of the women had had more than one previous spontaneous preterm delivery. Despite random allocation, more women in the placebo group had had more than one preterm delivery. Adjustment of the analysis controlling for the imbalance found that the treatment effect remained significantly different than the placebo. A majority of the women were of African-American ethnicity, and the treatment with 17P showed equal efficacy in the African-American women and in the non-African-American subjects.

In 2003, the ACOG Committee on Obstetric Practice published a Committee Opinion about the use of progesterone to reduce preterm birth.[3] The opinion recognized the benefit shown in the two trials for women with a prior spontaneous preterm delivery. The opinion cautioned that progesterone should not be recommended for women with other high-risk conditions (twin gestation, shortened cervix etc.) outside of randomized trials.

In 2005, Sanchez-Ramos et al[8] published a meta-analysis of trials of progestational agents to prevent preterm births. They included the two recent trials for a total of 10 trials which met the search criteria. The analysis found that 'compared with women randomized to the placebo, those who received progestational agents had lower rates of preterm delivery (26.2 versus 35.9%, OR 0.45, 95% CI 0.25–0.80).' However, the comparison of rates of perinatal mortality did not reach a statistically significant difference (OR 0.69, 95% CI 0.38–1.26).

Trials of progestational agents to halt the birth process of patients after labor have commenced have not been successful. Four published trials have employed a progestational drug for patients in preterm labor, and one trial in an attempt to prolong pregnancy in patients close to term.[17–21] Although the design of these trials, and the drugs employed, varied none of these studies have demonstrated any efficacy in prolonging pregnancy.

Thus, the use of progesterone as a tocolytic drug, or as an adjunct to tocolytic agents for patients in preterm labor, is to be discouraged outside of randomized trials. It is likely that once the physiologic or pathologic processes (such as the formation of gap junctions, or activation of the inflammatory cascade), have occurred, which precede labor, treatment with progestational agents is not effective in halting this process.

Currently, evidence exists to recommend treatment with a progestational drug for women with a history of a prior spontaneous preterm delivery. The preponderance of this evidence of efficacy relates to 17P, with only one successful trial reported to the present time which used progesterone suppositories. While this indication for use (a history of a prior preterm delivery) is valuable for the women concerned, this application has only modest potential impact on the problem of preterm birth in total, as demonstrated by Petrini et al.[7] These authors reported an interesting analysis of the potential impact of 17P treatment of women at risk for recurrent preterm delivery. Their calculations assumed a 33% reduction of preterm births (based on the results of the MFMU Network trial). By their calculations, if all women at risk for recurrent preterm delivery in the US were treated with 17P, 10 000 spontaneous preterm births would be prevented. However, the overall rate of preterm birth in the US would be reduced only from 12.1 to 11.8%.

We are aware of trials currently in progress using either 17P or progesterone vaginal cream to treat women with other high-risk problems, including women with a twin or triplet pregnancy. The results of these trials may broaden the indications for use of progestational agents to prevent preterm birth.

REFERENCES

1. Corner BW, Allen WA. Physiology of the corpus luteum. Am J Physiol 1929; 88: 326–46.
2. Papiernik E. Double blind study of an agent to prevent pre-term delivery among women at increased risk. In: Edition Schering, Serie IV, fiche 3. 1970; 65–8.
3. ACOG Committee Opinion No. 291. Use of progesterone to reduce preterm birth. Obstet Gynecol 2003; 102: 1115–16.
4. Meis PJ, Connors N. Progesterone treatment to prevent preterm birth. Clin Obstet Gynecol 2004; 47: 784–95.
5. Meis PJ, Aleman A. Progesterone treatment to prevent preterm birth. Drugs 2004; 64: 2463–74.
6. Meis PJ. For the Society for Maternal Fetal Medicine. 17 Hydroxy-progesterone for the prevention of preterm delivery. Obstet Gynecol 2005; 105: 1128–35.
7. Petrini JR, Callaghan WM, Klebanoff M et al. Estimated effect of 17 alpha-hydroxyprogesterone caproate on preterm birth in the United States. Obstet Gynecol 2005; 105: 267–72.
8. Sanchez-Ramos L, Kaunitz AM, Delke I. Progestational agents to prevent preterm birth: a meta-analysis of randomized controlled trials. Obstet Gynecol 2005; 105: 273–9.
9. Armstrong J, Nageotte M. For the Society of Maternal Fetal Medicine. Can progesterone prevent preterm birth? Contemp Ob Gyn 2005; 31–41.
10. da Fonseca EB, Bittar RE, Carvalho MHB et al. Prophylactic administration of progesterone by vaginal suppository to reduce the incidence of spontaneous preterm birth in women at increased risk: a randomized placebo-controlled double-blind study. Am J Obstet Gynecol 2003; 188: 419–24.
11. Meis PJ, Klebanoff M, Thom E et al. Prevention of recurrent preterm delivery by 17 alpha-hydroxyprogesterone caproate. N Engl J Med 2003; 348: 2379–85.
12. Goldstein P, Berrier J, Rosen S et al. A meta-analysis of randomized control trials of progestational agents in pregnancy. Br J Obstet Gynaecol 1989; 96: 265–74.
13. Daya S. Efficacy of progesterone support for pregnancy in women with recurrent miscarriage. A meta-analysis of controlled trials. Br J Obstet Gynaecol 1989; 96: 275–80.
14. Keirse MJNC. Progesterone administration in pregnancy may prevent pre-term delivery. Br J Obstet Gynaecol 1990; 97: 149–54.
15. Hobel CJ, Ross MG, Bemis RL et al. The West Los Angeles Preterm Birth Prevention Project I. Program impact on high-risk women. Am J Obstet Gynecol 1994; 170: 54–62.
16. da Fonseca EB. Progesterone and preterm birth. Am J Obstet Gynecol 2004; 190: 1801–2 (letter reply).
17. Fuchs F, Stademann G. Treatment of threatened premature labor with large doses of progesterone. Am J Obstet Gynecol 1960; 79: 172–6.
18. Kaupilla A, Hartikainen-Sorri A-L, Olli J et al. Suppression of threatened premature labor by administration of cortisol and 17 alpha-hydroxyprogesterone caporate: a comparison with ritodrine. Am J Obstet Gynecol 1980; 138: 404–8.
19. Erny R, Pigne C, Prouvost M et al. The effects of oral administration of progesterone for premature labor. Am J Obstet Gynecol 1986; 154: 525–9.
20. Noblott G, Audra P, Dargent D et al. The use of micronized progesterone in the treatment of menace of preterm delivery. Eur J Obstet Gynecol Reprod Biol 1991; 40: 203–9.
21. Brenner WB, Hendricks CH. Effect of medroxyprogesterone acetate upon the duration and characteristics of human gestation and labor. Am J Obstet Gynecol 1962; 83: 1094–8.

17

Antenatal corticosteroid treatment

John P Newnham and Timothy JM Moss

INTRODUCTION

Preterm birth is one of the world's major unsolved problems in health care. In developed countries, preterm births account for approximately 70% of newborn deaths and up to 75% of neonatal morbidity. The high cost of modern neonatal intensive care may also be followed by lifelong disability, with profound consequences for the individual, their family and the community.

Despite many years of research effort, strategies aimed at preventing preterm birth have, in general, been unsuccessful. Rates of preterm birth in different countries are either unchanged or rising. In the USA, the rate of preterm birth reached 12.1% in 2002, representing a 29% increase over the previous two decades.[1]

While our collective efforts to prevent preterm birth may have been unsuccessful, methods to reduce the risks that follow this complication of pregnancy have been far more rewarding. One of the greatest successes has resulted from the discovery that the fetal lungs may be matured by maternal injection of antenatal corticosteroids.

HISTORY

The discovery that corticosteroids may be used to mature the fetal lungs before preterm birth arose from experiments in Auckland, New Zealand, in the late 1960s. Professor Graham (Mont) Liggins was investigating, in sheep, the factors involved in initiation of labor.[2,3] He observed that administration of (adrenocorticotrophic hormone, ACTH) to fetal lambs through an indwelling catheter implanted into the peritoneal cavity resulted in preterm labor.[2] Dexamethasone infusion by the same route had a similar result, and

addition of deoxycorticosterone did not add to the effect, indicating the preterm labor had resulted from glucocorticoid rather than mineralocorticoid activity.[3] He noted that six of ten preterm lambs born vaginally after dexamethasone infusion had partial aeration of their lungs, and one of these lambs survived for 2 h. Lambs born by elective Cesarean section at such at an early gestational age would not otherwise survive without artificial ventilation and their lungs would not be aerated. From these observations, it was proposed that fetal exposure to dexamethasone had matured the fetal lungs, possibly by stimulating surfactant activity.

Professor Liggins and Dr RN Howie then investigated this hypothesis further by conducting a randomized controlled trial in which 282 women at high risk of preterm birth were allocated at random to receive an intramuscular injection of betamethasone or a control solution.[4] The betamethasone injection consisted of 6 mg betamethasone phosphate and 6 mg betamethasone acetate, and a second injection was given 24 h later if delivery had not occurred. The women in the control group received similar injections of 6 mg cortisone acetate, which had a glucocorticoid potency one-seventieth that of the betamethasone preparation. Early newborn death was observed in 3.2% of the treated group and 15% of controls. In those babies born before 32 weeks of gestation, and who were delivered >24 h after the first dose, the rate of respiratory distress syndrome was 11.8% in treated babies and 69.6% in controls. There were no deaths from respiratory distress syndrome in babies of women who had received betamethasone treatment >24 h before delivery. This series of animal studies, followed by the randomized controlled trial, led to one of the most useful discoveries in perinatal medicine. Professor Mont Liggins has since received a knighthood for his work.

HYPOTHALAMIC–PITUITARY–ADRENAL (HPA) AXIS

Until late in gestation, the fetus develops and grows in an environment characterized by low levels of glucocorticoids.[5] Circulating levels of cortisol in the mother are three-fold those in the fetus, and the enzyme 11β-hydroxysteroid dehydrogenase (11βHSD) type 2 in the placenta converts most cortisol passing from the mother to inactive cortisone. The fetal HPA axis is quiescent, and most cortisol that is to be found in the fetal circulation is of maternal origin. Late in pregnancy, levels of cortisol circulating in the fetus rise substantially. In sheep, this rise begins 10–15 days before term with a further rapid increase in the last 3–5 days. Most of this cortisol is of fetal origin. In sheep and baboons, this activation of the fetal HPA axis is manifest by increased mRNA encoding corticotrophin-releasing hormone (CRH) in the paraventricular nucleus of the fetal hypothalamus, resulting in stimulation of mRNA encoding proopiomelanocortin (POMC) in the fetal pituitary pars distalis. POMC is the precursor of ACTH. Elevated circulating levels of ACTH increase responsiveness of the fetal adrenal to ACTH stimulation, and in sheep this has been shown to include an increased number of ACTH receptors. The resulting increase in cortisol secretion has a variety of effects that are vital for the fetus to be prepared for extrauterine life. These effects include: structural changes to the lung and increased production of surfactant to allow for breathing; changes to enzymes regulating glucose metabolism in the liver that allow for a ready supply of glucose after birth; proliferation of intestinal villi, and induction of enzymes that allow the newborn to switch to enteral feeding; and inducing the switch from fetal to adult hemoglobin production in the bone marrow.

In sheep, the increased circulating levels of cortisol before birth induce changes in placental steroidogenesis that are a necessary prelude to the initiation of parturition. In primates, including humans, the sequence of events is not so simple and both fetal adrenal cortisol and C_{19} estogen precursors are linked to the onset of labor. As a result, birth in sheep is a process that follows maturation of the fetus while humans are more prone to the delivery of newborns that may not have received the full benefit of cortisol-induced fetal maturation.

SINGLE-COURSE TREATMENT

Effectiveness

Since publication in 1972 of the first randomized controlled trial of betamethasone to prevent respiratory distress syndrome of the preterm newborn, a further 17 trials of single-course treatment have been reported.[6,7] In general, these trials were based on treatment over a 48 h period either with 24 mg betamethasone, 24 mg dexamethasone or 2 g hydrocortisone. A total of 3700 babies were involved. Meta-analysis of these 18 trials has shown that such treatment is associated with a significant reduction in newborn mortality [odds ratio (OR) 0.6, 95% confidence interval (CI) 0.48–0.75] and respiratory distress syndrome (OR 0.53, 95% CI 0.44–0.63). Together, these findings confirm that a single course of corticosteroids given over a 48 h treatment period will halve the rate of death and respiratory distress syndrome of the preterm newborn. Some of these trials included cases in which the corticosteroids were administered on a repeated basis, but the study designs and presentation of data do not allow determination of the effects of repeated courses as distinct from single courses.[7]

REPEATED TREATMENTS

The success of antenatal corticosteroids to improve outcomes after preterm birth led clinical practice to evolve toward multiple treatments. This clinical practice was not supported by evidence from randomized controlled trials, and was based on incomplete evidence that the effect of treatment may dissipate if the pregnancy continues for 1 week or more after initial treatment.[4] Experimental studies on the question of whether treatments should be repeated if the pregnancy continued but the risk of preterm birth persisted were incomplete. In sheep, it had been shown that postnatal lung responses to antenatal betamethasone treatment remained unchanged between 48 h and 7 days after treatment.[8] Re-treating the ewe 6 days after the initial treatment did not add to the improvements in newborn lung function that occur after a single treatment.[9]

Surveys of obstetricians over the last decade have shown high rates of prescription of repeated courses. In a survey of obstetric units in UK in 1997, 98% reported the use of repeated courses.[10] Eighty-five percent of Australian obstetricians in 1998 prescribed multiple courses if the risk of preterm birth was persistent,[11] and more recently a survey of 641 European obstetricians in 14 countries revealed that a similar percentage still used multiple courses.[12] These surveys were conducted in response to new evidence that repeated and prolonged exposures to antenatal corticosteroids may be associated with untoward effects which could potentially carry lifelong problems for the child. The evidence was obtained from experimental studies with animals and clinical studies with humans, which included well-described cohorts, although with methodologies that fell short of the rigor of randomized controlled trials.

Possible harm from repeated antenatal corticosteroids

Birthweight

In studies of sheep, repeated doses of betamethasone to the ewe at weekly intervals (104, 111, 118, and 124 days) followed by delivery at 125 days (term is 150 days) resulted in reduced birthweight.[13] This reduction in birthweight was 15% after one dose, 19% after two doses, and 27% after three of four doses when compared with saline-treated controls. The effect continued if the pregnancy was extended to term gestation. Weights of all major organs were decreased, including the heart, liver, kidneys and placenta.[14] If sheep exposed to repeated maternal betamethasone treatments were left to deliver spontaneously at term gestation, body weights remained less than controls at 3 months postnatal age, but were restored to levels in controls by 6 months and remained as such through to adulthood.[15]

Birthweight has also been shown to be reduced after maternally administered corticosteroids in rabbits,[16] mice,[17] and rats.[18] Studies with monkeys, however, have not shown consistent effects on fetal growth;[19] some studies showed an increased weight of the fetal liver[20] associated with a four-fold increase in glycogen content.[21]

The effect of repeated courses of antenatal corticosteroids on birthweight in humans is less certain. In a prospective cohort study of 477 singleton newborns born <33 weeks of gestation in Western Australia, the birthweight ratio declined with increasing numbers of courses that the child had experienced before birth.[22] Multivariate analysis revealed that birthweight was reduced as much as 9% by prior exposure to repeated courses. In a comparison of 961 dexamethasone-treated infants compared with 2808 matched controls and an overall population of 122,629 infants in Texas, USA, the average birthweight of corticosteroid-exposed infants was smaller by 12 g at 24–26 weeks, 63 g at 27–29 weeks, 161 g at 30–32 weeks, and 80 g at 33–34 weeks.[23] A nonrandomized post-hoc analysis of 710 newborns born at 25–32 weeks of gestation, who had been enrolled in the North American Thyrotropin Releasing Hormone Trial, showed that newborns who had received two or more antenatal courses of antenatal corticosteroids had lower birthweights.[24] Expected birthweight, calculated by multiple linear regression, was decreased by 39 g after more than one course of antenatal corticosteroids and 80 g after more than two courses. Not all retrospective studies, however, have found effects of repeated courses of corticosteroids on fetal growth. A secondary analysis of a randomized controlled trial performed to determine whether antenatal treatment with phenobarbital and vitamin K would prevent intracranial hemorrhage in premature newborns did not observe an effect of repeated courses of corticosteroids on birthweight in the sample of 414 infants.[25]

There is some information available from randomized controlled trials. Guinn et al[26] colleagues reported in 2001 the results of a randomized controlled trial of repeated courses of corticosteroids that had been terminated mid-way through its planned recruitment. The study was of 502 pregnant women at high risk of preterm birth at 13 academic centers in USA. Women who had received a single course of antenatal corticosteroids and had not delivered 1 week later were allocated at random to receive weekly courses of corticosteroids until 34 weeks of gestation, or similarly administered placebo. There were no significant differences in mean birthweight between the two treatment groups, nor in gestational age at birth. If further results from randomized controlled trials show a similar lack of effect on birthweight, it may indicate that the statistical adjustments in the previous cohort studies which had suggested a negative effect had been unable to account for the biases that are inherent in nonrandomized studies. In such cases, pregnancies that had been exposed to repeated courses of antenatal corticosteroids may have been inherently at higher risk of growth restriction independent of any treatment. A lack of an effect of repeated courses of corticosteroids on birthweight in humans would also highlight considerable differences in glucocorticoid responses between species.

Head and brain growth

There are many studies of humans and other animals that suggest head growth may be affected by repeated doses of antenatal corticosteroids. In a seminal series of studies published by Johnson et al[27] more than two decades ago, treatment of pregnant rhesus monkeys with 2 mg betamethasone intramuscularly from day 120 to day 133 (term is 165 days) resulted 1 month later in a 20% reduction in brain weight. In sheep, repeated doses of betamethasone given at weekly intervals decreased weight of the preterm brain by approximately 10% and this effect was even more pronounced if the pregnancy was left to continue to term gestation (Figure 17.1).[14,28]

The reduction in brain growth did not include weights of the cerebellum and brain-stem. A major effect of antenatal corticosteroids on development of the fetal sheep brain is delayed myelination. Four weekly maternal

Control   Single dose   Repeated doses

Preterm

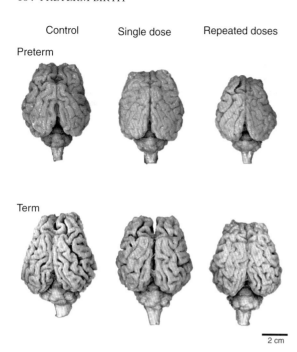

Term

2 cm

Figure 17.1 Dorsal views of representative brains of newborn lambs that had received saline, single betamethasone or repeated betamethasone treatments, and delivered at a preterm or term gestational age. The figure displays the reduction in fetal brain growth which follows maternal administration of intramuscular corticosteroids in the third trimester of pregnancy in sheep. (Reproduced with permission from Huang et al, Obstet Gynecol 1999; 94: 213–18.)

injections of betamethasone to the pregnant ewe inhibited myelination in the optic nerve by approximately 40%, probably resulting from effects on oligodendrocytes that are known to produce myelin and are sensitive to corticosteroids.[29] Axon numbers were not affected. Myelination was also reduced in the corpus callosum.[30] Recently, it has been shown that brain weights of adult sheep are reduced by exposure to single or repeated antenatal corticosteroid injections.[31] Indeed, the reduction in growth that results from prenatal corticosteroid treatment in sheep is followed after birth by catch-up in weight of all major organs except the brain.

In humans, multivariate analysis of a cohort of 477 infants born in Western Australia before 33 weeks of gestation revealed a reduction in head circumference of up to 4% in association with a history of three or more antenatal courses of corticosteroids.[22] A reduction in head circumference of 4% equates in simple geometric calculations to a decrease in cranial volume

of nearly 11%. In a retrospective multivariate analysis of 13 670 infants from 100 neonatal intensive care units in North America, Thorp et al[32] observed an effect of antenatal corticosteroids on head circumference of -3.1 ± 0.4 mm. Birthweight was also reduced, but the effect on head circumference persisted when birthweight was controlled for, suggesting there is a predilection for reduced brain growth relative to somatic growth. The antenatal corticosteroid use in this study was defined as incomplete or complete according to the full 48 h of treatment, and details of any repeated use were not provided. In the randomized controlled trial reported by Guinn et al,[26] in which weekly courses (n = 256) were compared with a single course (n = 246), no effect on head circumference was observed.[26]

Effects on neurological development

In the short term, antenatal corticosteroids protect the fetal brain from intraventricular hemorrhage. Nonrandomized studies have shown substantial reductions in the risk of newborn cerebral ventriculomegaly[33] and periventricular leucomalacia.[34] It is unknown how much of this protection from hemorrhage results from a direct effect on the developing brain, and how much can be attributed to improved stability of blood pressure and respiratory function. In later life, the risk of cerebral palsy is reduced by antenatal corticosteroids.[35,36]

Reassurance as to the long-term neurological safety of a single course of antenatal corticosteroids up to 31 years of age has been provided by data from follow-up of participants in the original Auckland trial that was published in 1972.[4,37] The evaluation involved 192 adults still living in Auckland, representing 69% of the eligible cohort in that region of New Zealand. No differences between the treated and control groups were found in measures of health-related quality of life and psychological functioning, including intelligence, working memory, psychiatric morbidity, state-trait anxiety and handedness.

There are, at this time, no data describing child or adult behavior from randomized controlled trials of repeated treatment. Data are available from a large geographic-based cohort of children born in Western Australia at early preterm gestational ages with follow-up at 3 and 6 years of age.[36] Three or more courses of antenatal corticosteroids were associated with significant increases in externalizing behavioral disorders. There were no effects on intelligence and the rate of cerebral palsy was decreased. However, measures of aggression, destructibility, distractibility and hyperactivity were greater in those who had received repeated treatments before birth. It is speculated this behavior may represent an adaptation resulting from early exposure to corticosteroids, programming the child for a world perceived to be 'stressful' or hostile. These findings highlight the need for follow-up studies of participants in the current randomized trials of repeated treatments to include tests of behavior.

Lung development

The 50% decrease in rates of respiratory distress syndrome that result from antenatal corticosteroid treatment is most likely due to anatomical changes rather than enhanced surfactant production.[38] In sheep, a single injection of betamethasone 48 h before operative preterm delivery doubles the functional volume of the newborn lung, as determined by calculation of a pressure–volume curve.[13,39] Morphometric studies have shown average alveolar volumes are increased by approximately 20% and the alveolar walls are significantly thinned.[40] The total alveolar number in control preterm lambs averaged 550 million, and this number was decreased almost 30% in the betamethasone-treated newborn group. Increases in pulmonary surfactant do not occur until >4 days after antenatal corticosteroid treatment in sheep.[13,41]

Studies of respiratory function up to 4 weeks of postnatal age in lambs exposed to single or repeated antenatal betamethasone have shown no ongoing effects in terms of blood gas values, minute ventilation, lung volumes or compliance.[42]

Glucose metabolism

In adult life, exposure to excessive levels of glucocorticoids predisposes to glucose intolerance and diabetes, whether the exposure results from pharmacological treatment or Cushing syndrome. Experiments with sheep have shown that repeated maternal treatments to the pregnant ewe disturb glucose tolerance in the offspring, but the pattern of responses is not straight forward. After one or four weekly antenatal betamethasone treatments, offspring at 6 months of age had elevated insulin levels both in the basal state and after a glucose challenge.[15] At 1 year of age, sheep that had been exposed to four weekly antenatal corticosteroid treatments had elevations in glucose and insulin levels both before and after a glucose challenge. Basal insulin:glucose ratios were elevated in 2-year-old sheep born after one or four weekly antenatal betamethasone treatments; this effect persisted until 3 years of age after four weekly antenatal injections. There is also an increase in hepatic glucose-6-phosphatase activity that persists into adulthood, potentially contributing to long-term alterations in glucose metabolism.[43]

Investigations of participants in the Auckland Steroid Trial have shown that antenatal corticosteroid exposure alters responses to glucose challenge at 30 years of age.[44] After a 75 g oral glucose challenge, betamethasone-exposed individuals had higher insulin levels at 30 min and lower glucose levels at 120 min. Further, there was a suggestion that the increase in insulin levels at 30 min was greater in those participants who had been exposed to a higher dose of betamethasone. These findings suggest that antenatal corticosteroid treatment may predispose to insulin resistance in later life, and ongoing follow-up of participants in such trials is warranted.

Blood pressure

Adults who have Cushing syndrome, or are treated pharmacologically with glucocorticoids, are prone to hypertension. In baboons, maternal glucocorticoid administration in doses comparable to those used in clinical practice is followed by significant increases in fetal blood pressure which persist throughout the duration of treatment.[45] In adulthood, prenatal exposure to glucocorticoids can predispose to hypertension, but the response is dependent on the gestational age at exposure. In sheep, treatment of the pregnant ewe with dexamethasone from day 22 to day 29 of gestation (term is 150 days) results in increased blood pressure in later life.[46] If sheep are treated with single or repeated doses of betamethasone during the third trimester, however, the offspring do not develop increased blood pressure when compared with controls at 6 months,[15] 1 year or 2 years of age.[31] From these experiments with sheep, it is suggested that single or repeated antenatal corticosteroid treatments would not be expected to predispose the offspring to adult hypertension.

Follow-up at 30 years age of people who had been participants in the original Auckland Steroid Trial has provided strong evidence that single-course treatment does not have deleterious effects on cardiovascular risk factors at that age.[44] There were no significant differences in socioeconomic status, body size, blood pressure, plasma lipids or use of antihypertensive therapy.

HPA axis function

The dose of glucocorticoid administered to enhance fetal lung maturation is not inconsiderable and carries the potential to cause long-term alterations in HPA axis function.[5,47] The effects of antenatal betamethasone treatment on subsequent function of the HPA axis of the offspring have been studied in sheep.[48] At 6 months of postnatal age, prior exposure to antenatal betamethasone did not alter ACTH or cortisol responses to challenge by intravenous infusion of CRH and arginine vasopressin (AVP). However, at 1 year of age, a single prenatal exposure to maternally administered betamethasone resulted in significant elevations in basal and stimulated cortisol levels. Repeated treatments did not produce this effect. At 2 years of age, cortisol levels in sheep that had been exposed prenatally to single or repeated maternal doses of betamethasone were no different from levels in saline-exposed controls, but by 3 years of age the betamethasone-exposed animals showed signs of adrenal suppression. Basal ACTH and cortisol levels were increased, and stimulated cortisol levels were attenuated in betamethasone-exposed sheep relative to levels in controls.[49] These findings suggest the postnatal HPA axis may respond to prenatal corticosteroid therapy by evolving from hyperresponsiveness in early life to hyporesponsiveness in later life. Although these studies were conducted in sheep and not humans, they provide clear evidence that participants in the randomized controlled trials of single or repeated courses of corticosteroids currently in progress will need to be followed well into their adult life.

Follow-up at 30 years of age of participants in the Auckland Steroid Trial revealed that early morning cortisol levels were 7% higher in the betamethasone-exposed group than in the cortisone-exposed group.[44] This difference, however, was abolished by allowance for a variety of potential confounding variables. Outcome data following repeated antenatal corticosteroids on the response of the adult HPA axis to stimulation or other consequences in later life are not available from humans.

Potential benefits of repeated courses

In sheep, three or four weekly doses of betamethasone before preterm Cesarean delivery improves lung function.[13] Where a single injection doubles functional lung volume in 48 h, four weekly injections quadruples that volume. This effect reflects anatomical changes which include increased size of alveoli, a decrease in tissue between the airspaces, and increases in surfactant phospholipid and surfactant protein-A, -B and -C levels.

In the randomized controlled trial reported by Guinn et al,[26] 502 pregnant women between 24 and 32 weeks of gestation were allocated at random to receive weekly courses of antenatal corticosteroids until 34 weeks of gestation, or a placebo. The principal endpoint under investigation was a composite neonatal morbidity score, defined as the presence of any of the following: severe respiratory distress syndrome, bronchopulmonary dysplasia, severe intraventricular hemorrhage, periventricular leucomalacia, necrotozing enterocolitis, proven sepsis, or death between randomization and discharge from the nursery. The sample size necessary to determine a significant effect was calculated to be 1000 women. After recruiting approximately one third

of the sample, the investigating team observed that rates of the composite neonatal morbidity score were similar in the two groups (24% in the repeated courses group and 27% in the single-course group). In view of this finding, combined with their awareness of increasing concerns as to the safety of repeated antenatal corticosteroids, the investigators elected to terminate the study. The final sample size in the treated and control groups were 256 and 246, respectively, and rates of the composite morbidity in these two groups were 22.5 and 28% respectively (P = 0.16). When subdivided by gestational age at birth, the composite morbidity score was significantly less in the repeated treatment group within the 24–27 weeks of age [relative risk (RR) 0.80, 95% CI 0.65–0.98], and this difference was the result of fewer cases of severe respiratory distress syndrome in the repeated courses group. There were no significant differences in the other gestational age groups. Cranial ultrasound examinations were available for some, but not all, of the newborns. There were more cases of severe intraventricular hemorrhage in the repeated courses group (nine cases) than in the single-course group (two cases), a difference that did not reach statistical significance (P = 0.06). There was also a nonsignificant trend to a higher rate of chorioamnionitis in the repeated courses group (24.1%) than in the single-course group (17.8%) (P = 0.09).

The decision to terminate this trial before reaching its full sample size has been the subject of debate. To cease such a trial before reaching its full sample size, because of the lack of a treatment effect, risked missing vital findings that may have emerged if the full recruitment had been achieved.[50] Premature cessation of this trial has also compromised interpretation of the significant benefit that was observed in the 24–27 weeks of gestational age group. The authors concluded that their data did not support use of weekly courses of antenatal corticosteroids, but it remains entirely feasible that an expanded sample may have produced compelling evidence of benefit in this high-risk group. Further, if the scientific community were to accept their reasons for terminating their trial, it may be inherently unethical to continue the other randomized controlled trials currently in progress, despite comments from the investigators themselves that the other trials in this field should continue.[51]

EFFECTS OF OBSTETRIC COMPLICATIONS

Infection

Since the introduction of antenatal corticosteroids for the purpose of enhancing fetal maturation, there have been lingering uncertainties as to whether the treatment could diminish the pregnant woman's immune response and exacerbate or cause infection. There also have been doubts as to whether the fetal response to spontaneous rupture of the membranes may involve maturation that diminishes any additional benefit that may arise from the corticosteroid treatment. Data from the original trial published in 1972 suggested that antenatal corticosteroid treatment in the presence of ruptured membranes did reduce the rate of respiratory distress syndrome in the preterm newborn, but this trend did not reach statistical significance.[52] More recently, analysis of the combined data from 15 controlled trials involving >1400 women with ruptured membranes has provided strong evidence that, in this setting, antenatal corticosteroids reduce the rate of respiratory distress syndrome, intraventricular hemorrhage and necrotizing enterocolitis.[52] The authors concluded that clinical decision-making in cases of antenatal corticosteroid therapy should not be altered by the presence of ruptured membranes.

There has also been a further analysis of the data from the randomized controlled trial of repeated treatments reported by Guinn et al[26] involving those women who had experienced preterm prelabor rupture of membranes.[53] Eighty-one women with preterm ruptured membranes and not in labor were allocated at random to receive weekly courses of corticosteroids, and 80 women to a single course. There were no significant differences between the two groups, suggesting that repeated weekly courses of antenatal corticosteroids are of no additional benefit when compared with a single course if the membranes have ruptured. There was however an increased rate of chorioamnionitis in those allocated to receive weekly courses [39/81 cases (49.4%)] when compared with those allocated to a single course [25/80 cases (31.7%)]. The authors concluded that the apparent lack of benefit, and possible increased risk of infection, preclude the use of repeated courses of antenatal corticosteroids in cases of preterm prelabor rupture of the membranes.

The recent realization that chorioamnionitis is present in many cases of preterm birth,[54] coupled with clinical[55] and experimental[56] evidence of preterm lung maturation in such cases, raises questions about the effectiveness of antenatal corticosteroids in cases of intrauterine inflammation/infection. In sheep, lung maturation induced by intra-amniotic lipolysaccharide (LPS) injection (which causes intrauterine inflammation) is augmented by preceding maternal betamethasone treatment.[57] Observational data from humans, however, suggest that the reduced risk of respiratory distress syndrome associated with chorioamnionitis is not further reduced by corticosteroid treatment.[58]

Fetal growth restriction

The vast majority of pregnancies enrolled in randomized controlled trials of antenatal corticosteroids have been complicated by preterm labor or preterm prelabor rupture of membranes. In recent years there has been interest in whether the fetus suffering from severe growth restriction and placental vascular insufficiency can tolerate corticosteroids just as well as a normally grown fetus. In sheep, corticosteroid administration increases fetal blood pressure and vascular resistance,[59] decreases cerebral blood flow and oxygen delivery,[60] and almost doubles fetal lactate levels.[61] Clinical studies have shown that antenatal corticosteroid treatment causes transient reductions in fetal heart rate variability and movements.[62] Together, these observations suggest that corticosteroid treatment may cause a transient reduction in the acid–base balance, which is not meaningful in most cases but may be a problem if the fetus has little placental reserve.

Contemporary evaluation of pregnancies complicated by fetal growth restriction includes evaluation of blood-flow patterns by Doppler ultrasound. In its most severe form, fetal growth restriction may be accompanied by the finding of absent or reversed diastolic flow in an umbilical artery, reflecting very high downstream resistance in the fetoplacental vasculature. Wallace and Baker[63] observed that antenatal corticosteroid therapy, in cases of absent or reversed diastolic flow, resulted in the appearance of diastolic flow within 24 h of treatment in more than half their cases, suggesting a decrease in umbilical arterial resistance. The median duration of the effect was 3 days. It was speculated the decrease in resistance may result from corticosteroid-induced secretion of CRH from the placenta.[63] Similar findings have been reported by others, but there is uncertainty as to the clinical significance. Simchen et al[64] observed that those cases in which diastolic flow did not appear in response to antenatal corticosteroids were at increased risk of death or severe acidosis. These authors suggested that monitoring diastolic flow in the days after treatment may identify those cases that would benefit from immediate delivery because the fetus has not tolerated the corticosteroid challenge. In those cases in which diastolic flow appears after treatment, it remains uncertain as to whether this finding indicates a net benefit in terms of improving placental perfusion, or whether the shunting of flow towards the placenta may compromise perfusion of other major organs.

Multiple pregnancy

The National Institutes of Health (NIH) Collaborative Study published more than two decades ago suggested that the beneficial effects of antenatal corticosteroids do not extend to multiple pregnancies.[65] Further, while dexamethasone did not reduce the incidence of respiratory distress syndrome in twins, there was a trend indicating selective effectiveness in female infants, twin pairs with first-born females and Black infants. The authors suggested the circulating levels achieved in multiple pregnancies may be less than in single pregnancies and that re-consideration should be given to the dosage of drug to be administered. Other investigators have provided further evidence that antenatal corticosteroids may be less effective in multiple pregnancies.[66] In an observational study of 4754 singleton infants, 2460 twin infants and 906 triplet infants, Blickstein et al[67] observed that the incidence of respiratory distress syndrome after a complete course of antenatal corticosteroids increased with increasing plurality (OR 1.4 and 1.8 for twins and triplets, respectively).[67] None of the randomized controlled trials of antenatal corticosteroid therapy specifically targeted multiple pregnancies, and at this time the issue of whether effectiveness is lessened by plurality remains unresolved.

IMPROVING THE EFFECTIVENESS OF ANTENATAL CORTICOSTEROIDS

Route of administration

The standard of practice in antenatal administration of corticosteroids is maternal intramuscular injection. An alternative is to inject the fetus directly under ultrasound guidance, thus allowing a much smaller dose than is required when treatment is given to the mother. Fetal intramuscular injection of betamethasone has been studied in sheep and the results have provided evidence that, when compared with maternal intramuscular injection, the treatment produces similar lung maturation, but birthweight is not affected and any effects on the developing brain are less.[14,41,68] This differential effect appears to arise from a shorter duration of exposure with half-lives in the fetal circulation of 8.5 h after maternal injection and of 1 hour after fetal injection (Figure 17.2).[69] Direct fetal intramuscular injection in humans however would not be without risk. Potential problems may include exacerbation of preterm labor and injury to surrounding structures such as the sciatic nerve if a thigh were the chosen target. Since single-course maternal intramuscular treatment has not been shown to result in any long-term adverse effects in humans, it would appear at the present time that direct fetal injection could not be justified as a potential alternative. This approach may, however, have merit in cases of maternal diabetes in which maternal injection may cause difficulty in

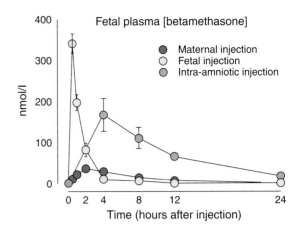

Figure 17.2 Fetal plasma betamethasone concentrations after maternal, fetal or intra-amniotic injection. Serial plasma samples were collected from catheterized fetal sheep after maternal intramuscular injection (0.5 mg/kg maternal weight), fetal intramuscular injection (0.5 mg/kg estimated fetal weight) or intra-amniotic injection (2 mg/kg estimated fetal weight). The duration of the exposure was greatest after intra-amniotic injection.

glycemic control, but direct fetal treatment would need rigorous evaluation within the context of randomized controlled trials with sufficient sample size to uncover any potential harm as well as benefit.

Direct injection of betamethasone into the amniotic cavity has also been evaluated in sheep.[70] This technique effectively improves preterm lung maturation, but is associated with high rates of mortality and morbidity, rendering this approach unsuitable for clinical use. It is suggested this morbidity results from prolonged exposure to a continuing pool of corticosteroid in the amniotic fluid (Figure 17.2).

Alternative preparations

The corticosteroid preparation employed in the original controlled trial was a combined preparation of betamethasone phosphate and acetate.[4] The phosphate ester provides short-term release of betamethasone into the circulation from the intramuscular site, while the acetate ester provides a more sustained release. Together, these two preparations result in maternal levels after maternal injection that have a half-life of approximately 6 h in humans[71] and 4.8 h in sheep.[69] We have investigated in sheep the hypothesis that the betamethasone phosphate alone may be as effective as the combined preparation and, because of its shorter half-life, have fewer risks of adverse outcomes. These studies have shown that the betamethasone phosphate preparation does indeed mature the fetal lung, but the effect is not as great as with the combined preparation.[72] To date, there have been no pharmacological preparations found to be superior to, or even comparable to, the combined betamethasone preparation proposed by Liggins and Howie in 1972.[4]

RECOMMENDATIONS

At this time, available evidence continues to support the recommendations of the USA NIH and the Royal College of Obstetricians and Gynaecologists published in 2001 and 2004, respectively.[73,74] In essence, these learned groups have recommended that single-course treatment remains the standard of practice, but that any use of repeated or 'rescue' courses should be confined to randomized controlled trials.

There are, however, many ways in which individual practitioners can refine their clinical care. It needs to be remembered that calculations of the 'number needed to treat' indicate we need to treat 13 women at risk of preterm birth with antenatal corticosteroids to prevent one case of respiratory distress syndrome.[75] After 34 weeks of gestation, the number needed to treat increases to 145. The data that underpin these calculations came from clinical environments that preceded introduction of surfactant therapy, and in which respiratory distress syndrome was more likely to have been fatal than it is today. Further, the diagnosis of true preterm labor has been refined by the availability of fetal fibronectin testing. Together, our evolving capabilities and changes in other aspects of clinical practice, should lead to care based on a thorough knowledge of the evidence of potential benefit and harm which may arise from antenatal corticosteroid treatment, and the need to restrict their use wherever possible to those cases in which the risk of early birth is real.

REFERENCES

1. Green NS, Damus K, Simpson JL et al. Research agenda for preterm birth: recommendations from the March of Dimes. Am J Obstet Gynecol 2005; 193(3 Pt 1): 626–35.
2. Liggins G. Premature parturition after infusion of corticotrophin or cortisol into foetal lambs. J Endocrinol 1968; 42: 323–9.
3. Liggins GC. Premature delivery of foetal lambs infused with glucocorticoids. J Endocrinol 1969; 45(4): 515–23.
4. Liggins GC, Howie RN. A controlled trial of antepartum glucocorticoid treatment for prevention of the respiratory distress syndrome in premature infants. Pediatrics 1972; 50(4): 515–25.
5. Challis JR, Sloboda D, Matthews SG et al. The fetal placental hypothalamic–pituitary–adrenal (HPA) axis, parturition and post natal health. Mol Cell Endocrinol 2001; 185(1–2): 135–44.
6. Crowley P. Prophylactic corticosteroids for preterm birth. Cochrane Library 2001; 4.
7. Newnham JP, Moss TJ. Antenatal glucocorticoids and growth: single versus multiple doses in animal and human studies. Semin Neonatol 2001; 6(4): 285–92.
8. Ikegami M, Polk DH, Jobe AH et al. Effect of interval from fetal corticosteriod treatment to delivery on postnatal lung function of preterm lambs. J Appl Physiol 1996; 80(2): 591–7.
9. Polk DH, Ikegami M, Jobe AH et al. Preterm lung function after retreatment with antenatal betamethasone in preterm lambs. Am J Obstet Gynecol 1997; 176(2): 308–15.
10. Brocklehurst P, Gates S, McKenzie-McHarg K, Alfirevic Z, Chamberlain G. Are we prescribing multiple courses of antenatal corticosteroids? A survey of practice in the UK. Br J Obstet Gynaecol 1999; 106(9): 977–9.
11. Quinlivan JA, Evans SF, Dunlop SA, Beazley LD, Newnham JP. Use of corticosteroids by Australian obstetricians – a survey of clinical practice. Aust NZ J Obstet Gynaecol 1998; 38(1): 1–7.
12. Empana JP, Anceschi MM, Szabo I et al. Antenatal corticosteroids policies in 14 European countries: factors associated with multiple courses. The EURAIL survey. Acta Paediatr 2004; 93(10): 1318–22.
13. Ikegami M, Jobe AH, Newnham J et al. Repetitive prenatal glucocorticoids improve lung function and decrease growth in preterm lambs. Am J Respir Crit Care Med 1997; 156(1): 178–84.
14. Newnham JP, Evans SF, Godfrey M et al. Maternal, but not fetal, administration of corticosteroids restricts fetal growth. J Matern Fetal Med 1999; 8(3): 81–7.
15. Moss TJ, Sloboda DM, Gurrin LC et al. Programming effects in sheep of prenatal growth restriction and glucocorticoid exposure. Am J Physiol Regul Integr Comp Physiol 2001; 281(3): R960–70.
16. Pratt L, Magness RR, Phernetton T et al. Repeated use of betamethasone in rabbits: effects of treatment variation on adrenal suppression, pulmonary maturation, and pregnancy outcome. Am J Obstet Gynecol 1999; 180(4): 995–1005.
17. Stewart JD, Gonzalez CL, Christensen HD, Rayburn WF. Impact of multiple antenatal doses of betamethasone on growth and development of mice offspring. Am J Obstet Gynecol 1997; 177(5): 1138–44.
18. Frank L, Roberts RJ. Effects of low-dose prenatal corticosteroid administration on the premature rat. Biol Neonate 1979; 36(1–2): 1–9.
19. Aghajafari F, Murphy K, Matthews S et al. Repeated doses of antenatal corticosteroids in animals: a systematic review. Am J Obstet Gynecol 2002; 186(4): 843–9.
20. Johnson JW, Mitzner W, London WT, Palmer AE, Scott R. Betamethasone and the rhesus fetus: multisystemic effects. Am J Obstet Gynecol 1979; 133(6): 677–84.
21. Epstein MF, Farrell PM, Sparks JW et al. Maternal betamethasone and fetal growth and development in the monkey. Am J Obstet Gynecol 1977; 127(3): 261–3.
22. French NP, Hagan R, Evans SF, Godfrey M, Newnham JP. Repeated antenatal corticosteroids: size at birth and subsequent development. Am J Obstet Gynecol 1999; 180(1 Pt 1): 114–21.
23. Bloom SL, Sheffield JS, McIntire DD, Leveno KJ. Antenatal dexamethasone and decreased birth weight. Obstet Gynecol 2001; 97(4): 485–90.
24. Banks BA, Cnaan A, Morgan MA et al. Multiple courses of antenatal corticosteroids and outcome of premature neonates. North American Thyrotropin-Releasing Hormone Study Group. Am J Obstet Gynecol 1999; 181(3): 709–17.
25. Thorp JA, Jones AM, Hunt C, Clark R. The effect of multidose antenatal betamethasone on maternal and infant outcomes. Am J Obstet Gynecol 2001; 184(2): 196–202.
26. Guinn DA, Atkinson MW, Sullivan L et al. Single vs weekly courses of antenatal corticosteroids for women at risk of preterm delivery: a randomized controlled trial. JAMA 2001; 286(13): 1581–7.

27. Johnson JWC, Mitzner W, Beck JC et al. Long-term effects of betamethasone on fetal development. Am J Obstet Gynecol 1981; 141: 1053–64.

28. Huang WL, Beazley LD, Quinlivan JA et al. Effect of corticosteroids on brain growth in fetal sheep. Obstet Gynecol 1999; 94(2): 213–18.

29. Dunlop SA, Archer MA, Quinlivan JA, Beazley LD, Newnham JP. Repeated prenatal corticosteroids delay myelination in the ovine central nervous system. J Matern Fetal Med 1997; 6(6): 309–13.

30. Huang WL, Harper CG, Evans SF, Newnham JP, Dunlop SA. Repeated prenatal corticosteroid administration delays myelination of the corpus callosum in fetal sheep. Int J Dev Neurosci 2001; 19(4): 415–25.

31. Moss TJ, Doherty DA, Nitsos I et al. Effects into adulthood of single or repeated antenatal corticosteroids in sheep. Am J Obstet Gynecol 2005; 192(1): 146–52.

32. Thorp JA, Jones PG, Knox E, Clark RH. Does antenatal corticosteroid therapy affect birth weight and head circumference? Obstet Gynecol 2002; 99(1): 101–8.

33. Leviton A, Dammann O, Allred EN et al. Antenatal corticosteroids and cranial ultrasonographic abnormalities. Am J Obstet Gynecol 1999; 181(4): 1007–17.

34. Canterino JC, Verma U, Visintainer PF et al. Antenatal steroids and neonatal periventricular leukomalacia. Obstet Gynecol 2001; 97(1): 135–9.

35. Gray PH, Jones P, O'Callaghan MJ. Maternal antecedents for cerebral palsy in extremely preterm babies: a case-control study. Dev Med Child Neurol 2001; 43(9): 580–5.

36. French NP, Hagan R, Evans SF, Mullan A, Newnham JP. Repeated antenatal corticosteroids: effects on cerebral palsy and childhood behaviour. Am J Obstet Gynecol 2004; 190(3): 588–95.

37. Dalziel SR, Lim VK, Lambert A et al. Antenatal exposure to betamethasone: psychological functioning and health related quality of life 31 years after inclusion in randomised controlled trial. BMJ 2005; 331(7518): 665.

38. Jobe AH, Ikegami M. Lung development and function in preterm infants in the surfactant treatment era. Annu Rev Physiol 2000; 62: 825–46.

39. Jobe AH, Polk D, Ikegami M et al. Lung responses to ultrasound-guided fetal treatments with corticosteroids in preterm lambs. J Appl Physiol 1993; 75(5): 2099–105.

40. Willet KE, Jobe AH, Ikegami M et al. Antenatal endotoxin and glucocorticoid effects on lung morphometry in preterm lambs. Pediatr Res 2000; 48(6): 782–8.

41. Jobe AH, Newnham J, Willet K, Sly P, Ikegami M. Fetal versus maternal and gestational age effects of repetitive antenatal glucocorticoids. Pediatrics 1998; 102(5): 1116–25.

42. Moss TJ, Harding R, Newnham JP. Lung function, arterial pressure and growth in sheep during early postnatal life following single and repeated prenatal corticosteroid treatments. Early Hum Dev 2002; 66(1): 11–24.

43. Sloboda DM, Moss TJ, Li S et al. Hepatic glucose regulation and metabolism in adult sheep: effects of prenatal betamethasone. Am J Physiol Endocrinol Metab 2005; 289(4): E721–8.

44. Dalziel SR, Walker NK, Parag V et al. Cardiovascular risk factors after antenatal exposure to betamethasone: 30-year follow-up of a randomised controlled trial. Lancet 2005; 365(9474): 1856–62.

45. Koenen SV, Mecenas CA, Smith GS, Jenkins S, Nathanielsz PW. Effects of maternal betamethasone administration on fetal and maternal blood pressure and heart rate in the baboon at 0.7 of gestation. Am J Obstet Gynecol 2002; 186(4): 812–17.

46. Dodic M, May CN, Wintour EM, Coghlan JP. An early prenatal exposure to excess glucocorticoid leads to hypertensive offspring in sheep. Clin Sci (Lond) 1998; 94(2): 149–55.

47. Newnham JP. Is prenatal glucocorticoid administration another origin of adult disease? Clin Exp Pharmacol Physiol 2001; 28(11): 957–61.

48. Sloboda DM, Moss TJ, Gurrin LC, Newnham JP, Challis JR. The effect of prenatal betamethasone administration on postnatal ovine hypothalamic–pituitary–adrenal function. J Endocrinol 2002; 172(1): 71–81.

49. Sloboda DM, Moss T, Nitsos I et al. Antenatal glucocorticoid treatment in sheep results in adrenal suppression in adulthood. J Soc Gynecol Invest 2003; 10: 435.

50. Jenkins TM, Wapner RJ, Thom EA, Das AF, Spong CY. Are weekly courses of antenatal steroids beneficial or dangerous? JAMA 2002; 287(2): 187–8; author reply 189–90.

51. Murphy KE, Hannah M, Brocklehurst P. Are weekly courses of antenatal steroids beneficial or dangerous? JAMA 2002; 287(2): 188; author reply 189–90.

52. Harding JE, Pang J, Knight DB, Liggins GC. Do antenatal corticosteroids help in the setting of preterm rupture of membranes? Am J Obstet Gynecol 2001; 184(2): 131–9.

53. Lee MJ, Davies J, Guinn D et al. Single versus weekly courses of antenatal corticosteroids in preterm premature rupture of membranes. Obstet Gynecol 2004; 103(2): 274–81.

54. Goldenberg RL, Hauth JC, Andrews WW. Intrauterine infection and preterm delivery. N Engl J Med 2000; 342(20): 1500–7.

55. Watterberg KL, Demers LM, Scott SM, Murphy S. Chorioamnionitis and early lung inflammation in infants in whom bronchopulmonary dysplasia develops. Pediatrics 1996; 97(2): 210–15.

56. Jobe AH, Newnham JP, Willet KE et al. Endotoxin-induced lung maturation in preterm lambs is not mediated by cortisol. Am J Respir Crit Care Med 2000; 162(5): 1656–61.

57. Newnham JP, Kallapur SG, Kramer BW et al. Betamethasone effects on chorioamnionitis induced by intra-amniotic endotoxin on sheep. Am J Obstet Gynecol 2003; 189: 1458–66.

58. Foix-L'helias L, Baud O, Lenclen R, Kaminski M, Lacaze-Masmonteil T. Benefit of antenatal glucocorticoids according to the cause of very premature birth. Arch Dis Child Fetal Neonatal Ed 2005; 90(1): F46–8.

59. Derks JB, Giussani DA, Jenkins SL et al. A comparative study of cardiovascular, endocrine and behavioural effects of betamethasone and dexamethasone administration to fetal sheep. J Physiol 1997; 499(Pt 1): 217–26.

60. Schwab M, Roedel M, Anwar MA et al. Effects of betamethasone administration to the fetal sheep in late gestation on fetal cerebral blood flow. J Physiol 2000; 528(Pt 3): 619–32.

61. Bennet L, Kozuma S, McGarrigle HH, Hanson MA. Temporal changes in fetal cardiovascular, behavioural, metabolic and endocrine responses to maternally administered dexamethasone in the late gestation fetal sheep. Br J Obstet Gynaecol 1999; 106(4): 331–9.

62. Mulder EJ, Derks JB, Zonneveld MF, Bruinse HW, Visser GH. Transient reduction in fetal activity and heart rate variation after maternal betamethasone administration. Early Hum Dev 1994; 36(1): 49–60.

63. Wallace EM, Baker LS. Effect of antenatal betamethasone administration on placental vascular resistance. Lancet 1999; 353(9162): 1404–7.

64. Simchen MJ, Alkazaleh F, Adamson SL et al. The fetal cardiovascular response to antenatal steroids in severe early-onset intrauterine growth restriction. Am J Obstet Gynecol 2004; 190(2): 296–304.

65. Effect of antenatal dexamethasone administration on the prevention of respiratory distress syndrome. Am J Obstet Gynecol 1981; 141(3): 276–87.

66. Quist-Therson EC, Myhr TL, Ohlsson A. Antenatal steroids to prevent respiratory distress syndrome: multiple gestation as an

effect modifier. Acta Obstet Gynecol Scand 1999; 78(5): 388–92.

67. Blickstein I, Shinwell ES, Lusky A, Reichman B. Plurality-dependent risk of respiratory distress syndrome among very-low-birth-weight infants and antepartum corticosteroid treatment. Am J Obstet Gynecol 2005; 192(2): 360–4.

68. Quinlivan JA, Beazley LD, Braekevelt CR et al. Repeated ultrasound guided fetal injections of corticosteroid alter nervous system maturation in the ovine fetus. J Perinat Med 2001; 29(2): 112–27.

69. Moss TJ, Doherty DA, Nitsos I, Harding R, Newnham JP. Pharmacokinetics of betamethasone after maternal or fetal intramuscular administration. Am J Obstet Gynecol 2003; 189(6): 1751–7.

70. Moss TJM, Mulrooney NP, Nitsos I et al. Intra-amniotic corticosteroids for preterm lung maturation in sheep. Am J Obstet Gynecol 2003; 189(5): 1389–95.

71. Ballard PL, Granberg P, Ballard RA. Glucocorticoid levels in maternal and cord serum after prenatal betamethasone therapy to prevent respiratory distress syndrome. J Clin Invest 1975; 56(6): 1548–54.

72. Newnham JP, Moss TJM, Nitsos I, Ikegami M, Jobe AH. Determining the optimal dose and pharmacological preparation of betamethasone for the enhancement of fetal maturation in sheep. J Soc Gynecol Invest 2005; 12: 676.

73. Antenatal corticosteroids revisited: repeat courses – National Institutes of Health Consensus Development Conference Statement, August 17–18, 2000. Obstet Gynecol 2001; 98(1): 144–50.

74. Antenatal corticosteroids to prevent respiratory distress syndrome. Royal College of Obstetricians and Gynaecologists 2004; Guideline No. 7.

75. Sinclair JC. Meta-analysis of randomized controlled trials of antenatal corticosteroid for the prevention of respiratory distress syndrome: discussion. Am J Obstet Gynecol 1995; 173(1): 335–44.

18

Monitoring the growth-restricted fetus during the preterm period

Gerard HA Visser

INTRODUCTION

This chapter deals with monitoring of the high-risk fetus. Given the context of this book, data are restricted to the preterm fetus, with emphasis on the intrauterine growth restricted (IUGR) fetus.

RANK ORDER OF CHANGES OCCURRING WITH PROGRESSIVE DETERIORATION OF THE FETAL CONDITION

There are a number of antenatal assessment techniques which are suitable to identify the abnormal pregnancy: assessment of the fundal height, kick-chart, ultrasound biometry, Doppler examination of the uterine artery, measurement of maternal blood pressure, etc. Having thus identified the fetus with inadequate growth as a result of impaired uteroplacental function, a number of tools are available to monitor fetal wellbeing. All of these techniques can contribute to our understanding of the fetal condition, and one is not superior to another. Combining information obtained from a number of tests is superior to the use of a single technique, since it reduces the risk of false positives leading to inappropriate intervention.

With progressive deterioration of the fetal condition a certain rank order can be determined in which test results become abnormal. It is useful to be informed about the rank order of these changes. It helps us to understand the gradual process of compensation and adaptation through decompensation. Awareness of the rank order may be helpful in determining the degree of deterioration, the timing of delivery, and assessing the effect of treatment modalities.

Figure 18.1 shows the rank order in which changes occur in the various assessment tests, with progressive deterioration of the condition of the IUGR fetus.

This rank order is based on longitudinal and cross-sectional studies in which the results of tests for fetal wellbeing were related to blood gases obtained by cordocentesis or from cord blood, immediately after Cesarean section. The sequence of events shown in Figure 18.1 applies to the entire population of IUGR fetuses studied, and it is wise to consider that individual fetusus may show different patterns. The rank order holds especially for the preterm period. Near term, Doppler waveform patterns are not particularly useful. The various studies that have formed the basis of the rank order proposed have been reviewed in detail previously,[1,2] and will not be discussed here.

DOPPLER WAVEFORM PATTERNS

Abnormalities of Doppler flow velocity waveforms (FVW) of the fetal umbilical artery are usually the first signs of impending deterioration of the fetal condition.[3] Abnormal waveform patterns probably reflect inadequate development of the placenta, and are most likely an indication of increased impedance to blood flow due to abnormalities in the small capillaries of the terminal villi.[4] About 2–3 weeks later changes can be observed in the FVW forms of fetal cerebral vessels[5] with reduced impedance to flow, suggesting a compensatory mechanism known as 'redistribution of the fetal circulation'. During the preterm period, changes in umbilical and cerebral artery waveform patterns precede the onset of fetal hypoxemia,[6] and in the presence of a normal fetal heart rate (FHR) pattern the pO_2 in fetal cord samples will usually be in the lower part of the normal range.[7]

In IUGR fetuses the interval between the first abnormal Doppler finding and the onset of FHR abnormalities/hypoxemia varies considerably. The interval is shorter in late than in early gestation, and also shorter in IUGR

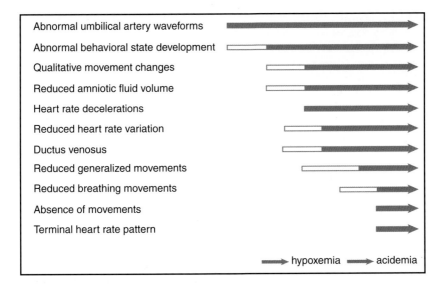

Figure 18.1 Suggested order in which blood velocity waveform, amniotic fluid volume, movement and heart changes occur in growth-retarded human fetuses with progressive deterioration of the fetal condition. Interfetal variation in the first occurrence of an abnormal test result is indicated by the unshaded part of the arrow. (Adapted from Visser and Stiger, in Asphyxia and Fetal Brain Damage, 1998[2] and the PhD theses of DJ Bekedam and LSM Ribbert.)

complicated by pre-eclampsia (Figure 18.2).[1,3,8,9] Apparently, a tiny fetus in early gestation can cope with a reduced placental supply for much longer than a bigger IUGR fetus later in pregnancy. This seems logical, taking into account the higher oxygen requirements in the latter. From these findings, one may also conclude that in pre-eclampsia the deterioration of the placental function occurs more rapidly than in IUGR fetuses without pre-eclampsia. The clinical implication of these observations is that once Doppler waveforms become abnormal, FHR monitoring should be carried out more frequently beyond 30 weeks, and in all cases complicated by pre-eclampsia.

Around and after term, Doppler examinations are no longer useful, since fetal hypoxemia will generally precede Doppler changes. So, at term we still have to rely on assessments of amniotic fluid, FHR and fetal movements.

Doppler waveform patterns of the umbilical artery may deteriorate from decreased to absent, and finally to reversed end-diastolic velocities. This sequence is not indicated in Figure 18.1, since its occurrence in relation to changes in other tests varies substantially (see also Figure 18.2).

Prior to 30 weeks of gestation, most fetuses with FHR abnormalities will have had absent end-diastolic velocities of the umbilical artery for a considerable period; after 36 weeks, absent end-diastolic velocities are a rare phenomenon, and are associated with signs of severe

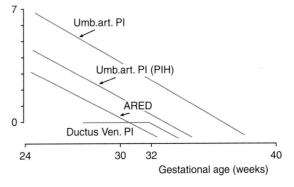

Figure 18.2 Interval (in weeks) between first abnormal Doppler result and the occurrence of fetal hypoxemia (=abnormal fetal heart rate pattern), according to gestational age (in weeks). This interval is longer at early gestation and longer in intrauterine growth restricted fetuses without pregnancy induced hypertension. Shortest intervals occur for absent or reversed end diastolic velocities and abnormal ductus venosus waveforms.

fetal compromise. Reversed end-diastolic flow in the umbilical artery probably reflects fetal cardiac failure, since cardiac contractility decreases concomitantly.[10] It is associated with the occurrence of a terminal FHR pattern (which is indicative of myocardial hypoxemia),[11] and outcome is poor. With progressive deterioration of the fetal condition, the changes in waveform patterns of cerebral vessels (e.g. middle cerebral artery) follow a biphasic pattern. Initially there is a progressive increase in end-diastolic velocities (and a decrease in pulsatility index). Later, a plateau occurs and finally end-diastolic velocities decrease again.[5] The latter may be due to a decrease in cardiac contractility, the occurrence of cerebral edema, or both. It has been reported that this decrease in end-diastolic velocities precedes the occurrence of FHR abnormalities,[5] but in my opinion it may be a very late and rare sign of impairment coinciding with fetal acidemia.

Since abnormal umbilical artery Doppler waveforms occur rather early in the process of deterioration, this technique has been shown to be useful in a high-risk population to identify fetuses at risk of becoming hypoxemic, and to distinguish 'low-risk' small-for-gestational-age fetuses from 'high-risk' IUGR fetuses.[12,13] A meta-analysis of randomized trials has shown that Doppler investigation of the umbilical artery reduces perinatal mortality in high-risk populations.[14] In low-risk populations, no benefits have been shown thus far.[15]

In fetuses before 32 weeks of gestation, changes in ductus venosus FWV occur more or less at the same time as FHR abnormalities, and are therefore likely to coincide with fetal hypoxemia.[9] Thereafter, FHR abnormalities, usually occur first. This suggests that ductus venosus examinations are only useful at early gestation (i.e. <32 weeks).

FETAL HEART RATE (FHR)

Abnormalities of the FHR coincide with the occurrence of fetal hypoxemia. This applies to a reduction of FHR variation below the normal range and to the occurrence of late FHR decelerations.[7,16,17] FHR variation usually decreases gradually during the weeks preceding the appearance of late decelerations (and fetal hypoxemia).[18] Longitudinal FHR recordings may, therefore, indicate a gradual deterioration of the fetal condition, even before the onset of hypoxemia. However, a single recording will not identify the small fetus at risk of becoming hypoxemic, since FHR variation is still within the normal range. This indicates that antenatal FHR monitoring is not a useful screening test. It should be applied longitudinally in a high-risk population. The best indication for serial FHR monitoring is the IUGR fetus with abnormal Doppler waveform patterns, in whom hypoxemia is likely to occur in due course. Trends in FHR variation can best be obtained by using a computerized FHR system (see ref 18).

AMNIOTIC FLUID VOLUME

In IUGR fetuses, oligohydramnios is most likely due to a reduced renal blood flow (caused by blood flow redistribution) and decreased urine output.[19] In most third-trimester IUGR fetuses, oligohydramnios occurs before the onset of FHR abnormalities (and hypoxemia).[11] Therefore, its occurrence is an important finding which warrants intensive fetal monitoring. Also, during the preterm period oligohydramnios usually occurs before the onset of FHR abnormalities.[9]

FETAL BEHAVIOR AND MOVEMENTS

Disturbances in the development of fetal behavioral (sleep) states usually precede the occurrence of FHR abnormalities by some weeks.[20,21] With advancing gestation, fetal behavioral states normally become more organized, demonstrated by a decrease in percentage of no-coincidence, i.e. a decrease in the percentage of time that FHR patterns, and eye and body movement patterns, do not fit within a particular state. In IUGR fetuses which eventually become hypoxemic, this decrease in no-coincidence does not take place.[21] Monitoring of fetal behavioral states is clinically not feasible, since it is time consuming and requires considerable experience. However, these data indicate that in IUGR fetuses, disturbances in brain function antedate the occurrence of fetal hypoxemia. Apart from these disturbances in development of sleep states, there is also a redistribution in the incidence of occurrence of the different states, with an increase of state 1F (quiet sleep) and a decrease of state 2F (active sleep).[22] The latter phenomenon may be considered as a sign of fetal adaptation. Abnormalities in the quality of fetal movements (monotonous, reduced speed and amplitude) also precede the occurrence of FHR decelerations.[23] These disturbances of the functioning of the fetal nervous system in IUGR fetuses could well be the result of prolonged malnutrition rather than merely an effect of fetal hypoxemia. This is in line with observations from cord blood analysis in IUGR fetuses where hypoglycemia and abnormally low levels of essential amino acids were shown even before the occurrence of hypoxemia.[7,24]

The incidence of fetal movements usually only falls below the normal range after the occurrence of FHR abnormalities, and this reduction is associated with impending acidemia.[25,26] Longitudinal observations of fetal movements in IUGR fetuses have also shown that the incidence of body movements declines when FHR variation has reached the lower limit of the normal range, i.e. at the time the fetus is likely to have become hypoxemic.[11] Thereafter, FHR variation usually remains constant over a certain period of time, during which the incidence of body movements continues to fall. Eventually, FHR variation is reduced further, and body and breathing movements disappear: the fetus becomes progressively hypoxemic and acidemic. These data suggest that a constant level of fetal pO_2 is maintained for some time by the reduction in body movements. Reduction of fetal movements when oxygen supply is limited aids in maximizing delivery of oxygen to vital organs and may be considered a sign of fetal adaptation. In the fetal sheep it has been shown that oxygen consumption fell by 17% after neuromuscular blockade,[27] while pO_2 values rose by a similar percentage.[27,28]

It is also known, from subjective fetal movement records kept by pregnant women, that before the sudden decline in movements which may indicate impending fetal death, the movement incidence is still within the normal range.[29,30] Recording of movements by pregnant women ('kick chart') does not have a high sensitivity or specificity with regard to fetal compromise; however, it is cheap and may identify the small and compromised fetus that was not identified by routine prenatal care.

TIMING OF DELIVERY

There is evidence that IUGR fetuses delivered when severe waveform abnormalities of fetal vessels are present have a greater morbidity and mortality than those with end-diastolic frequencies still present. Growth-retarded fetuses that had antepartum FHR decelerations are more likely to develop a severe degree of intraventricular hemorrhage, or show abnormal neurological signs, during the newborn period than those that had been delivered before decelerations had occurred. Fetuses delivered before 34 weeks of gestation have poorer cognitive development at age 2 years when antenatal FHR abnormalities had been present than when only abnormal Doppler results had been obtained. Moreover, IUGR fetuses who were acidemic at cordocentesis or at elective Cesarean section have a poorer neonatal, and subsequent neurological, development than nonacidemic fetuses (see ref 2 for a review). These data may lead to the conclusion that IUGR fetuses shoud be delivered before antenatal test results become severely abnormal.[31] However, in none of these studies were patients randomized, and gestational age was lower and growth retardation more severe in the populations with the poorest outcome. When we matched IUGR fetuses with and without end-diastolic velocities in the umbilical artery for gestational age and birthweight, no differences in outcome were found.[3] This seems to indicate that absence of end-diastolic velocities is a marker of early and severe IUGR – which by itself has an effect on outcome – rather than a marker purely related to outcome.

So, when should the growth-restricted fetus be delivered, taking into account the fact that delivery at an earlier age may increase the risk of prematurity-related neonatal complications? A small fetus with an estimated weight of 900 g at 31 weeks is bound to be at risk of neurological handicap. The obstetrician may decide to deliver this fetus before signs of hypoxemia occur, say at about 29 or 30 weeks, but handicap may then result from pulmonary problems during the neonatal period. It may be decided to leave the fetus in utero longer, in the hope of improving maturation; but then the impact of prolonged malnutrition, particularly on the brain, may offset these benefits.

First randomized data on the timing of delivery of the preterm IUGR fetus have come from the Growth Restriction Intervention Trial (GRIT).[32,33] Before birth, 588 babies were randomly assigned to immediate delivery or delayed delivery, in case there was clinical uncertainty whether immediate delivery was indicated. The median difference between immediate delivery and defer was (only) 4.5 days. There was no difference in perinatal or infant death. Direct morbidity was somewhat lower in the defer group [need for ventilation odds ratio (OR) 1.9, 95% confidence internal (CI) 1.3–2.7; necrotizing enterocolitis OR 1.5, CI 0.7–3.2; periventricular haemorrhage OR 1.9, CI 0.8–4.6). Outcome at 2 years of age was better in the defer group, but only for infants born before 30 weeks of gestation (severe impairment in 6 versus 16%). So, from these data we can conclude that when there is clinical uncertainty whether or not to deliver the preterm IUGR fetus, immediate delivery or some delay does not affect outcome after 30 weeks of gestation. Before 30 weeks some delay may be beneficial for the infant, since gestational age and fetal maturation are essential for outcome at such an early age.[34,35]

In the GRIT trial no management guidelines had been given as to when to deliver the IUGR fetus. Each clinician had to make his/her own judgement. So this study did not result in clear advice as to management. Currently, a randomized management study is recruiting patients; in this study delivery is either based on reduced FHR variation, or on early or late ductus venosus abnormalities (TRUFFLE study).[36] This study has been based on observational longitudinal data, which show that perinatal mortality in preterm IUGR fetuses was lower when only FHR variation or ductus venosus velocities were abnormal, when compared to fetuses in which both parameters were abnormal.[9,37,38] Until the results of this management study are available, one may decide to deliver the preterm IUGR fetus after 30 weeks of gestation if either FHR or ductus venosus is abnormal (based on the GRIT and on the quoted longitudinal observational studies). Before 30 weeks, expected management may prove beneficial, but only if one of the two parameters is abnormal.

Small for gestational age fetuses, and probably also IUGR fetuses, do not seem to be protected against respiratory distress syndrome (RDS).[39,40] There are no studies on the effects of antenatal corticosteroids on the incidence of RDS in these fetuses. Moreover, side effects of corticosteroids (reduced cell devision) may be greater in IUGR than in appropiate-for-dates fetuses. Therefore, I would like to promote (re)introduction of amniocentesis to determine fetal lung maturation when early delivery is pending. Between 30 and 32 weeks half of IUGR fetuses have a mature lecithin/sphingomyelin ratio (data derived from ref 41). This may help in determining the timing of delivery and prevent the administration of corticosteroids in half of cases.

CONCLUSIONS

Monitoring of the high-risk IUGR fetus during the preterm period is facilitated by the fact that most assessment techniques work properly during that period. This holds especially for Doppler FVW, which usually precede the occurrence of fetal hypoxemia and may therefore be used to identify the fetuses at risk (in contrast to term pregnancies). Results from the ongoing TRUFFLE trial are awaited to find out if delivery can best be based on abnormal FHR patterns and/or on abnormal ductus venosus FVW. Results from the GRIT study have shown that <30 weeks of gestation a more conservative approach towards delivery is associated with a more favorable perinatal outcome than a more aggressive approach. FHR variation is much lower at early gestation than at term, which hampers its assessment. Analysis of FHR variation can, therefore, best be based on computerized assessment of heart rate variation.

REFERENCES

1. Visser GHA. Assessment of fetal well being in growth retarded fetuses. In: Hanson MA, Spencer JAD, Rodeck CH, eds. Fetuses and Neonate, Volume 3: Growth. Cambridge: Cambridge Univerity Press, 1995: 327–45.
2. Visser GHA, Stigter RH. Monitoring the growth retarded fetus. In: Maulik B, ed. Asphyxia and Fetal Brain Damage. New York: Wiley-Lin, 1998: 333–43.
3. Bekedam DJ, Visser GHA, Van der Zee AGJ, Snijders RJM, Poelmann-Weesjes G. Abnormal velocity waveforms of the umbilical artery in growth retarded fetuses. relationship to antepartum late heart rate decelerations and outcome. Early Hum Dev 1990; 24: 70–90.
4. Krebs C, Macara LM, Leiser R et al. Intrauterine growth restriction with absent end-diastolic flow velocity in the umbilical artery

5. Arduini D, Rizzo G, Romanini C. Changes of pulsatility index from fetal vessels preceding the onset of late decelerations in growth retarded fetuses. Obstet Gynecol 1992; 79: 605–10.
6. Bilardo CM, Nicolaides KH, Campbell S. Doppler measurements of fetal and uteroplacental circulation: relationship with umbilical venous blood gases measured at cordocentesis. Am J Obstet Gynecol 1990; 163: 115–20.
7. Pardi G, Cetin I, Marconi AM et al. Diagnostic value of blood sampling in fetuses with growth retardation. New Engl J Med 1993; 328: 692–6.
8. Arduini D, Rizzo G, Romanini C. The development of abnormal heart rate patterns after absent end-diastolic velocity in umbilical artery. Am J Obstet Gynecol 1988; 168: 43–8.
9. Hecher K, Bilardo CM, Stigter RH et al. Monitoring of fetuses with intrauterine growth restriction: a longitudinal study. Ultrasound Obstet Gynecol 2001; 18: 564–70.
10. De Vore GR. Examination of the fetal heart in the fetus with intrauterine growth retardation. Semin Perinat 1988; 12: 66–79.
11. Ribbert LSM, Visser GHA, Mulder EJH, Zonneveld MF, Morssink LP. Changes with time in retal heart rate variation, movement incidences and haemodynamics in intrauterine growth retarded fetuses; a longitudinal approach to the assessment of fetal wellbeing. Early Hum Dev 1993; 31: 195–208.
12. Reuwer PHJM, Rietman GW, Sijmons EA, van Tiel MWM, Bruinse HW. Intrauterine growth retardation: prediction of perinatal distress by Doppler ultrasound. Lancet 1987; 1: 415–18.
13. Beattie RB, Dordan JC. Antenatal screening for intrauterine growth retardation with umbilical artery Doppler ultrasonography. Br Med J 1989; 298: 631–5.
14. Divon MY. Randomized controlled trials of umbilical artery Doppler velocimetry: how many are too many. Ultrasound Obstet Gynecol 1995; 6: 377–9.
15. Goffinet F, Paris-Llado J, Nisand I, Bréart G. Umbilical artery Doppler velocimetry in unselected and low risk pregnancies: a review of randomised controlled trials. Br J Obstet Gynaecol 1997; 104: 425–30.
16. Bekedam DJ, Visser GHA, Mulder EJH, Poelmann-Weesjes G. Heart rate variation and movements incidence in growth-retarded fetuses: the significance of antenatal late heart rate decelerations. Am J Obstet Gynecol 1987; 157: 126–33.
17. Visser GHA, Sadovsky G, Nicolaides KH. Antepartum heart rate patterns in small-for-gestational-age third trimester fetuses: correlations with blood gas values obtained at cordocentesis. Am J Obstet Gynecol 1990; 162: 698–703.
18. Snijders RJM, Ribbert LSM, Visser GHA, Mulder EJH. Numeric analysis of heart rate variation in intrauterine growth-retarded fetuses: a longitudinal study. Am J Obstet Gynecol 1992; 166: 22–7.
19. Arduini D, Rizzo G. Fetal renal artery velocity waveforms and amniotic fluid volume in growth-retarded and past-term fetuses. Obstet Gynecol 1991; 72: 370–3.
20. Van Vliet MAT, Martin CB, Nijhuis JG, Prechtl HFR. Behavioural states in growth-retarded fetuses. Early Hum Dev 1985; 12: 183–98.
21. Arduini D. Rizzo G, Caforio L. Boccolini MR, Romanini C, Mancuso S. Behavioural state transitions in healthy and growth retarded fetuses. Early Hum Dev 1989; 19: 155–65.
22. Gazzolo D, Visser GHA, Santi F et al. Behaviourral development and Doppler velocimetry in relation to perinatal outcome in small for dates fetuses. Early Hum Dev 1995; 43: 185–95.
23. Sival DA, Visser GHA, Prechtl HFR. The effect of intrauterine growth retardation on the quality of general movements in the human fetus. Early Hum Dev 1992; 28: 119–32.
24. Cetin I, Ronzoni S, Marconi AM et al. Maternal concentrations and fetal-maternal concentration differences of plasma amino

acids in normal and intrauterine growth-retarded pregnancies. Am J Obstet Gynecol 1996; 174: 1575–83.

25. Ribbert LSM, Snijders RJM, Nicolaides KH, Visser GHA. Relationship of fetal biophysical profile and blood gas values at cordocentesis in severely growth-retarded fetuses. Am J Obstet Gynecol 1990; 163: 569–71.

26. Ribbert LSM, Nicolaides KH, Visser GHA. Prediction of fetal acidaemia in intrauterine growth retardation: comparison of quantified fetal activity with biophysical profile score. Br J Obstet Gynaecol 1993; 100: 653–56.

27. Rurak DW, Gruber NC. Effect of neuromuscular blockade on oxygen consumption and blood gases in the fetal lamb. Am J Obstet Gynecol 1983; 145: 258–62.

28. Nathanielsz PW, Yu HK, Calabum TC. Effect of abolition of fetal movements on intravascular PO_2 and incidence of tonic myometrial contractures in the pregnant ewe at 114 and 134 days gestation. Am J Obstet Gynecol 1982; 144: 614–18.

29. Sadovsky E, Yaffe H, Polishuk WZ. Fetal movement monitoring in normal and pathologic pregnancy. Int J Obstet Gynecol 1974; 12: 75–9.

30. Pearson JF, Weaver JB. Fetal activity and fetal well-being; an evaluation. Br Med J 1976; 1: 1307.

31. Hackett GA, Campbell S, Gamsu H et al. Doppler studies in the growth retarded fetus and prediction of neonatal necrotising enterocolitis, haemorrhage and neonatal morbididty. Br Med J 1987; 294: 13–16.

32. GRIT study group. A randomised trial of timed delivery for the compromised preterm fetus: short term outcomes and Bayesian interpretation. Br J Obstet Gynecol 2003; 110: 27–32.

33. Thornton JG, Hornbuckle J, Vail A, Spiegelhalter DJ, Levene M; GRIT study group. Infant wellbeing at 2 years of age in the Growth Restriction Intervention Trial (GRIT): multicentred randomised controlled trial. Lancet 2004; 364: 513–20.

34. Yu VYH, Loke HL, Bajuk B et al. Prognosis for infants born at 23 to 28 weeks' gestation. Br Med J 1986; 293: 1200–3.

35. Bilardo CM, Wolf H, Stigter RH et al. Relationship between monitoring parameters and perinatal outcome in severe, early intrauterine growth restriction. Ultrasound Obstet Gynecol 2004; 23: 119–25.

36. http://wwwthelancet.com/info/info.isa?n1=authorinfo&n2=Protocol+reviews&uid=27361.

37. Baschat AA, Gembruch U, Weiner CP, Harman CR. Qualitative venous Doppler waveform analysis improves prediction of critical perinatal outcomes in premature growth-restricted fetuses. Ultrasound Obstet Gynecol 2003; 22: 240–5.

38. Ferrazzi E, Bozzo M, Rigano S et al. Temporal sequence of abnormal Doppler changes in the peripheral and central circulatory systems of the severely growth-restricted fetus. Ultrasound Obstet Gynecol 2002; 19: 140–6.

39. Tyson JE, Kennedy K, Broyles S, Rosenfeld CR. The small for gestational age infant: accelerated or delayed pulmonary maturation? Increased or decreased survival? Pediatrics 1995; 95: 534–8.

40. Ley D, Wide-Swensson D, Lindroth M, Svenningsen N, Marsal K. Repiratory distress syndrome in infants with impaired intrauterine growth. Acta Paediatr 1997; 86: 1090–96

41. Wijnberger LD, de Kleine M, Voorbij HA et al. The effect of clinical characteristics on the lecithin/sphingomyelin ratio and lamellar body count: a cross-sectional study. J Matern Fetal Neonatal Med 2003; 14: 373–82.

Index